Textbook of

Human
Parasitology

Protozoology and Helminthology

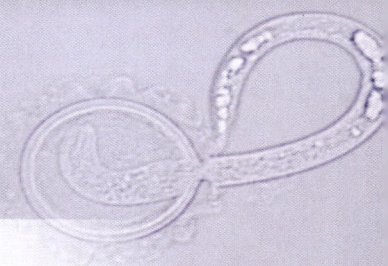

Textbook of
Human
Parasitology
Protozoology and Helminthology

Ramnik Sood MD
Consultant Pathologist/Molecular Pathologist
Speciality Diagnostic Labs, Panaji, Goa, India

and

Consultant Pathologist/Histopathologist/
Cytopathologist/Molecular Pathologist
Avivo Group, Dubai, UAE

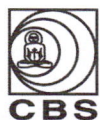

CBS Publishers & Distributors Pvt Ltd

New Delhi • Bengaluru • Chennai • Kochi • Kolkata • Mumbai
Bhopal • Bhubaneswar • Hyderabad • Jharkhand • Nagpur • Patna • Pune
Uttarakhand • Dhaka (Bangladesh) • Kathmandu (Nepal)

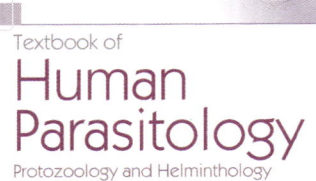

Textbook of

Human Parasitology

Protozoology and Helminthology

ISBN: 978-93-89261-78-3

Copyright © Author and Publisher

First Edition: 2020

Published by Satish Kumar Jain and produced by Varun Jain for

CBS Publishers & Distributors Pvt Ltd

4819/XI Prahlad Street, 24 Ansari Road, Daryaganj, New Delhi–110 002, India.
Ph: 23289259, 23266861, 23266867   Website: www.cbspd.com
Fax: 011-23243014   e-mail: delhi@cbspd.com; cbspubs@airtelmail.in

Corporate Office: 204 FIE, Industrial Area, Patparganj, Delhi–110 092
Ph: 4934 4934   Fax: 4934 4935 e-mail: publishing@cbspd.com; publicity@cbspd.com

Branches

- **Bengaluru:** Seema House 2975, 17th Cross, K.R. Road, Banasankari 2nd Stage, Bengaluru-560 070, Karnataka, India
  Ph: +91-80-26771678/79   Fax: +91-80-26771680   e-mail: bangalore@cbspd.com

- **Chennai:** 7, Subbaraya Street, Shenoy Nagar, Chennai–600 030, Tamil Nadu, India
  Ph: +91-44-26680620, 26681266   Fax: +91-44-42032115   e-mail: chennai@cbspd.com

- **Kochi:** 42/1325, 1326, Power House Road, Opposite KSEB Power House, Ernakulam–682 018, Kochi, Kerala, India
  Ph: +91-484-4059061-65   Fax: +91-484-4059065   e-mail: kochi@cbspd.com

- **Kolkata:** 6/B, Ground Floor, Rameswar Shaw Road, Kolkata–700 014, West Bengal, India
  Ph: +91-33-22891126, 22891127, 22891128   e-mail: kolkata@cbspd.com

- **Mumbai:** 83-C, Dr E Moses Road, Worli, Mumbai–400018, Maharashtra, India.
  Ph: +91-22-24902340/41   Fax: +91-22-24902342   e-mail: mumbai@cbspd.com

Representatives

• **Bhopal**	0-8319310552	• **Bhubaneswar**	0-9911037372	• **Hyderabad**	0-9885175004
• **Jharkhand**	0-9811541605	• **Nagpur**	0-9421945513	• **Patna**	0-9334159340
• **Pune**	0-9623451994	• **Uttarakhand**	0-9716462459		
• **Dhaka (Bangladesh)**	01912-003485	• **Kathmandu (Nepal)**	977-9818742655		

Printed at HT Media Ltd., Greater Noida, UP, India

to
all students and teachers
related to the vast field of
human parasitology

Preface

A nyone would loathe, detest, abhor and hate the word 'parasite'. Reason? Parasites live in other living beings. While doing so they occupy space within the host, utilise its resources for their own growth and propagation and release their wastes and toxins within the host's body. Result? Evolution of horrendous parasites has been an important reason for minor morbidity and sometimes fatalities in humans. There are hundreds of parasites on our mother earth, some known and others unknown as yet. As human is undertaking development and disturbing the natural balances that were 'meant to be'—newer parasites attack human, adding to the ever expanding list of these abominable organisms.

As medical science progresses, so do its diagnostic tools and capabilities, this trend has also evolved in relation to parasitic diseases. Unfortunately, the same statement cannot be logged on to their therapeutic aspects. Many parasitic infestations, till date, have either no or largely ineffective cures and sadly enough they terminate in death. As human (in the name of advancement, development and progress) is invading habitat of wild animals and keeping newer species as pets—many parasites of these animals are attacking human, finding as an easy prey. "Prevention is better than cure,", this universal statement applies aptly to parasitic diseases. Prevention is possible only if we know the life cycles and portals of entry of the concerned parasites, implication being that parasitology can no longer be overlooked or brushed aside. With the arrival of AIDS, the otherwise innocuous parasites have become agents of death, e.g. pneumocystis.

Although, by definition, fungi, bacteria and viruses are also parasites, however, traditionally, they have been kept outside the domain of parasitology.

This book covers most parasites that affect human intentionally or accidentally. The rarer ones have also been included. A more or less uniform format has been retained for description—starting from historical aspects to their therapeutics. Line diagrams and flow sketch diagrams are provided for all parasites discussed and wherever felt necessay colour pictures have been provided. The book begins with a colour atlas to give you a preview of what you are going to study about in pages to come. It is an easily digestible and assimilable way. This book should prove useful for undergraduates and practitioners alike. Diagnostic parasitology and therapy of parasitic infections have been discussed at the end. Every effort has been made to weed out any mistake, typographical or otherwise, at the time of going to press, the author or the publishers, however, undertake no responsibility for any errors that may have crept in indavertently. Latest diagnostic platforms have not been forgotten. You will find polymerase chain reactions (PCRs), nucleic acid technologies wherever applicable and available.

Wishing you all the best.

Ramnik Sood

Contents

Preface   *vii*

Colour Plates (I–VIII)

1. Introduction to Parasitology   1

2. Phylum Protozoa   11

3. Ciliates   67

4. Sporozoa (Subphylum)   71

5. Protozoa of Uncertain Status   106

6. Helminthology   108

Colour Plates (IX–XVI)

7. Phylum Nemathelminthes   109

8. Phylum Platyhelminthes Class Trematoda   202

9. Practical Parasitology   235

10. Immunodiagnostics in Parasitology   251

11. PCRs—an Aid to Diagnose Parasitic Diseases   270

12. Therapy of Parasitic Infections   287

Remembering What Has Been Learnt   299

Index   315

Plate I

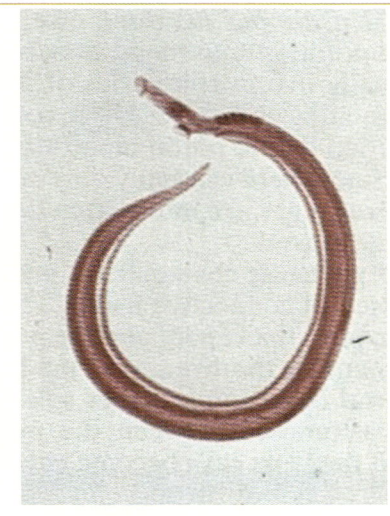 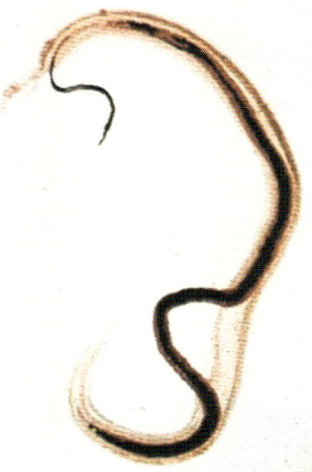 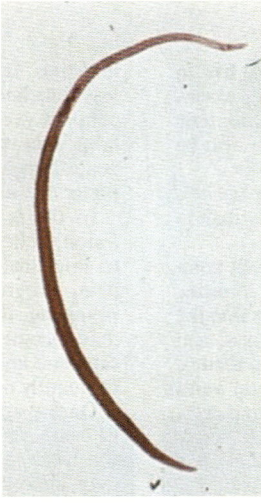

S. mansoni (male)

- 8–10 mm long
- Has gynaecophoric canal
- Dorsal surface covered with tubercle

S. mansoni (male and female)

S. mansoni (female)

- 14 mm long
- Taller and thinner
- Vitelline glands occupy 2/3 of the body

Male and female S. mansoni

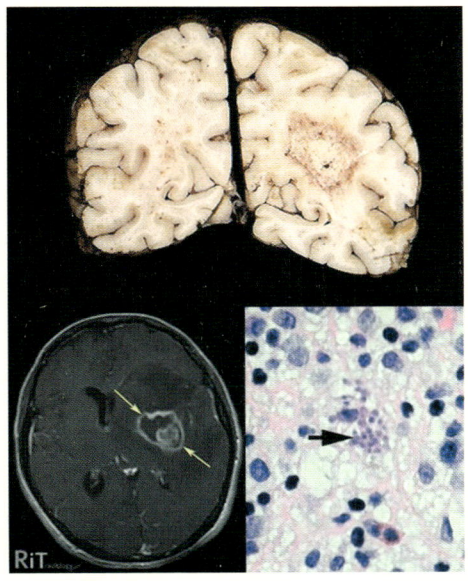

Cerebral toxoplasmosis

Toxoplasma gondii

CT/MRI: Multiple ring-enhancing lesions

Morphology:

- Multiple abscesses
- Acute lesions—necrosis surrounded by acute/ chronic inflammation and vascular proliferation
- Free tachyzoites and encysted bradyzoites

Brain in acute toxoplasmosis

Plate II

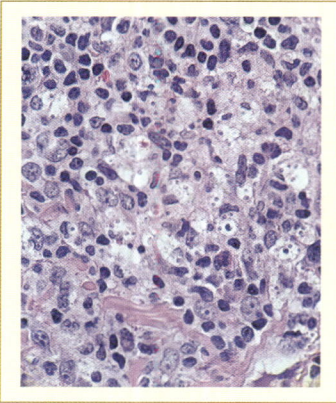

Cutaneous leishmaniasis

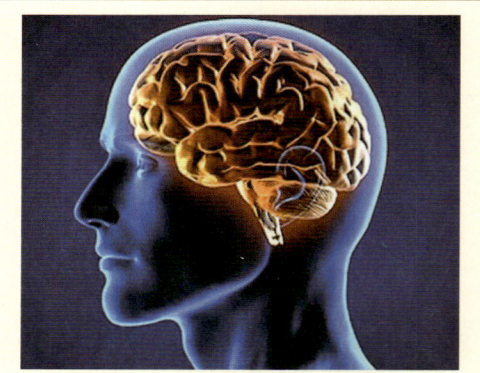

Abscess of hepatic amoebiasis

Amoebic liver abscess

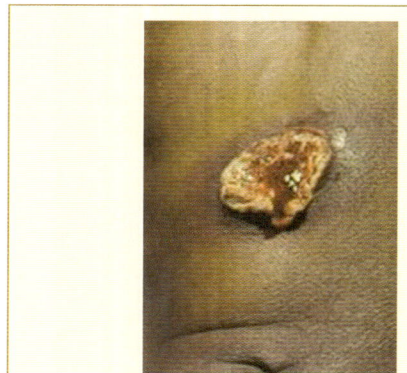
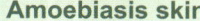

Amoebiasis skin

Brain

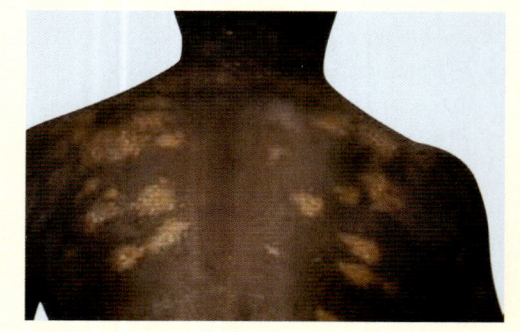

Post kala-azar dermatitis

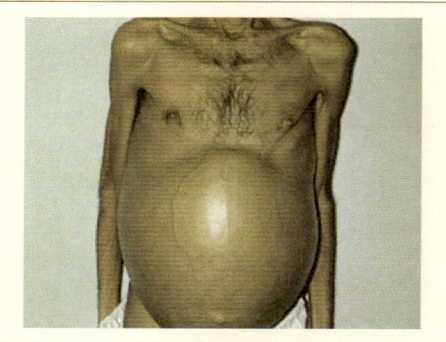

Splenomegaly in schistosomiasis

Plate III

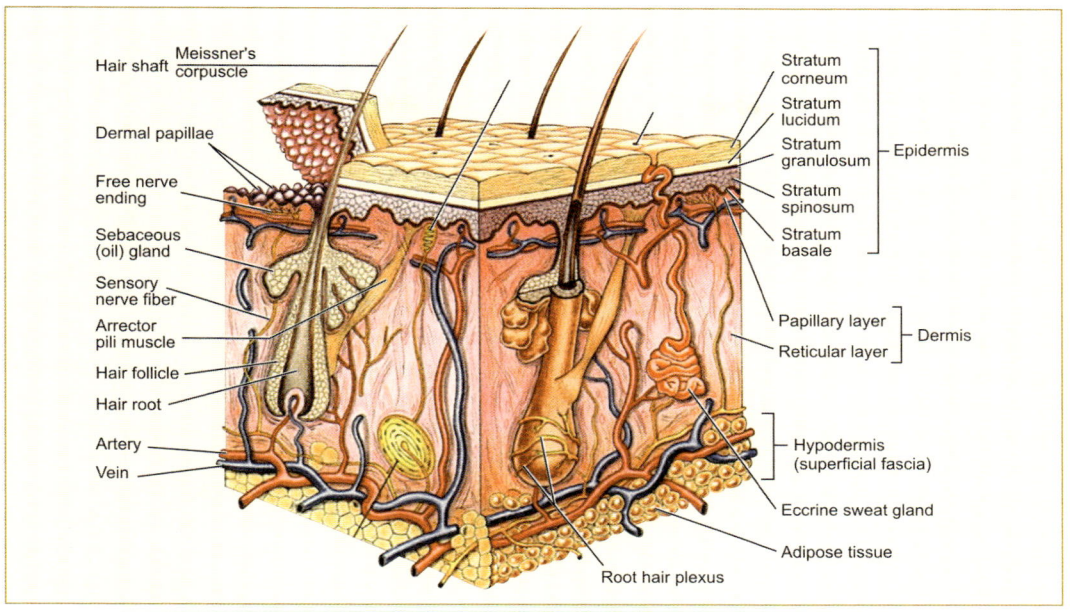

Hair shaft
Meissner's corpuscle
Dermal papillae
Free nerve ending
Sebaceous (oil) gland
Sensory nerve fiber
Arrector pili muscle
Hair follicle
Hair root
Artery
Vein

Stratum corneum
Stratum lucidum
Stratum granulosum
Stratum spinosum
Stratum basale
Epidermis

Papillary layer
Reticular layer
Dermis

Hypodermis (superficial fascia)

Eccrine sweat gland
Adipose tissue
Root hair plexus

Skin

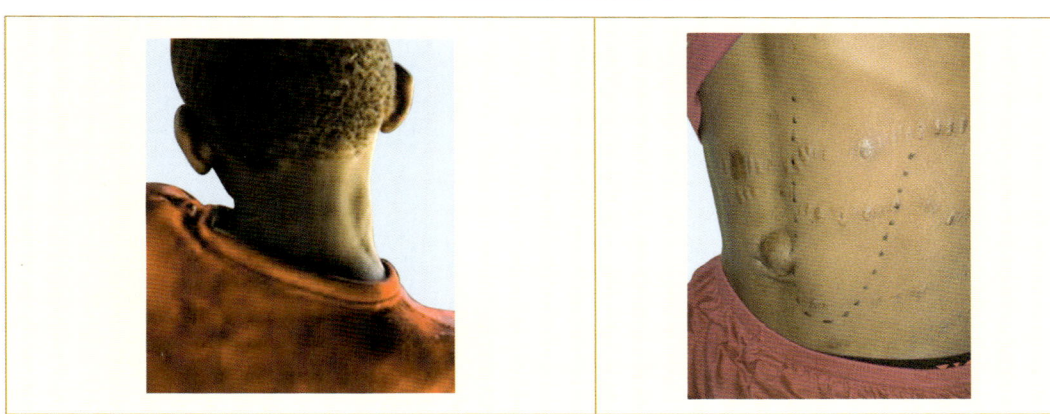

Lymphadenopathy in *T. brucei* infestation

Splenomegaly in chronic malaria

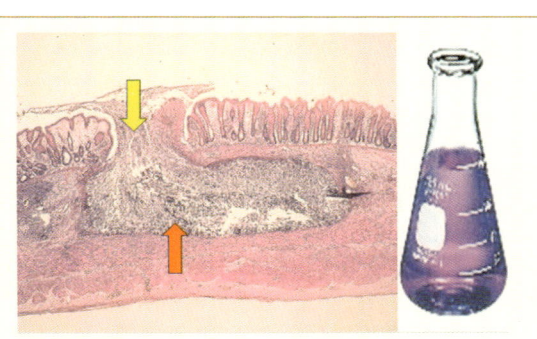

Histopathology of typical flask-shaped ulcer of intestinal amoebiasis

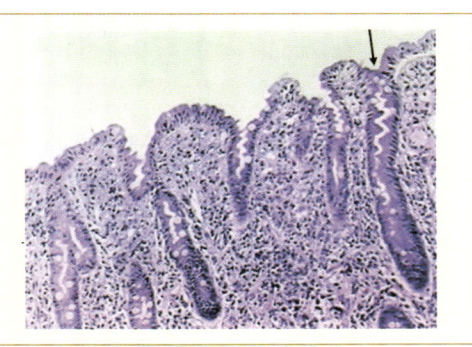

Villous atrophy in duodenojejunal giardiasis

Plate IV

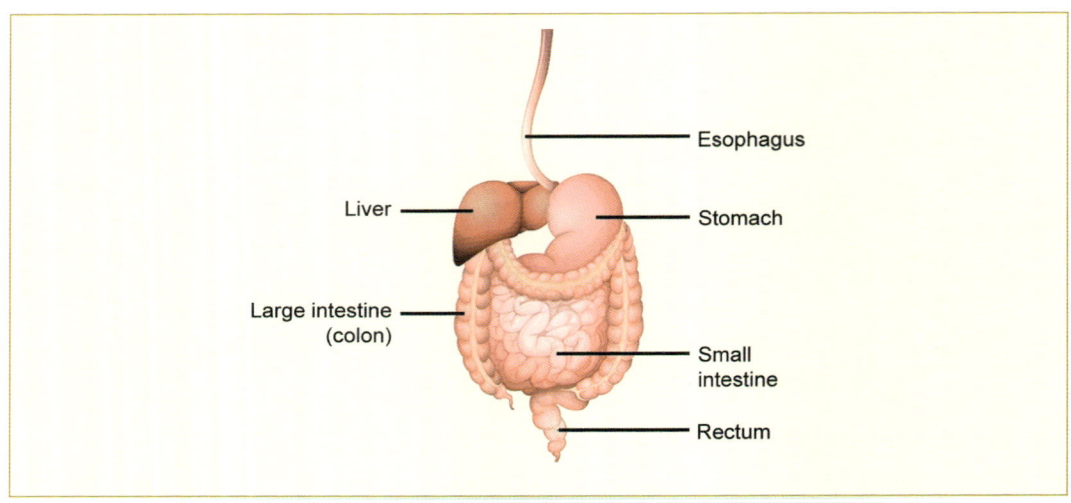

Esophagus

Liver

Stomach

Large intestine
(colon)

Small
intestine

Rectum

Gastrointestinal tract

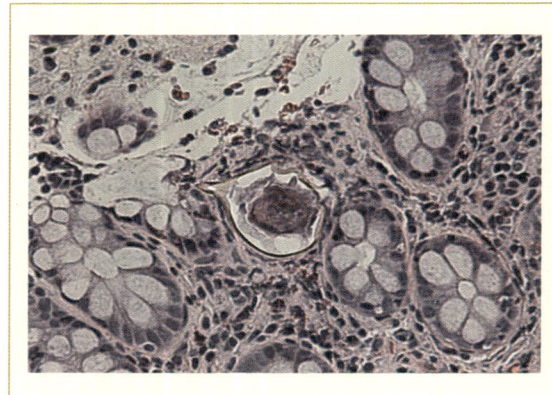

S. japonicum **eggs in colon**

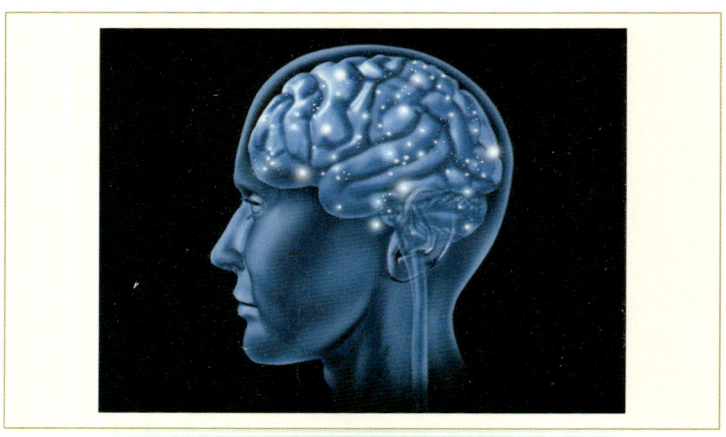

Trypanosome in lymph fluid

Brain

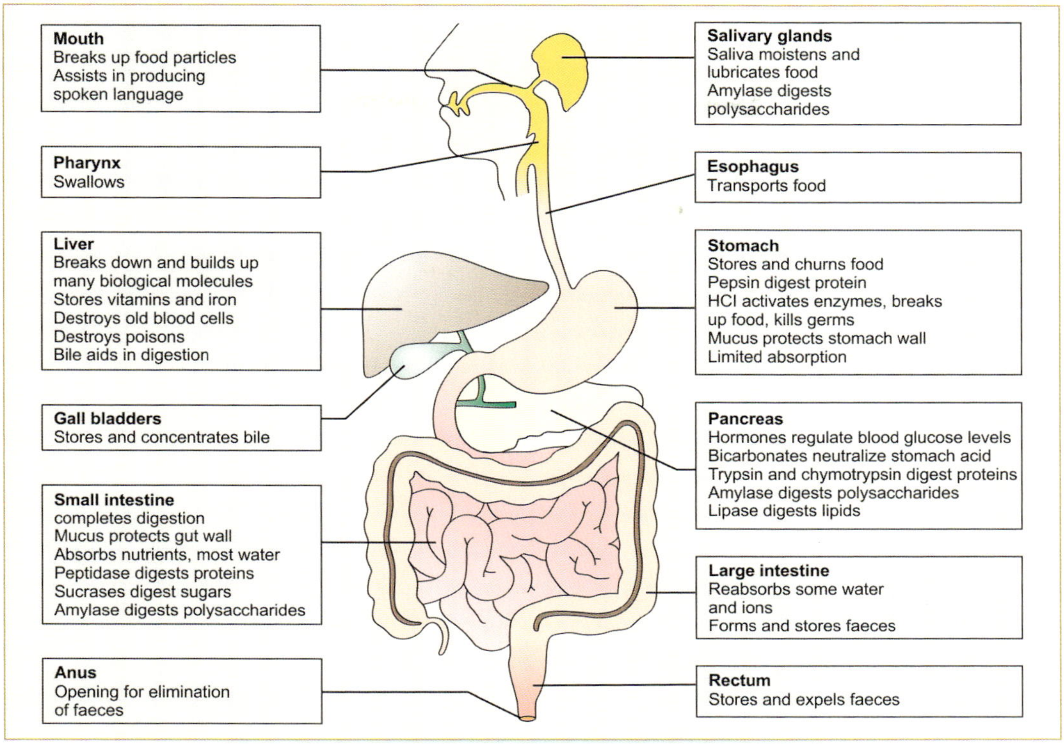

Plate V

Mouth
Breaks up food particles
Assists in producing
spoken language

Salivary glands
Saliva moistens and
lubricates food
Amylase digests
polysaccharides

Pharynx
Swallows

Esophagus
Transports food

Liver
Breaks down and builds up
many biological molecules
Stores vitamins and iron
Destroys old blood cells
Destroys poisons
Bile aids in digestion

Stomach
Stores and churns food
Pepsin digest protein
HCl activates enzymes, breaks
up food, kills germs
Mucus protects stomach wall
Limited absorption

Gall bladders
Stores and concentrates bile

Pancreas
Hormones regulate blood glucose levels
Bicarbonates neutralize stomach acid
Trypsin and chymotrypsin digest proteins
Amylase digests polysaccharides
Lipase digests lipids

Small intestine
completes digestion
Mucus protects gut wall
Absorbs nutrients, most water
Peptidase digests proteins
Sucrases digest sugars
Amylase digests polysaccharides

Large intestine
Reabsorbs some water
and ions
Forms and stores faeces

Anus
Opening for elimination
of faeces

Rectum
Stores and expels faeces

Gastrointestinal system

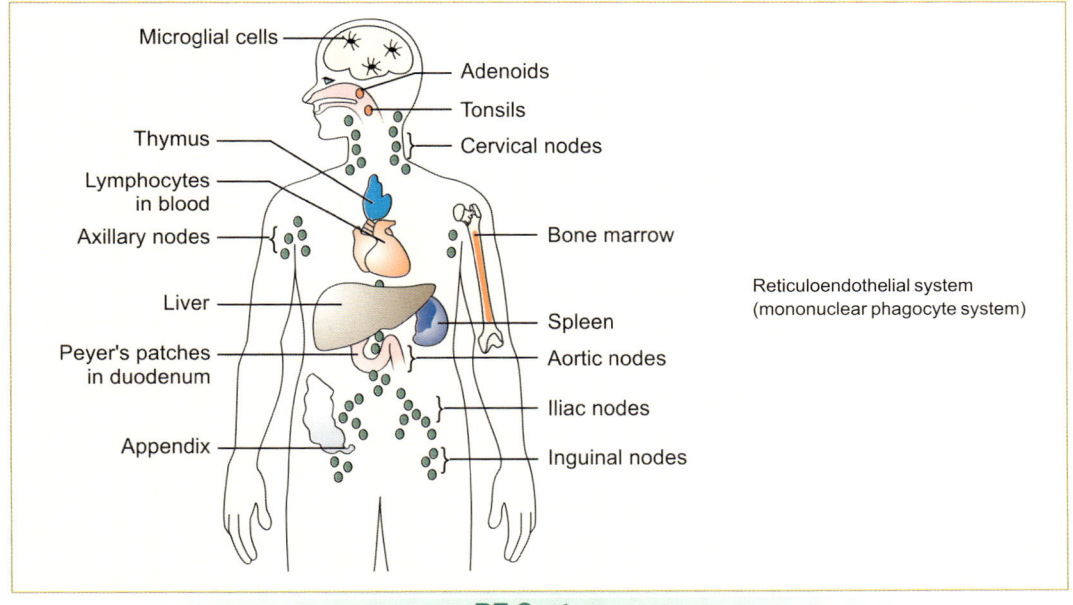

Microglial cells

Adenoids

Tonsils

Thymus

Cervical nodes

Lymphocytes
in blood

Axillary nodes

Bone marrow

Liver

Spleen

Peyer's patches
in duodenum

Aortic nodes

Iliac nodes

Appendix

Inguinal nodes

Reticuloendothelial system
(mononuclear phagocyte system)

RE System

Plate VI

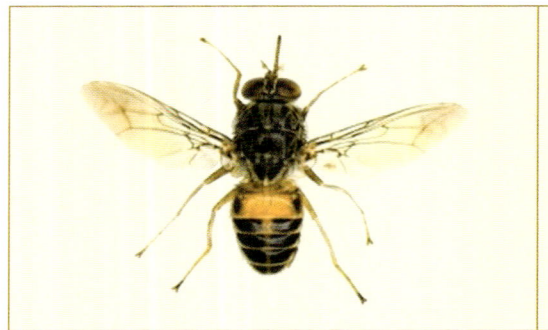

Tsetse fly

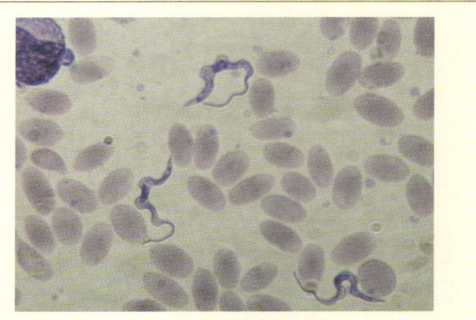

Trypanosome in human blood

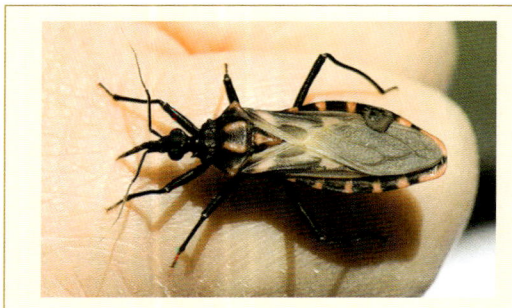

Reduviid bug

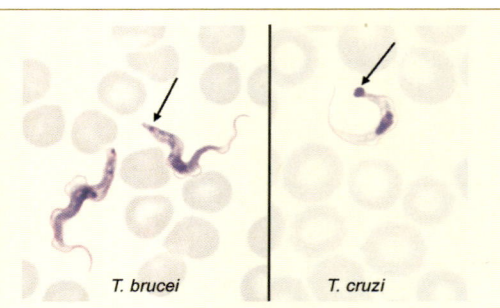

T. cruzi and T. brucei

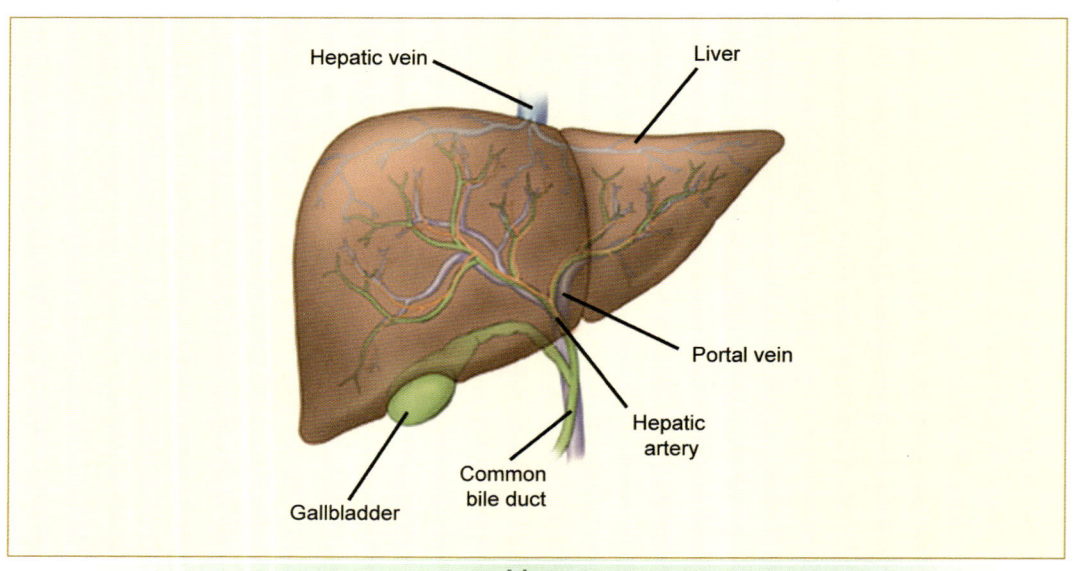

Liver

Plate VII

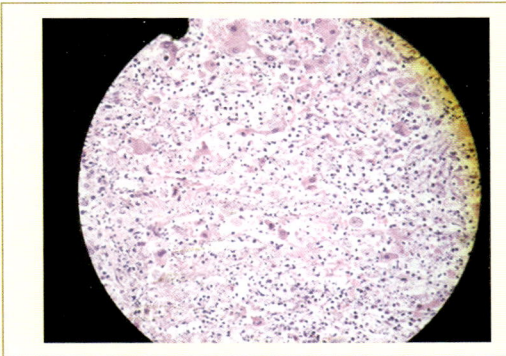

Amoebic liver abscess

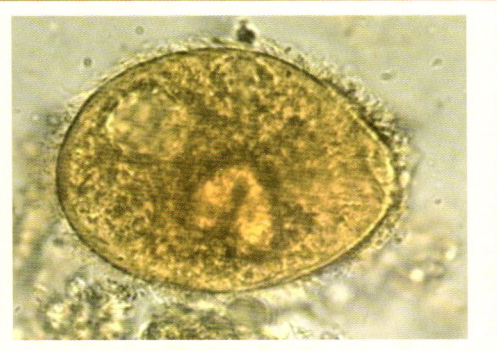

Balantidium coli

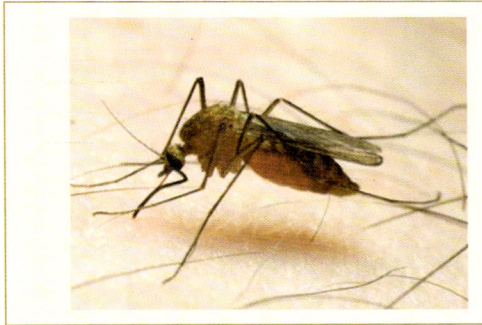

Anopheles mosquito

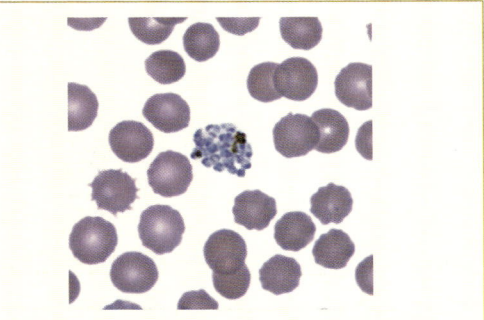

Vivax malaria schizont

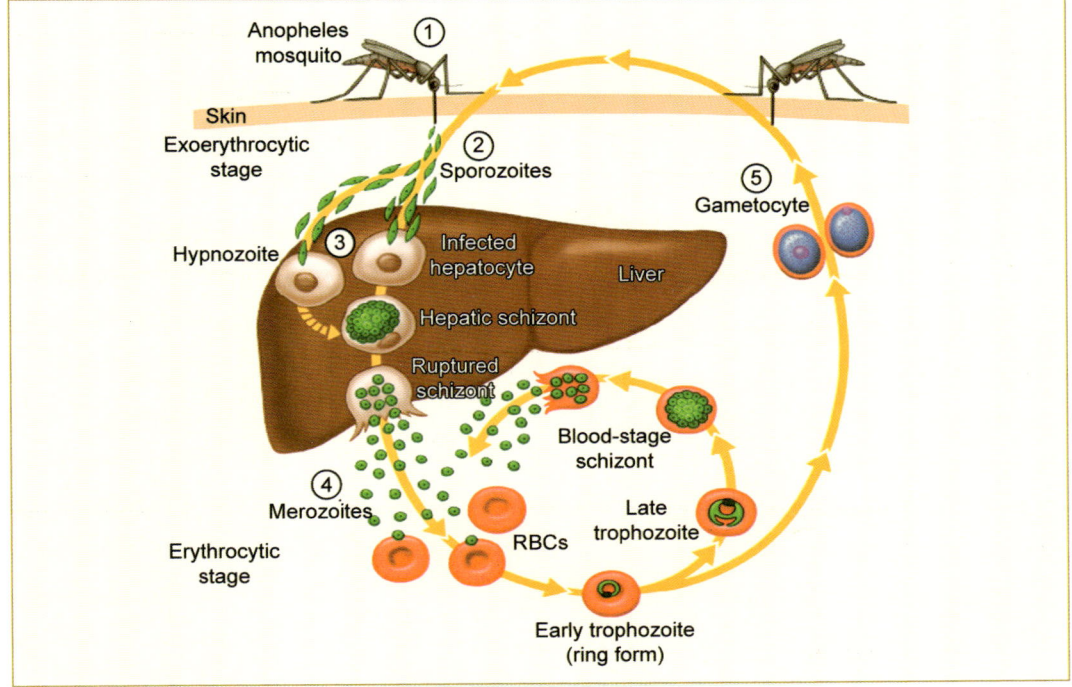

Liver in malaria and life cycle

Plate VIII

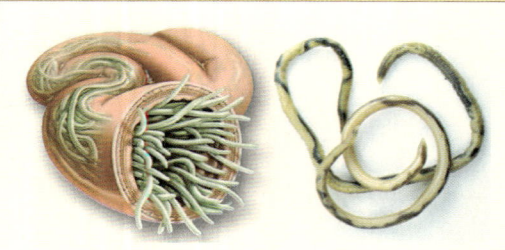

Intestine filled with roundworms

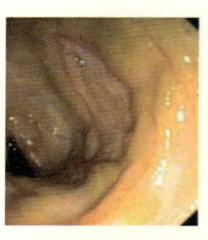

Cecal ulcer in amoebiasis

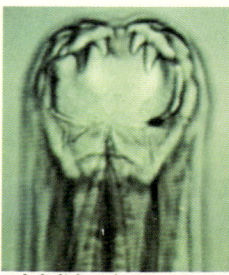

Adult hookworms
note teeth

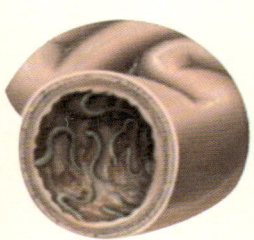

Hookworms living
inside the intestines

Adult hookworms in intestine

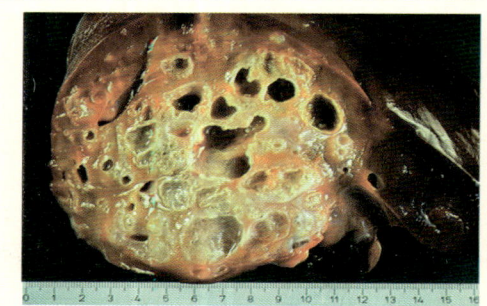

Hydatidosis liver

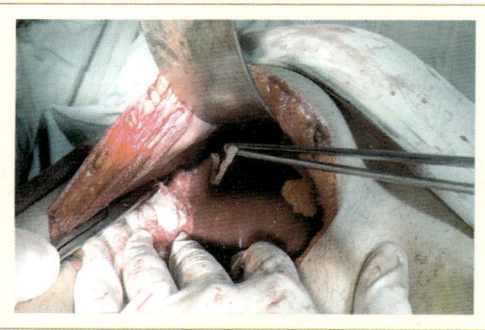

Ascariasis liver

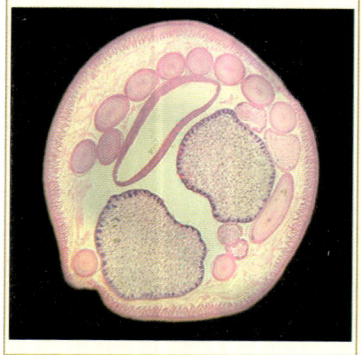

Enlarged lymph node in filariasis

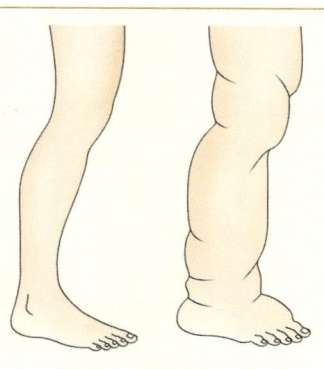

Elephantiasis leg

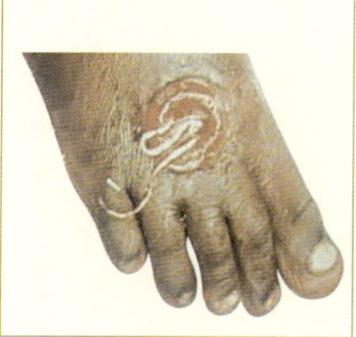

Adult guinea worm in skin

Introduction to Parasitology

Commonly Employed Terminology

Parasite is described as a living organism which derives its nourishment from another organism and adapts itself to live in it. The english dictionary meaning of 'parasite' is to eat from someone else's table.

Host is an organism which harbors the parasite.

Classification of Relationships Between two Living Organisms

Symbiosis is a relationship between two organisms whereby both are dependent upon each other and no harm is caused to either of them as a result of the association. Organisms are designated as symbionts.

Commensalism is association where the parasite benefits from the host without causing injury or disease to it. A commensal can live on its own too, e.g. *Entamoeba coli.*

Parasitism is an association whereby the parasite derives benefit from the host and also produces disease or injury in the host, however, insignificant that may be. The host usually does offer some resistance but may sometimes adapt to exist with the parasite, i.e. develop tolerance. Parasites that produce disease are also designated as 'pathogens'. A parasite is not capable of independent existence without the host, e.g. *Entamoeba histolytica.*

Zoonosis is development of a disease in human beings naturally acquired from an infection that is primarily restricted to vertebrate animals. 'Zoonosis' literally means a disease of animals, e.g. leishmaniasis, sleeping sickness, trichinelliasis and echinococcosis (hydatid cyst).

Classification of Parasites

Ectoparasite: Lives outside or on the surface of the body of the host.

Endoparasite: Lives within the body of the host.

Temporary parasite: Enters the host for a short period.

Permanent parasite: Leads a parasitic life throughout its existence.

Facultative parasite: Lives as a parasite when it gets an opportunity to do so.

Obligatory parasite is destined to live only a parasitic life.

Occasional or accidental parasite: Attacks an unusual host.

Wandering or aberrant parasite: The parasite arrives at a place where it cannot survive.

Classification of Hosts

Definitive host is a host that either harbors the adult stage of the parasite or where the parasite undergoes the sexual method of reproduction. By and large in most human parasitic infections, man is the definitive host.

Intermediate host: Such a host harbors the larval stages of the parasite. Sometimes two different intermediate hosts may be required to complete larval stages—here the hosts are designated as first and second intermediate hosts respectively. In malaria and hydatid cyst—man acts as an intermediate host.

Paratenic host is described as a transport or a carrier host. The parasite remains viable without further development.

Scheme of Study Observed in this Book

Medical parasites have been described in this book by and large as per the sequence mentioned below:
1. Historical aspects as related the parasite.
2. Geographical distribution.
3. Habitat within the human host.
4. Morphology and life cycle.
5. Modes of infection.
6. Effects of the parasite.
7. Immunological responses.
8. Laboratory diagnosis.
9. Treatment.
10. Prophylaxis.

Brief Description of Headings

History: Year of discovery, name of discoverer and any relevant or important facts pertaining to discovery or acquisition of knowledge regarding the parasite being discussed.

Geographical distribution: Temperature, humidity (environmental factors), social customs and personal habits influence the distribution of parasites; hence each parasite has specific geographic distribution.

Habitat: As per needs of a particular parasite, it occupies a particular place of residence in the host. A parasite may reach elsewhere in the body—a place ideal for its growth to sexual maturity or it may often taking a circumroutous path arrive at its original portal of entry (as happens in the case of *Ascaris lumbricoides*). In some cases the parasite may mature at one place and then migrate elsewhere to an appropriate location to enable its progeny to be transferred to a second host (as in Schistosoma), or it may discharge its larvae which are carried to some distant place either to be taken up by an intermediate host (as in Wuchereria) or stay encysted in a striped muscle (as in Trichinella). The sites of localisation, therefore, determine the pathogenic effects and the channels through which the progeny may come out of the human host.

Morphology and life cycle: The general structure of the parasite and the various phases through which it passes are studied under this heading. The parasite may have one or more hosts.

Modes of infection: Infective stages of the parasite are responsible for transmission of the parasite from one host to another. The means and avenues made use of by infecting agents need closer look. An endemic area usually has humans or animals serving as an intermediate host (vector) in dissemination of the disease, its bionomics should be examined too.

Infection reservoirs by and large man is the main reservoir and works as a carrier (symptoms not manifested), the parasite evolves certain resistant forms which assist in further spread of the disease, e.g. gametocytes of malarial parasite and cysts of *E. histolytica*. In certain species of parasites, both men and lower animals are infected, the latta serving as reservoirs of infection, e.g. Oriental sore (dog), Kala-azar in China and Mediterranean region (dog), balanticliasis (pig), trichnellasis (pig and rat), hydatid cyst (sheep and cattle) and *Rhodesian trypanosomiasis* (antelope).

Source of Infection and Portal of Entry (Table 1.1)

Given below are the way by which a parasite may reach a human host:

I. Through digestive tract via contamination of food or drink

    A. Cysts of *E. histolytica* and ova of *A. lumbricoides* that contaminante the food or drink.

    B. The infective form may reside in the flesh of same intermediate hosts, which are consumed as food, e.g.

        (i) Beef containing the larval stages of *T. saginata (Cysticercus bovis)*;

        (ii) Pork containing the larval form of *T. solium (Cysticercus cellulosae)* and the larval forms of *T. spiralis*;

        (iii) Fish containing the plerocercoid larvae of *D. latum* and metacercarial form of *C. sinesis*;

        (iv) Crab or crayfish containing metacercarial forms of *P. westermani*.

    C. Sometimes the intermediate host may be consumed as a whole, e.g. cyclops infected with the larval forms of *D. medinesis* are ingested with water.

    D. The infective forms may come out of its intermediate host and encyst in aquatic plants, eaten as food by humans, e.g. metacercarial forms of *F. buski* and *F. hepatica*.

II. Contamination of skin or mucous membrane

    A. Filariform larvae of *A. duodenale*, *N. americanus* and *S. stercoralis* which are often found it moist soil may penetrate the intact skin of an individual walking barefooted on such soil (as happens with gardeners).

    B. The cercarial forms of *S. haematobium*, *S. mansoni* and *S. japonicum* in infected water, may pierce through the skin of a person coming in contact with such water.

III. Via an insect host. An infected blood-sucking arthropod may introduce the organism straight into the bloodstream or into the integumentary layers (skin) at the time of sucking a blood-meal, e.g. Plasmodia (malarial parasites) by Anopheline mosquitoes, Trypanosoma by Glossina (Tsetse fly), Leishmania by Phlebotomus (Sandfly) and Wuchereria by Culcine mosquitoes. In the group the parasites undergo morphological development for a certain period before becoming infective to human beings.

Table 1.1: Spread of parasitic infections			
Source of infection	Infective forms situation	Entry portal	Involved parasite
Through water			
Infective forms released from snail	Cercaria of Schistosome released in water	Direct cutaneous penetration	S. haematobium S. mansoni S. japonicum
Infected cyclops	Drancunculus larvae present in cyclops	Ingestion, alimentary tract	D. medinesis
Through soil			
Polluted with human faeces	A. Embryonated ova or Ascaris, Trichuris	Ingestion, alimentary tract	A. lumbricoides T. trichiura
	B. Filariform larvae of hookworm and Stronglyloides	Direct cutaneous penetration	A. duodenale N. americanus
Polluted with faeces	Embryonated egg of A. caninum and A. brazilense	Infestation, alimentary skin	Larva migrans (cutaneous)
Through human faeces			
Contamination of food	A. Ova of Enterobius, Hymenolepis nana and T. solium	Ingestion, alimentary tract	E. vermicularis H. nana
	B. Cyst of E. histolytica & B. coli.	Ingestion, alimentary tract	E. histolytica B. coli
Through arthropod			
Crab of crayfish	Metacerariae in fish	Ingestion, alimentary tract	P. westermani
Cyclops	A. Larvae inside the body cavity	Ingestion, alimentary tract	D. medinesis
	B. Proceroid larvae inside the body	Ingestion, alimentary tract	Plerocercoid larvae spirometra
Reduvid bug	Metacyclic form in hind gut	Contamination, skin	T. cruzi
Tsetse fly (glossina)	Metacyclic forms of trypomastigotes in salivary gland	Inoculation, skin	T. brucei
Sandfly (Phlebotomus, Lutzomyia)	Promastigotes in pharynx and buccal cavity	Inoculation, skin L. tropica	L. donovani
Mosquitoes	Sporozoites in salivary glands	Inoculation, skin	Malarial parasites
Culex	Larvae in proboscis	Dropped on skin	W. bancrofti
Mansonioides	Larvae in proboscis	Dropped on skin	B. malayi
Chrysops	Larvae in proboscis	Dropped on skin	L. loa

Contd.

Table 1.1: Spread of parasitic infections (*Contd.*)			
Source of infection	*Infective forms situation*	*Entry portal*	*Involved parasite*
Simulium	Larvae in proboscis	Dropped on skin	*O. volvulus*
Housefly	Cyst in alimentary canal, food contamination	Ingestion, alimentary tract	*E. histolytica*
Through mollusca (Snail)	Cercariae encysted in aquatic vegetation	Ingestion, alimentary tract	*F. buski* *F. hepatica*
	Cercariae liberated in water	Cutaneous penetration	*Schistosomes*
Through piscine host			
Freshwater fish	Plerocercoid larvae in fish-flesh	Ingestion, alimentary tract	*D. latum*
	Metacercariae in fish-flesh	Ingestion, alimentary tract	*C. sinensis*
	B. Procercoid larvae inside the body	Ingestion, alimentary tract	*Plerocercoid larvae*
			Spirometra *H. heterophyes* *M. Yokogawai*
Through mammalian	*C. bovis* in muscles	Ingestion, alimentary tract	*T. saginata*
Cow pig	A. *C. cellulosae* in muscles	Ingestion, alimentary tract	*T. solium*
	B. Encysted larvae in muscles	Ingestion, alimentary tract	*T. spiralis*
	C. Plerocercoid larvae in muscles	Ingestion, alimentary tract	Spirometra (larval stage)
	D. Cyst of *B. coli* in faeces	Ingestion, alimentary tract	*B. coli*
Dog	Ova of *E. granulosus* and *T. canis* in faeces, food contamination	Ingestion, alimentary tract	*Larva migrans* (visceral)
Cat	Oocystis in faeces	Ingestion, alimentary tract	*T. gondii*
Man	Autoinfection—finger to mouth	Ingestion	Pinworm

Effects of Parasite

Pathogenic effects: Vary with different parasites. In *protozoal* infection, the lesions are significantly influenced by proliferation, multiplication and metastasis to distant organs. In *Entamoeba histolytica,* the trophozoites secrete a powerful histolytic enzyme, thereby causing destruction of surrounding tissues. In malaria, the parasite while undergoing erythrocytic schizogony, causes haemolyses of erythrocytes.

In *Helminthic* infections, the adult parasites are found inside the human body and no multiplication occurs except in cases of strongyloidiasis and hymenolepiasis. The number of invading organisms during primary infection or re-infection determine the clinical manifestations in helminthiasis. The effects caused therefore depend upon their habitat, i.e. the locations where the parasites attack the tissues and also on the pattern of laying eggs or larvae. In certain helminthic infections, the normal secretions and excretions of the growing larvae and the products liberated after the death of the parasites behave as foreign proteins and elicit various allergic responses. Various skin tests, therfore, are employed in diagnosis of these infections.

Miscellaneous Pathogenic Effects

Certain parasitic infections induce an immunosuppressive state, thereby making the patient vulnerable to bacteria (both pathogenic and otherwise), e.g. trypanosomiasis, kala-azar and malaria. Compromised immunological state (owing to infections or drugs) may help parasitic multiplication, resulting in fulminant parasitemia, as in falciparum malaria or may favour extensive invasion of tissue, as in strongyloidiasis or may help 'opportunistic infections', as in toxoplasmosis.

Parasites may cause chronic irritation and be responsible for development of a neoplastic lesion:

   (i) Fascioliases and Clonorchiasis may lead to development of adenocarcinoma of bile duct and hepatocellular carcinoma.

   (ii) Schistosomiasis may lead to carcinoma of colon, rectum, liver or urinary bladder.

  (iii) Malarial infection may be responsible for Burkitt's lymphoma.

The migrating larvae may carry with them bacteria or viruses from intestine to blood or other tissues—as may occur in Strongyloidisis, Trichinosis and Ascariasis.

Immunological responses of the host may also be responsible for the pathological effects, e.g.

   (i) Tropical splenomegaly syndrome (TSS) and nephrotic syndrome in malaria.

   (ii) Autoimmune haemolytic anaemia observed in kala-azar and malaria.

  (iii) Granulomatous reaction with subsequent fibrosis in schistosomiasis—consequent to cell-mediated immune responses.

  (iv) Manifestations seen in occult filariasis.

Immunological Responses and Parasites

Akin to other infectious agents, parasites also elicit immune responses in the host, both humoral as well as cellular. But immunological protection against parasites is far less effective when one compares it with that of bacterial or viral infections. These are two main types of immunity: Innate and acquired. *Innate immunity* does not depend upon previous exposure to the infective agent and does not arise out of specific responses of immunocompetent cells. Genetic constitution of the host determines the innate immunity, e.g. Central/West Africans are more resistant than the white westerners to hookworm infection and vivax malaria. It is also well known that African children carrying the sickle-cell anaemia trait (HbS heterozygotes) are relatively resistant to *P. falciparum* infection. Acquired immunity may be gradually developed after a natural infection (following clinically apparent or a subclinical infection) or may be artifi-cially induced, as in cutaneous leishmaniasis (Oriental sore). This is known as active immunity. Immunoglobulins may be passively transferred to a neonate via placenta or milk (colostrum) of an immune pregnant woman called *Passive immunity.* In endemic malarious regions the infants born to immune mothers are thus protected for the first 6 months of life against *P. falciparum* infections. Subsequently, the child may suffer from malarial attacks for 2–5 years when acquired immunity takes over with further development of tolerance as the child grows (i.e. child may or may not show signs and symptoms to reinfections).

ACQUIRED ACTIVE IMMUNITY

Immune reactions in acquired active immunity may be humorally mediated or cell-mediated or may have both the components:

1. **Humoral factors:** Involves development/production of *specific immunoglobulins.* The antigens are first taken up by macrophages before being transferred onto the immunocompetent cells—'thymus dependent' lymphocytes and plasma cells. The antibody manufacturing plasma cells are derived from bone marrow stem cells and are not thymus dependent. Immunoglobulins are of 5 different classes, viz. IgG, IgM, IgA, IgD and IgE; the first two are most important. A significant level of specific immunoglobulins are found in many protozoal and helminthic infections. They may be protective and assist in recovery from infection, or they may be precipitating and may be made use of in various specific serological tests employed for immunodiagnosis of parasitic infections. Both IgG and IgM are increased in malaria, the former has antiplasmodial effect and latter asissts in phagocytosis. A nonspecific IgM is greatly increased in trypansomiasis, this immunoglobulin, however, has no affinity for the infecting organism. Likewise antibodies are demonstrable in kala-azar also but here too they do not assist in recovery from infection. Protective antibodies also develop in helminthic infections but only to a lesser extent they lower the worm load, e.g. in Strongyloidiasis, Ancylostomiasis and Ascariasis.

2. **Cellular factors:**

   A. *Induction of cell-mediated immunity (CMI):* Thymus derived lymphocytes dispersed to lymph nodes and spleen are necessary for CMI. They get sensitised and later play an important role in eliminating the parasites. This kind of immunity can be transferred by lymphocytes and can be hampered by immunosuppressive diseases or drugs. They also produce antibodies that tag onto cells and are not easily released, thereby behaving as specific antigen recognising mechanism of these sensitised cells. A significantly marked CMI develops in self-curing cutaneous leishmaniasis like Oriental sore—this can be demonstrated by a delayed type of hypersensitivity skin reaction. CMI also develops in trichinosis and schistosomiasis.

   B. *Development of non-specific cellular response:* Antigenic stimulus induces the cells of reticuloendothelial system (RES) to proliferate and actively phagocytose the antigen—this is especially observed in African Trypanosomiasis where macrophages help in eliminating the trypomastigotes. Macrophages, along with serum antibodies act synergistically to control malaria.

OTHER TYPES OF IMMUNE REACTIONS

A. **Autoimmune reaction:** Implies development of antibodies against one's own body tissues, e.g. autoimmune antibody development against RBCs and causing anaemia, as seen in kala-azar and malaria.

B. **Hypersensitivity reaction:** Immune reactions at times, besides being protective, can also be harmful (production of excessive/exaggerated response) and be responsible for various pathogical reactions. These may be of two types: Immediate or delayed.

(a) *Immediate hypersensitivity:* Resulting from antibody-mediated immunity. May occur from contact of antigen with antibody fixed to the cells, as in anaphylactic reaction or the antigen-antibody complexes may induce pathological alterations, as in nephrotic syndrome in quartan malaria.

(b) *Delayed hypersensitivity:* Resulting from CMI. Often made use of in intradermal tests for parasitological diagnosis as in Montenegro reaction in leishmaniasis and is also responsible for the granulomatous reaction provoked by Schistosome eggs.

(c) *Premunition* is described as concomitant immunity or infection immunity in which there is relative resistance to re-infection of host still haboring the infecting organism. It vanishes with the eradication of the parasitic infection, e.g. in schistosomiasis and malaria. In malaria as long as erythrocytic parasites exist, the 'premunition' persists but with total elimination of parasistes—it disappears. In schistosomiasis the adult worms resist immunological attacks and persist in the host for long periods. It has been attributed to the acquisition of a coating of host antigen which prevents their destruction by the immune responses excited by the adult worms themselves.

(d) *Tolerance:* Implies infection immunity whereby host-parasite adjustment takes place in such a way that the infection continues without producing any ill effects on the host and the individual concerned becomes resistant to reinfection. This explains increasing resistance to infection with advancing age.

Prophylactic immunisation has by and large been unsuccessful against human parasitic diseases except in a few protozoal infections, e.g. Oriental sore. *Plasmodium knowlesi* is being tried for developing a prophylactic immunisation agent against malaria.

Laboratory diagnosis: Depending upon the nature and habitat of the parasite involved—various materials can be obtained/utilised for establishing the diagnosis.

I. **Blood:** When the parasite normally resides and/or circulates during its life cycle in blood. Examination of peripheral blood smear can be done, e.g.

(i) In malaria, parasites are found within the RBCs.

(ii) In kala-azar, *L. donovani* are found inside monocytes of blood.

(iii) In African sleeping sickness and Chaga's disease, trypomastigotes are found in blood plasma.

(iv) In Bancroftian and Malayan filariasis microfilariae are found in blood plasma.

II. **Stool:** Stool examination is of great significance for diagnosing intestinal parasites (protozoal or helminths). Ducts draining into the intestinal tract may harbor helminths, which discharge their eggs into the intestine, these are ultimately diagnosed from stool examination.

In protozoal infections, trophozoites or cysts may be found in stool. Trophozoites during active phase and cysts during the chronic phase, e.g. in amoebiasis, giardiasis and balantidiasis.

In *helminthic infection* either the adult worm or their eggs may be found in stool. Rarely, as in roundworm infection, they may be vomitted out too.

(i) Eggs are observed in intestinal helminthiasis (ascariasis, ancylostomiasis, trichuriasis, fascilopsiasis, intestinal schistosomiasis, taeniasis, diphyllobo-thriasis, hymenolepiasis and diplydiasis) and also where the worms reside in the biliary tract (fascioliasis and clonorchiasis).

(ii) In *Enterobius veirmicularis* infection, eggs are rarely seen in stool because they are deposited on the perianal skin, therefore, anal swabs are used here for diagnosis.

(iii) In strongyloidiasis, larvae, and not eggs, are found in freshly-passed stool.

(iv) Adult worms may be observed in stool in ascariasis and after a vermifuge in hookworm infection and enterobiasis. Adult worm segments are observed in taeniasis, diphyllobothriasis and other intestinal tapeworm infections.

III. **Urine:** When parasites inhabit the uninary tract, urine examination is helpful in diagnosis:

(i) In vesical schistosomiasis, terminal-spined eggs of *E. haematobium* are found.

(ii) In chyluria caused by *W. bancrofti,* the microflariae are detected.

IV. **Sputum:** Sputum examination is useful in:

(i) Where the parasite resides in the respiratory tract, as in paragonimiasis, the eggs of *P. westermani* are found.

(ii) In amoebic lung abscess or liver abscess bursting into the lung—the tropho-zoites of *E. histolytica* (and not cysts) are detected in sputum.

(iii) In ruptured hydatid cyst of lung, scolices and hooklets of *E. granulosus* are obtained.

V. **Biopsy material/aspirates:** It varies with different parasitic infections:

(i) Splenic puncture in kala-azar.

(ii) Bone marrow aspirate in kala-azar and African trypansomiasis.

(iii) Lymph node puncture in cases of African sleeping sickness and filariasis; also in cases of kala-azar occurring in Mediterranean region and China.

(iv) Skin biopsy in dermal leishmanoid, espundia and onchocerciasis.

(v) Muscle biopsy in cases of cysticercosis, trichnelliasis and Chagas' disease.

(vi) Liver biopsy in visceral larva migrans and visceral schistosomiasis.

(vii) Rectal biopsy in cases of intestinal schistosomiasis.

(viii) *Aspiration of:*

(a) Hydatid fluid

(b) Anchovy sauce

(c) Fluid from hydrocele for revealing scolex of *E. granulosus,* trophozoite of *E. histolytica* and microfilaria of *W. brancrofti* respectively

(ix) Lumbar puncture. Cerebrospinal fluid may be collected for the diagnosis of African trypanosomiasis (sleeping sickness).

VI. **Indirect evidences:** Investigations that do not reveal parasites, but indicate their presence in the host.

(i) *Cytomorphological changes in blood: Eosinophilia* often indicates tissue invasion by a helminth, leucopenia is seen in kala-azar and neutrophilia is found in amoebic liver abscess. Anaemia is a feature of malaria and hookworm infestation.

(ii) *Biochemical alteration in blood:* Hypergammaglobulinemia is detected in cases of kala-azar, African trypanosomiasis, schistosomiasis and visceral larva migrans. Can be detected as formol gel test (aldehyde test of Napier) or as a precipitation reaction (Sia's test, antimony test of Chopra) or by doing immunoelectropho-resis or turbidometric estimation of immunoglobulins.

    (iii) *Serological tests*
        (a) Specific complement fixation test is used in many protozoal anal helminthic infections, such as Chagas' disease, amoebiasis, toxoplasmosis, filariasis, trichinelliasis, hydatid disease, schistosomiasis and clonorchiasis. Non-specific complement fixation test—as in kala-azar.
        (b) Specific precipitin test, as in schistosomiasis, hydatid disease and amoebiasis. Specific precipitin antibody may also be demonstrated by flocculation test, such as bentonite flocculation test conducted for trichnelliasis and hydatid disease.
        (c) Specific agglutination test, as in leishmaniasis.
        (d) Specific dye test of Sabin and Feldman, as in toxoplasmosis.
        (e) Immobilisation test, as in amoebiasis.
        (f) Fluorescent antibody technique (FAT). Reaction of the parasite with fluorescin-tagged homologous antibody, as in *E. histolytica* and Toxoplasma. The fluorescent antibody technique has also been used for the serological diagnosis of certain helminthic infections (Schistosomiasis, trichnelliasis, ascariasis and strongyloidiasis), and also in malaria and visceral leishmaniasis.
        (g) *Elisa/Clia:* Enzyme-linked immunosorbent assay. It is the latest amongst serological diagnostic techniques and is available for diagnosing amoebiasis, malaria, giardiasis, toxoplasmosis, echinococcosis, cysticercosis, leishmaniasis, etc.
        (h) Nucleic Acid Technology/PCR DNA DetectonTechnologies
    (iv) *Intradermal reaction (skin test):* This is positive in many helminthic infections, such as hydatid cyst (Casoni's test), schistosomiasis (Fairley's test), trichnelliasis, ascariasis and strongyloidiasis; it is also positive in certain protozoal infections, such as Chagas' disease, espundia, Oriental sore, amoebiasis and toxoplasmosis.

Treatment: Large number of parasitic infections can be cured by specific chemotherapeutic agents. Protozoal disease treatment has come a long way.

    For the treatment of intestinal helminthic infections, drugs are given orally for direct action on helminths. For a drug to be maximally useful, it should not be absorbed and should have no/negligible toxic effects.

    For somatic helminthiasis, drugs given orally should exert maximum effect on the parasite and least on other organs of the host. When given parenterally, the drugs must concentrate where the parasites are present. Effective medications are yet not discovered for somatic helminthiasis, some advances have been made in regards to paragonimiasis, clonorchiasis, schistosomiasis, fascioliasis and wuchereriasis.

Prophylaxis: Prophylactic measures employed include:
  (a) *Therapeutic prophylaxis:* Parasite is attacked within the host, thereby preventing the dissemination of the infecting agent.
  (b) *Drug prophylaxis:* Measures are employed not to prevent the infection but to abort the clinical manifestations by specific drug therapy, therefore, this method is also designated as clinical prophylaxis or suppressive therapy.
  (c) Eradication of the infection in the reservoir hosts and destruction of intermediate hosts. The infective agents may also be destroyed while they exist free outside the human body.
  (d) Personal prophylaxis may further be ensured by preventing the susceptible individuals coming in contact with infecting agents.

Phylum Protozoa

Table 2.1: Classification in brief of medically important protozoans				
Subphylum	*Class*	*Subclass or Group*	*Genus*	*Species*
Sporozoa		**Coccidia** Sexual and asexual cycle in same host, parasitise intestinal epithelium	*Isospora* *Eimeria*	*hominis* spurious parasites in man
		Haemosporidia Sexual and asexual cycles in different hosts. Parasitise fixed tissue and RBC, of vertebrate host	*Plasmodium*	*vivax* *falciparum* *malariae* *ovale*
			Sarcocystis Parasites striated muscle	*lindemanni*
Sarcodina move by pseudopodia have asexual reproduction	**Rhizopodea** Parasitic in GI tract usually, Encystment common		*Entamoeba* *Endolimax* *Iodamoeba* *Dientamoeba*	*coli* (commensal) *histolytica* *nana* *butschlii* *fragilis*
Mastigophora Flagellar movement	**Zoomasti-gophora**	Group A Habitat-GI tract and genitalia No biological vector needed Encystment frequent	*Cheilomastix* *Giardia* *Trichomonas*	*mesnili* *lamblia* *hominis*
		Group B Habitat—blood stream and tissues	*Leishmania*	*donovani* *tropica* *braziliensis* *gambiense*
		Biological vector needed	*Trypanosoma*	*rhodesiense* *cruzi*

Contd.

Subphylum	Class	Subclass or Group	Genus	Species
Ciliophora	**Ciliatea**		*Balantidium*	*coli*
Move by cilia Asexual and conjugate (sexual) reproduction			Habitat-GI tract	
Of uncertain status			*Toxoplasma*	*gondii*
No special locomotor apparatus			Parasitic in various organs	
No sexual stage			*Pneumocystis* Parasitic in respiratory passages	*carinii*

BASIC MORPHOLOGICAL FEATURES OF PROTOZOA

Definition: Protozoans consist of a single 'cell-like unit' that is complete in itself. Protozoans differ from metazoans in the following ways:

	Protozoa	Metazoa
Morphology	Unicellular	Multicellular
	A single cell-like unit	Consist of a number of cells making up a complex individual
Physiology	The single cell performs all necessary functions: Digestion, excretion, respiration and reproduction	Each specialised cell performs a particular function

Nucleus

May be single or multiple; necessary for life, genetic transmission and reproduction
consists of ⌈ Nuclear membrane
├ Nucleoplasm
└ Chromatin ──────────── ⌐ Compact

(Important in recognition   └ Scattered sometimes
of rhizopoda)   with karyosome

or

Particles throughout

or

Lining nuclear membrane

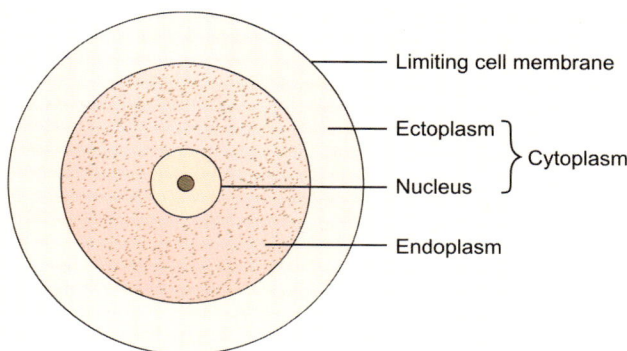

Fig. 2.1: Nucleus

Endoplasm: Moderately dense granular
      For synthesis of food and reproduction
      Food storage in vacuoles (undigested)
      As chromidial bars (glycogen or protein)

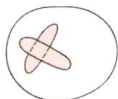

Ectoplasm is homogeneous external hyaline portion.
      For procumbent and ingestion of food
      Food may be absorbed anywhere or may enter through a specalised cell mouth
      (cytosome) ⎯⎯⎯⎯⎯⎯⎯⎯⎯⎯⎯⎯⎯⎯⎯⎯⎯⎯→

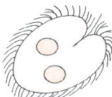

      Food obtained may be predigested or may need to be digested.
      For respiration that may be aerobic or anaerobic
      For discharging waste products—at any site
                        —may collect in vacuoles first
                        —may have specialised cell anus

    For protection
    May have contractile vacuoles in *B. coli* ⎯⎯⎯⎯⎯⎯⎯⎯⎯⎯⎯⎯⎯⎯⎯→

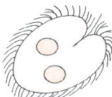

Limiting Cell Membrane

May have no constant shape

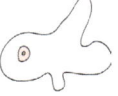

    or

maintain a more or less constant shape.

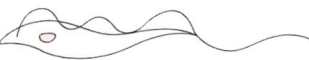

Locomotor Apparatus

No special structures or method,

Pseudopodia	(speed = 0.2–3 μm/second)
Flagella	(speed = 15–30 μm/second)

                  Parabasal body
Kinetoplast: Blepharophast
                  Axoneme
Sometimes connected to body by undulating membrane
Cilia   (speed = 400–2000 μm/second)

Locomotor Apparatus

No special structures or method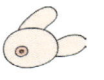

Pseudopodia 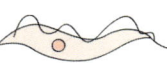   (speed = 0.2–3 µm/second)

Flagella   (speed = 15–30 µm/second)

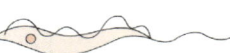

Kinetoplast: Parabasal body
               Blepharoplast
               Axoneme

Sometimes connected to body by undulating membrane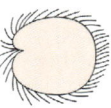

Cilia   (speed = 400–2000 µm/second)

Adaptation for Survival

Direct host to host transfer

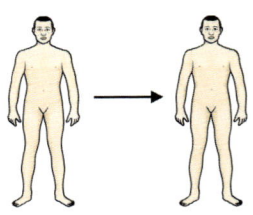

Cyst formation   Protective   Secretion of capsule

                      Reproductive   Nucleus divides

                                        Often store food

                                        (Chromidial tars)

Host to host transfer via intermediate host
(usually invertebrate)

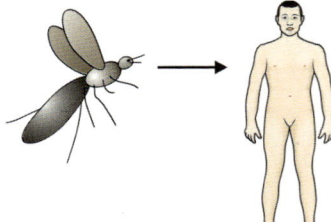

Sexual stages in life cycle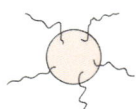

GASTROINTESTINAL TRACT AMOEBAE

Classification

Phylum	Protozoa

Subphylum	**Sarcodina** Sporozoa Mastigophora Ciliophora Uncertain status
	Move by pseudopodia
	Asexual reproduction by binary fission

Class	**Rhizopoda**
	Encystment common
	Parasitise intestinal tract
	Genera primarily differentiated by nuclear structure

Genera   *Entamoeba* ⟶ *histolytica/coli*
Generally one nucleus in trophozoite
Small karyosome at or near centre
Nuclear membrane lined wih chromatin granules
Forms cysts

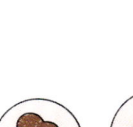

Endolimax nana
Generally one nucleus in trophozoite
Large irregular karyosome attached to nuclear membrane.
No peripheral chromatin
Forms cysts

Idamoeba butschlii
Generally one nucleus in trophozoite
Large karyosome surrounded by achromatic granules
No peripheral chromatin
Forms cysts

Dientamoeba fragilis
Minute
Generally binucleate
Central particulate karyosome
No peripheral chromatin
No cystic stage

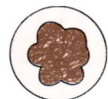

Pathogenic: Intestinal amoeba—*E. histolytica*
Nonpathogenic (Commensal)   Mouth—*E. gingivalis*
    Intestine—*E. coli, E. nana, I. butschlii, D. fragilis*

ENTAMOEBA HISTOLYTICA

Historical

Lambl (1859) discovered the parasite
    Losch (1875) proved its pathogenic nature
    Schaudinn (1903) differentiated pathogenic and non-pathogenic varieties of amoebae.

Geographical Distribution

Worldwide. More common in tropics and subtropics than in temperate zone.

Habitat

Trophozoites of the *E. histolytica* (tissue invading forms of the large race) live in the mucous and submucous layers of the large intestine.

Morphology

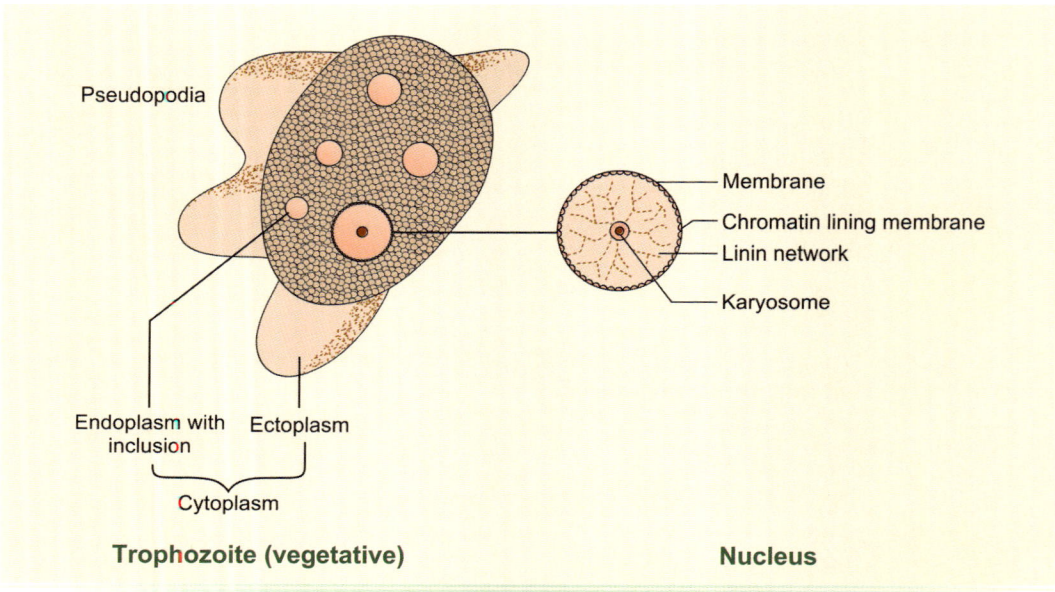

Trophozoite (vegetative)   **Nucleus**

Fig. 2.2: *E. histolytica* **trophozoite morphology**

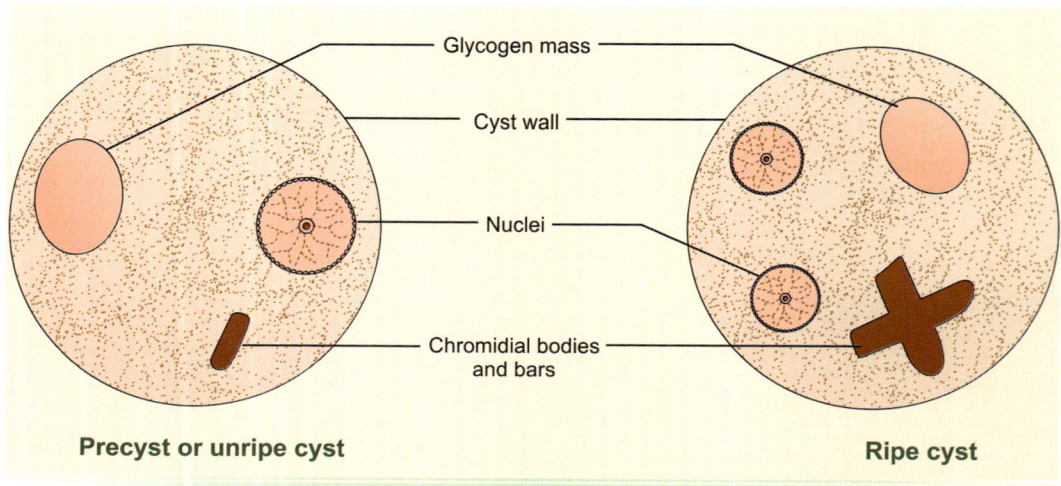

Precyst or unripe cyst   **Ripe cyst**

Fig. 2.3

UNSTAINED PREPARATIONS				
E. histolytica				***E. coli***

TROPHOZOITE

	E. histolytica		E. coli	
15–60 μ	Granular	Cytoplasm	Conspicuously granular	15–50 μ
	Clear finger-like	Pseudopodia	Blunt	
	Active—purposeful	Movement	Sluggish—not purposeful	
	Generally invisible	Nucleus	Ring refractile granules with eccentric karyosome	
	Red blood cells	Inclusions	Vacuoles. crystals, vegetable cells, bacteria, no RBCs	

PRECYST AND UNRIPE CYST

	E. histolytica		E. coli	
	Granular	Cytoplasm	Granular	
	May be refractile ring	Nucleus	Visible as refractile ring	
	Rod-like refractile chromidial bars	Inclusions	May be slender refractile chromidial bars	
	Glycogen masses		Glycogen masses	

RIPE CYST

	E. histolytica		E. coli	
3.5–20 μ	Round	Shape	Round	10–33 μ
	Refractile	Wall	Conspicuous refractile double outline	
	Difficult to see (1–4)	Nuclei	1–8 refractile nuclei with eccentric karyosomes	
	Refractile chromidial bars often	Inclusions	Only rudimentary slender chromidial bars	

NOTE: Small race cysts < 10 μ. May be commensal (*E. hartmanni*)
　　　　Large race cysts > 10 μ. Pathogenic

IODINE PREPARATIONS

TROPHOZOITE

	E. histolytica		E. coli	
	Finely granular yellow green	Cytoplasm	Conspicuous granularity	
	Red cells (yellow)	Inclusions	Bacteria etc. No RBC	
	Yellow ring with centre yellow dot (karyosome)	Nucleus	Nuclear membrane with eccentric karyosome easily recognised	

		PRECYST		
	Brown, diffuse As above	Glycogen Cytoplasm Nucleus	Brown, compact As above	

STAINED BY IRQN HAEMATOXYLIN

TROPHOZOITE

  	Purplish brown	Cytoplasm	Greyish blue
	Faintly granular		Coarsely granular
	RBC black	Inclusions	Vacuoles black, as are bacteria, etc.
	Lined with minute black granules	Nucleus membrane	Thick with plaques of black chromatin
	Small black central dot	Karyosome	Eccentric black dot or plaque
	Trace only seen	Linin network	More conspicuous may have chromatin plaques

PRECYST

	Round	Shape	Round
	As trophozoite	Cytoplasm nucleus	As trophozoite
	Black chromidia! bodies or bars	Inclusions	May have slender black chromidial bars
	Glycogen (dissolved) replaced by vacuoles		Glycogen (dissolved) replaced by vacuoles

CYST

	Grey-blue	Cytoplasm	Greyish blue, granular
	As precyst, less conspicuous or absent	Inclusions	As precyst, less conspicuous or absent in 2 nuclei stage glycogen vacuoles may be dumb-bell shaped
	Unstained, hyaline	Wall	Unstained, hyaline
	As trophozoite 1–4	Nuclei	As trophozoite 1–8

Method of Reproduction

A. **Excystation:** On reaching an appropriate climate (alimentary canal of man)—the trophozoites are transformed to cysts. Here a quadrinucleate cyst gives rise to eight amoebae and each one can develop into a trophozoite.

B. **Encystation** is the process of transformation of trophozoites to cysts and occurs in the intestinal lumen of an infected individual. Conversion occurs within hours and the mature cyst lives inside the intestinal lumen for about 2 days. Conversion to cyst *does not* take place in the human tissues, e.g. intestinal wall or in metastatic sites, but occurs in the intestinal lumen (this is basically a protective mechanism). Excystation and encystation may occur in the same host but once cysts are formed they need to enter another host to restart the cycle.

C. **Multiplication:** Occurs only in trophozoite phase. This occurs by simple binary fission, first of the nucleus which divides by a modified type of mitosis and then, of the cytoplasmic body of the organism.

Cultivation: Initially cultured by Boeck and Drbohlav in 1925 by using solidified blood agar or solidified egg slopes covered with Locke's solution. Growh of *E. histolytica* in cultures needs the presence of starch/ rice flour and some other metabolic associates, such as enteric bacteria or the parasitic flagellate such as *T. cruzi* (living or dead) or *organism t* (a nonpathogenic bacterium). Microcultures are prepared from a single washed amoeba in microtubes (measuring 4 × 50 mm) containing a medium of thioglycollate preparation, horse serum and an overlay of rich culture of *T. cruzi* (Philip's medium). *E. histolytica* has also been grown in a serum medium containing thioglycollate and penicillin inhibited streptobacilli which are living but not multiplying (Shaffer and Frye's medium).

Susceptible Animals: Experimentally, amoebic lesions may be reproduced in dogs, cats and monkeys. In kittens the infection is usually fatal while pups survive much longer.

Life cycle: *E. histolytica* completes its life cycle in only one host—man. There are mainly two stages (Fig. 2.4):

(a) Trophozoite

(b) Cyst, with a transitory stage of a precystic form.

Mature quadrinucleate cysts are the infective forms of the parasite. On gaining entry into the alimentary canal of a susceptible person—they pass unaltered in the stomach (not destroyed by the acidic environment), but the cyst wall is digested by trypsin of the intestine. The excystation occurs when the cyst reaches the caecum or the distal part of ileum (neutral or mildly alkaline medium). Here, the cytoplasmic body retracts from the cyst wall, vigorous amoeboid movements rupture the cyst wall through which a mass of cytoplasm and later the whole body comes out. Each cyst gives rise to a single amoeba with four nuclei (a tetranucleate amoeba) which forms eight amoebulae (metacystic trophozoites) by the division of nuclei with successive fission of cytoplasm. These actively mobile young amoebulae invade the tissues and ultimately lodge in the submucous tissue of the large gut. Hence, they grow and multiply by binary fission. The trophozoites are responsible for the production of the characteristic lesions of amoebiasis.

E. histolytica secretes histolysin (proteolytic enzyme) that destroys and brings about necrosis of surrounding tissue on which the parasite then survives. These invading amoebae gradually recede from the dead tissues towards the margin of fresh ones and wander in the gut wall. On entering into the deeper layers they may reach the radicles of the portal vein and be transported to liver via the bloodstream. In liver the trophozoites may live and survive but encystation does not occur.

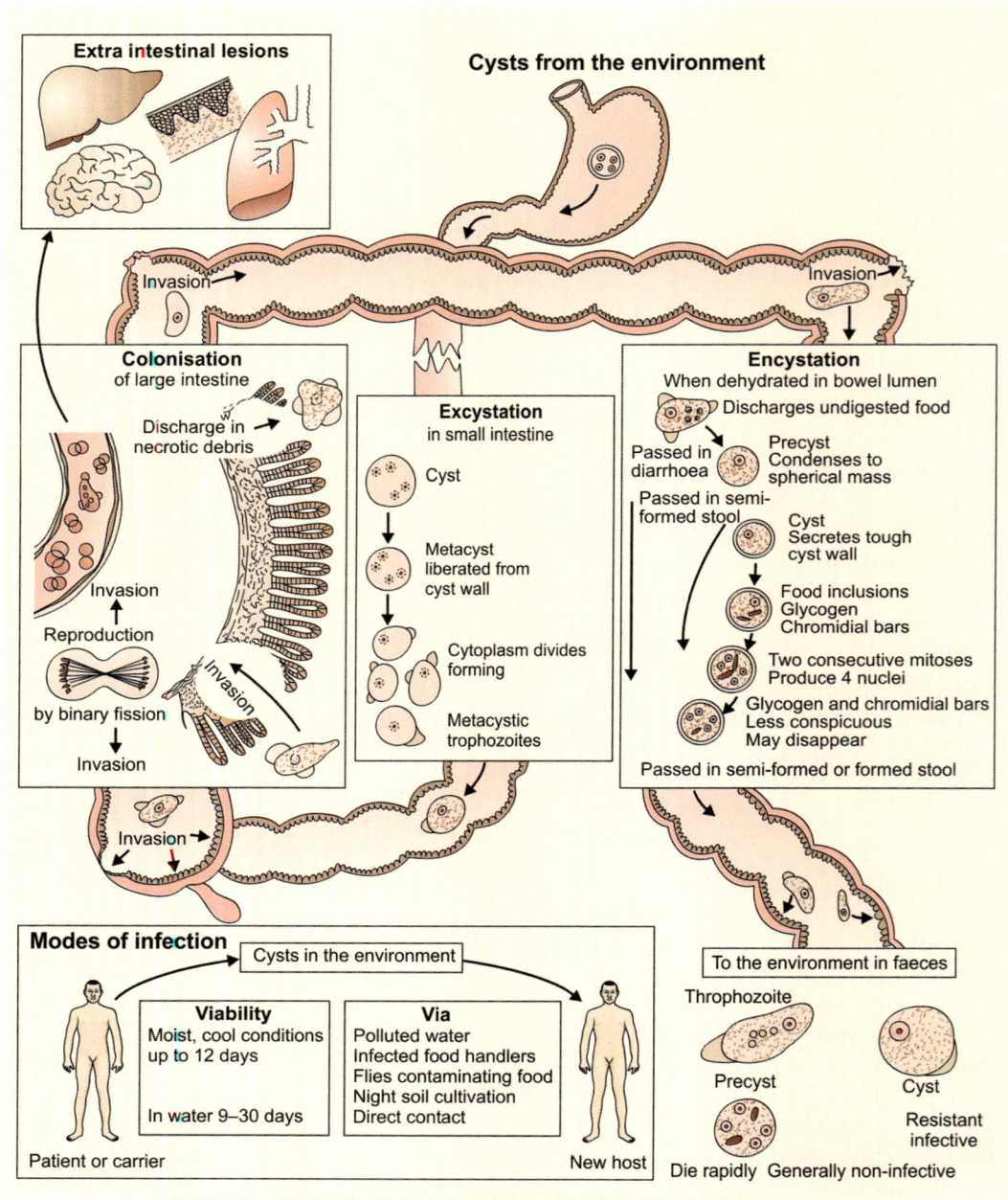

Fig. 2.4: Life cycle

Parasites that remain in the intestinal wall may cause an attack of acute dysentery (ulcerative colitis) in which large numbers of trophozoites are discharged with the slough. After some time when the effect of the parasite becomes gradually less and the host concomitantly increases its tolerance, the lesions become quiescent and start to heal. Now the parasite finds it difficult to survive and prepares for saving its own race. Some of the trophozoites discharged in the lumen of the bowel are transformed into the small precystic forms from which the cysts are developed.

If the parasite enters a resistant host, the injuries it produces are mild and superficial with discharge of precystic and cystic forms to propagate its species. These persons become a constant source of infection to others.

The fully mature quadrinucleate cysts are the most resistant and infective forms of the parasite and are developed when a state of equilibrium has been established between the host and the parasite. The cysts so produced have to reach another host to propagate the cycle and keep the race going.

Reservoirs of infection: Natural infection of E. histolytica is seen only among men and monkeys. Therefore, man is the commonest source of infection.

Modes of infection: Transmission takes place from man to man through its encysted stage and infection occurs through the ingestion of these cysts. Faecal contamination of drinking water, vegetables and food are the primary causes.

Role of carriers: Food handlers, if infected (cyst-passers or cyst carriers) transmit the disease to many individuals. Carriers may be classified into two types:
(a) 'Contact'—individuals who have never suffered from amoebic dysentery and are healthy.
(b) 'Convalescent'—those who have recovered from a clinical attack of acute amoebic dysentery.

The trophozoites that are passed with the slough in acute amoebic dysentery cannot survive for more than a couple of hours and are therefore an unlikely source of infection. Even if they are ingested, they are destroyed by the gastric juice. Houseflies may transmit cysts while passing from faeces to unprotected foodstuff, but seem usually to be of relatively little importance. The cysts of E. histolytica have been found in the droppings of cockroaches which also serve as a source of infection.

Pathogenicity (Fig. 2.5)

Incubation period: Though variable, is usually 4–5 days.

Clinical features and symptoms: Amoebiasis refers to and embraces all the different conditions that E. histolytica can produce in the human host. Amoebic dysentery is only a part of amoebiasis where stool is passed admixed with blood and mucous.

Pathogenic Lesions

1. **Primary or intestinal lesions:** The infection is limited entirely to the large intestine, the initial habitat of the parasite.
2. **Secondary or metastatic lesions:** The extracolonic regions where the trophozoites of E. histolytica can migrate and produce lesions include:
   (a) Liver
   (b) Lungs and
   (c) Brain

Apparent symbiosis		Offence		Defence
Many harbour *E. histolytica* with no apparent clinical disease. Some authorities say Small cysts. (<10 μ) commensal *E. hartmanni* Large cysts (>10 μ) pathogenic	DECREASED RESISTANCE ⇒	Cytolytic ferment Motility Invasion Secondary infection	⇒	Practically none Inflammatory reaction

Pathology
Site of Entry

1. Colonisation of the large intestine

Initially minute
Then irregular ulcer
shape typically flask-like
edges overhanging
Base Necrotic Lysed Tissue
Amoebae invading around
discharge necrotic debris,
    mucus and amoebae

Colonisation elsewhere
in large bowel

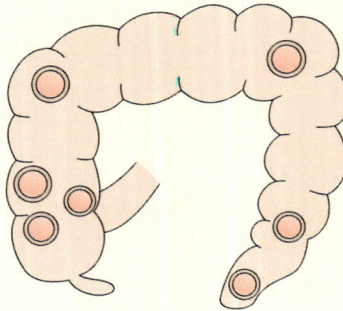

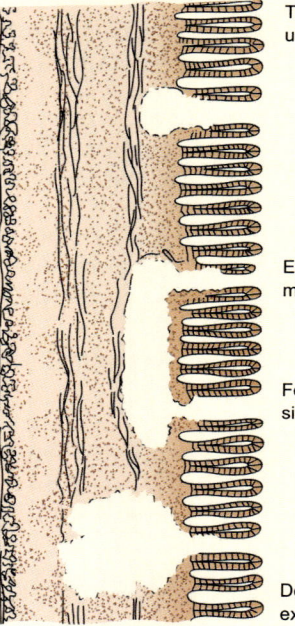

The primary ulcer — Invasion of mucosa via crypta
Repair may
Overtake necrosis with healing
Keep pace with necrosis persistent superficial lesions
Lag behind extension

Muscularis mucosae relatively resistant

Extension in mucosa — Accumulation of amoebae superficial to it.
Lateral extension of lytic necrosis

Formation of sinuses — Abscesses may coalesce under intact mucosae
Later mucoase may slough with widespread ulceration

Muscularis mucosae eventually pierced (directly or via vessels)

Deep extension — Deep necrosis of submucosa even muscle and subserosa

2. Complications and sequelae

Perforation

Haemorrhage (Rare)

Secondary infection

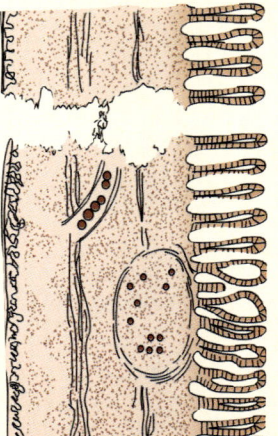

With peritonitis haemorrhage

With surrounding inflammatory reaction and fibroblastic proliferation

Amoeboma (Rare)
(Clinically simulates neoplasm)

A mass under oedematous mucosa with internal abscesses of necrotic tissue and amoebae.

Surrounding granulomatous tissue zone with eosinophils lymphocytes and fibroblasts

Invasion of blood vessels
Direct extension outside bowel

An outer firm nodular fibrous tissue

Fig. 2.5: Pathogenicity

Intestinal Lesions

Production of Intestinal lesions

The metacystic trophozoites enter through the crypt's of Lieberkühn and penetrate directly through the columnar epithelium of the mucous membrane by their amoeboid activity and also by dissolving the intestinal epithelium with a proteolytic ferment—histolysin. They keep burrowing deeper till they reach the submucous coat. Here they multiply rapidly and increase in number forming colonies and destroying surrounding tissue and using the material so produced as their food.

Next, the amoebae disperse in all directions further damaging more submucosa and undermining the mucous membrane above. The abscess so formed finally breakdown leading to ulceration.

ACUTE AMOEBIC DYSENTERY—INTESTINAL LESIONS

GROSS PATHOLOGY

Ulcer distribution: Largely confined to colon, the amoebic ulcers may be generalised or localised.
  A. **Generalised:** The whole length of the colon right down till the internal anal sphincter is involved.
  B. **Localised:** Two levels of involvement
     (i) *Ileocaecal region*—caecum, ascending colon, ileocaecal valve and appendix are involved.
     (ii) *Sigmoid-rectal region*—Involves sigmoid colon and rectum.
  Ileocaecal region involvement is commoner. The ulcers usually cannot be ascertained from the external aspect of the colon. They are best seen when the colon is cut open or examined from the lumen. The ulcers are discrete with presence of healthy mucous membrane in between the ulcers (even when the damage is extensive). The first changes seen are nodular elevations on the mucosa having an opening at the centre with hyperaemia and oedema of the marginal tissues. If one cuts open the nodule — brownish-yellow necrotic material comes out, the examination of which may reveal trophozoites. Liberation of the cytolysed tissue leads to formation of superficial ulcers.

An amoebic ulcer shows the undermentioned features.

Size: Variable from pin's head to an inch in diameter.

Shape: Round or oval; transverse in larger coalescing ulcers. Seen vertically—it is flask-shaped.

Margin: Ragged and undermined, being formed by the overhanging mucous membrane.

Base is formed by muscle coat and is filled by necrotic debris.

The superficial ulcers do not extend beyond muscularis muscosae. The deeper ulcers are restricted to the submucous coat but may extend laterally to communicate with adjacent ulcers. When the destruction is not limited to the submucosa but extends deeper into the muscular and even the serous layers—it may lead to local peritonitis, haemorrhage, perforation and generalised peritonitis, pericaecal or pericolic abscess, sloughing and gangrene of colon. When the slough separates, granulation tissue forms on the ulcer floor. Superficial small ulcers heal up completely with restoration and regeneration of mucous membrane. In large and deeper ulcers healing is accompanied by scar tissue formation over which re-epithelialisation does not occur and these areas can be detected as smooth depressed scars, the centers of which may or may not be pigmented. Excessive scarring may lead to strictures and obstruction.

MICROSCOPIC FEATURES

In early ulcers the lesion is limited above the muscularis mucosae and amoebae may be seen placed along the interglandular spaces causing cytolysis. At this stage the cells of crypts of Lieberkuhn show varying degrees of necrosis and subsequently with destruction of its basement membrane, the amoebae will be found to penetrate deeper. On seeing a section longitudinally, one would find:
  (a) A central necrosed area without any trophozoites in the necrotic material.
  (b) The periphery shows amoebic trophozoites in large numbers either singly or in groups, without much associated cellular infiltration.
   In advanced lesions the trophozoites may be seen further away from the actual ulcer and invading the intermuscular spaces to reach the peritoneal coat. The parasites may be seen burrowing into the venous radicles. Endothelial cells of the blood vessels may undergo hyperplasia leading to then obstruction and thrombosis. The thrombi may show *E. histolytica* trophozoites.

Chronic Intestinal Amoebiasis—Intestinal Lesions

The lesions reveal characters of ulcerative and regenerative changes and exhibit the undermentioned features.
  1. Small ulcers involving only the mucosa
  2. Extensive superficial ulceration with hyperaemia
  3. Marked scarring of intestinal wall with thinning, dilatation and sacculation.
  4. Severe adhesions with surrounding viscera.
  5. Localised thickening of intestinal wall leading to narrowing of lumen.
  6. Generalised thickening of the colon wall making it palpable per abdomen.
  7. Amoeboma formation—formation of tumour-like masses of granulation tissue. Diagnostic evidence is demonstration of *E. histolytica* trophozoites in sections of tissues obtained by biopsy or at autopsy.
   When superadded acute exacerbations occur, the ulcers may be seen extending deeply, even up to the peritoneal coat.

METASTATIC LESIONS IN AMOEBIASIS

Hepatic Amoebiasis (Amoebic Liver Abscess) (Fig. 2.6)

Incidence: In tropical regions, averaging about 5% of the individuals infected with *E. histolytica*, suffer from hepatic complications. Liver abscess is commoner among men and is rarely seen in children under ten years of age. About half of the cases may not give a history of amoebic dysentery. Usually, the hepatic lesions appear one to three months following an acute dysentery attack (however, rarely, these may develop simultaneously or years later after an acute attack).

Production of hepatic lesions: *E. histolytica* trophozoites are carried as emboli by the portal vein radicles from the base of an ulcer in the large intestine, usually from the caecum or the ascending colon. The trophozoites are held by the liver capillaries. Once established, they multiply and commence the cytolytic action. Subsequently, the portal venules are thrombosed causing further anaemic necrosis of the hepatocytes. The necrotic process proceeds in concentric layers around the primary focus. Initially solid, later the necrotic material liquefies on account of cytolytic action of amoebae and it extends radially. A fairly big-sized abscess forms by coalescence of these miliary abscesses.

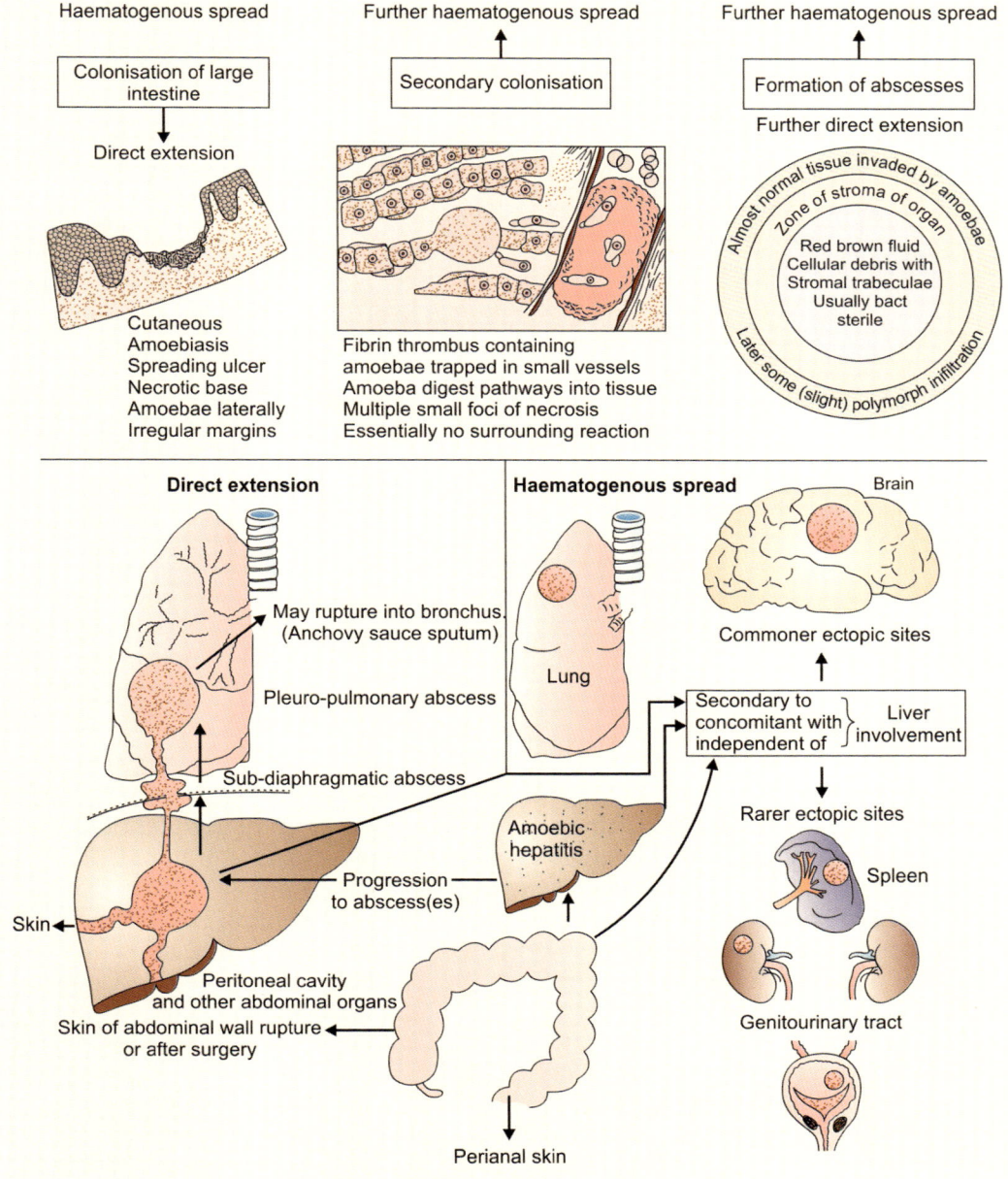

Fig. 2.6: Extraintestinal lesions

GROSS FEATURES

Amoebic liver abscesses vary in size and are usually confined to the posterosuperior surface of the right lobe. Usually a single large abscess is found. The abscess region appears to be reddish brown in colour with a semifluid consistency. Shreds of connective tissue may be seen in the abscess cavity. The abscess cavity wall is ragged and shaggy in appearance and is formed by the necrotic liver tissues merging into the healthy zones with intervening zone of hyperaemia. In an old abscess, however, the wall is smooth and composed of dense collagenous tissue. (Cases of multiple small abscesses or a single huge abscess are also seen sometimes.)

MICROSCOPIC FEATURES

From the centre towards the periphery—three zones can be identified.
  A. A central zone of cytolysed granular material with no amoebae.
  B. An intermediate zone of degenerated liver cells, a few leucocytes, connective tissue cells, RBCs and an occasional *E. histolytica* trophozoite.
  C. A peripheral zone of congested capillaries, varying degrees of necrosis of hepatocytes. Amoebic trophozoites can be seen to be multiplying in the area and invading the adjoining healthy liver tissue.

In an old abscess, the third zone may show walling by actively proliferating connective tissue cells, lymphocytes and monocytes.

Liver Abscess Pus (Fig. 2.6)

The pus produced is not of suppurative origin but is an admixture of sloughed liver tissue and blood. It is thick and chocolate brown in colour—called 'anchovy sauce pus.' Microscopically it reveals degenerated hepatocytes, few RBCs and occasional leucocytes. The trophozoites of *E. histolytica* are not seen in the freshly aspirated liver-pus but may appear in the escaping 'pus' four or five days after the initial aspiration.

AMOEBIC LIVER ABSCESS—CLINICAL FEATURES

Onset is insidious. *Pain and tenderness* in the right hypochondrium initially due to stretching of the liver capsule (pain is sometimes referred to the right shoulder due to irritation of the phrenic nerve which supplies the undersurface of the diaphragm). A dry cough may be present initially. Occasionally, the pain may be referred to the lower abdomen or the right iliac region. *Fever* with mild evening rise or low remittent temperature that later becomes quotidian and takes a hectic character. This is on account of pyrogenic effect of necrosed hepatocytes. *Jaundice* is unusual. The patient gradually gets emaciated. *On examination* liver is palpable and tender. Liver dullness extends upwards. Right-sided chest movement may be diminished or absent. There may be marked rigidity of the upper part of right rectus that interfere with liver palpation. The left liver lobe may undergo compensatory hypertrophy. *Lung signs* occur due to collapse of right lung caused by growing liver abscess, a right-sided pleural effusion may be present. *Apical pulse:* This may be displaced upwards and laterally by a large abscess. *Intestinal symptoms* such as diarrhoea or dysentery are absent. On abdominal palpation, colonic thickening areas may be felt.

Course of Liver Abscess

It may heal up spontaneously leaving an encysted mass, the contents of which may be dried up, fibrosed or even calcified.

If the abscess process continues, the abscess may grow into various directions as it comes into contact with adjacent tissues and organs into which the contents may be discharged.

A. A right-sided liver abscess may rupture
   1. *Externally:* A spontaneous rupture through the parieties, the skin in these cases may be secondarily infected with the trophozoites of *E. histolytica* forming granuloma cutis.
   2. *Into the lungs:* The 'pus' is expectorated with the sputum giving rise to haemoptysis. Such a sputum will have a viscid consistency and is chocolate brown in colour. Microscopically, hepatocytes and *E. histolytica* trophozoites may be seen.
   3. *Into the right pleural cavity:* Causing empyema-thoracis.
   4. *Below the diaphragm:* Causing a subphrenic abscess.
   5. *Into the peritoneal cavity:* Causing a generalised peritonitis.
B. A left-sided liver abscess may rupture into:
   1. *Stomach*—pus vomited out, leading to haematemesis.
   2. *Pericardial cavity*—causing purulent pericarditis (fatal).
   3. *Externally*—through the anterior abdominal wall in the epigastric region.
   4. *Left pleural cavity*—causing empyema-thoracis.
C. A liver abscess situated on the inferior surface may rupture into:
   1. *Bowel*—transverse colon or duodenum, causing diarrhoea and discharge of pus in the stool.
   2. *Peritoneal cavity*—causing a fatal peritonitis
D. A liver abscess situated posteriorly may rupture into:
   1. *Inferior vena cava*—although very rare, would be fatal.

Rarely a liver abscess may rupture into common bile duct, the pelvis of the kidney and the perinephric tissues of the lumbar region.

METASTATIC LESIONS IN OTHER ORGANS (FIG. 2.6)

A. **Pulmonary amoebiasis:** May be primary or secondary amoebic abscess.
   1. *Primary:* Occurs rarely, even in the absence of any hepatic lesion. In these cases *E. histolytica* trophozoites gain entrance from the gut-wall via the portal circulation into the pulmonary capillaries. Evolution of lung abscess either single of multiple, occurs in the same way as that of hepatic amoebic abscess.
   2. *Secondary:* Arises secondarily to a liver abscess by direct extension through the adhesion formed with the diaphragm, the liver and the base of the right lung. The abscess is usually single and large, in the lower lobe of right lung.
B. **Cerebral amoebiasis:** Rarely seen. Arise secondarily to hepatic and/or pulmonary abscess. Abscess is generally single and small and located mostly in the cerebral hemispheres.
C. **Cutaneous amoebiasis:** Usually found over an underlying visceral amoebic lesion, e.g. in the areas of drainage of liver abscess or colostomy wound, in the sites of ruptured appendicular and pericolic abscesses. Extensive sloughing of skin and necrosis of subcutaneous tissues is caused by trophozoites of *E. histolytica*. Besides these granulomatous ulcerations, a granulomatous mass simulating an epithelioma have been seen in the perianal region.

D. **Splenic abscess:** Found in association with hepatic abscess. Transmission of the trophozoites of *E. histolytica* occurs directly through an adherent splenic flexure of the colon.

Immunology

Serological tests, such as complement fixation test, ELISA, precipitin test, immobilisation test of *E. histolytica* with hyper-immune sera of rabbits and reaction of *E. histolytica* with fluorescin-tagged homologous antibody suggest the development of specific immune bodies in the sera of individuals suffering from amoebiasis especially invasive amoebiasis with tissue destruction. These humoral antibodies, however, do not protect the individual who has suffered/recovered from amoebiasis against re-infection. PCR/NucleicAcid Technologiesare also available cyrrently which are highly specific and sensitive.

LABORATORY DIAGNOSIS OF AMOEBIASIS

Primarily depends on demonstration of *E. Histolytica* in stool, can also employ PCR techniques
Aspirates, intestinal or other organs
Biopsy material: Pinch biopsy at proctoscopy or sigmoidoscopy
Surgical biopsy elsewhere

INTESTINAL

Stool examination including differentiation from stool in bacillary dysentery (Fig. 2.7)

Naked Eye	Amoebiasis	Shigellosis
Faecal matter	Always present	May be absent, blood and mucus only
Mucus	Not tenacious	Tenacious
	Not abundant	Abundant in acute stages
Microscopic		
(1) Bacteria	Numerous	May be scanty
(2) Pus cells	Scanty, well preserved	Very numerous, degenerate
(3) Red blood cells	Often in rouleaux	Scattered
(4) Large macrophages	Not a feature	May be numerous, may have ingested red cells (do not mistake for amoebae)
(5) Characot-Leyden crystals	May be present	Absent
(6) *E. histolytica*	Present	Absent

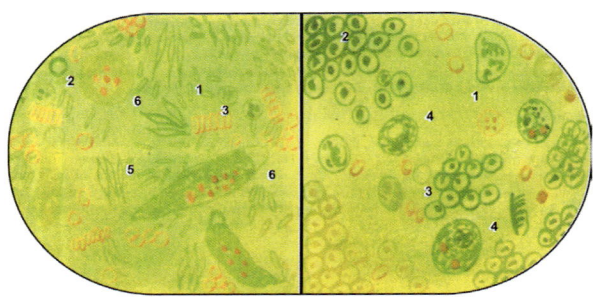

Fig. 2.7: Stool examination

Culture	Special methods for amoebae (Not employed as a routine)	Isolation of Shigella spp.
Do not forget	Vegetative *Entamoeba histolytica* in diarrhoea	Activity motile. Purposeful movement. Finger like clear pseudopodia. Ingested red cells, No nucleus seen
	Precyst or cysts in semi-formed or solid stool	Nuclear characteristics-number of nuclei (1–4), glycogen, chromidial bars

Serological Tests: CFT and ELISA of little value in uncomplicated intestinal amoebiasis.

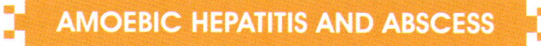

AMOEBIC HEPATITIS AND ABSCESS

Leucocytosis with neutrophilia
Stool examination—for *E. histolytica*
Serological tests—CFT using extract of culture of amoebae as antigen: Of doubtful value.
Elisa—confirmatory of tissue invasion.
Aspirated material—examination for *E. histolytica*
Biopsy material—histology
Radiological evidence: Raised right dome of diaphragm, ultrasound or scanning methods.

OTHER EXTRAINTESTINAL LESIONS

Along similar lines

Treatment

Anti-amoebics (amoebicides) may be grouped as follows:
1. **Tissue amoebicides:** Drugs acting on the trophozoites of *E. histolytica* in the tissues (invasive amoebae)
   A. In the intestinal wall, liver and other metastatic lesions—emetine and dehydro-emetine—given parenterally
   B. In the liver and lungs only—4 aminoquinoline—chloroquin
2. **Luminal amoebicides:** Drugs acting on trophozoites and cysts of *E. histolytica* in the lumen only:
   A. Direct acting luminal or contact amoebicides:
      (a) Halogenated hydroxyquinolines
         di-iodohydroxyquinoline—Diodoquin
         Idochlorhydroxyquinoline—Cliquinol
      (b) Dichloroacetamide group—Mebinol
         Diloxanide furoate—Furamide
         Chlorbetamide—Mantomide
      (c) Pentavaleat ansenicals
         Stovarsol
         Carbarsone
         Bismuth glycoloylarsanilate
      (d) Antibiotics
         Paromomycin—Humatin

    (e) Oral emetine
         Emetine bismuth iodide
         Dehydroemetine bismuth iodide
    B. Indirect acting luminal amoebicides—Antibiotic (tetracycline)
3. **Both luminal and tissue amoebicides:**
    Niridazole—Ambilhar
    Metronidazole—Flagyl
    Tinidazole—Tiniba

Various combinations of the above-mentioned amoebicides are also available.

Prophylaxis

Personal Prophylaxis

- Use of boiled drinking water
- Protection of all food and drink from contamination by flies, cockroaches and rats
- Avoidance of use of raw vegetables and fruit
- Personal cleanliness and elementary hygienic conditions are to be observed while taking of meal
- Food handlers to be screened and treated (applies to both—unit homes and mass eating places—like restaurants and hotels).

Community Prophylaxis

- Effective sanitary disposal of faeces
- Protection of water supplies from faecal pollution
- Avoidance of use of human excreta as manure
- Detection, isolation and treatment of carriers

PRIMARY AMOEBIC MENINGOENCEPHALITIS

This is a relatively newer disease entity, first reported in 1965 by Fowler and Carter. A few cases have been reported from India also.

It is labelled 'Primary' so as to differentiate it from that caused by E. histolytica secondary to lesion elsewhere in the body.

It is caused by free living amoebae that are found in fresh water, mud and moist soil. They belong to the genus Naegleria (have smaller trophozoites with a flagellate phase) and Hartmannella.

Morphological Features of the Amoeba

The trophic forms are briskly mobile at 21°C. Size varies from 6–15 μm in diameter. They have one pointed and one broad end. Nucleus is single and large (2 μm), has a large nucleolus and fine nuclear membrane. There is a perinuclear halo and is made up of 4 to 6 vacuoles.

Infections in Human Beings

These occur either from nasopharyngeal contamination during swimming in infected waters or other close contact, e.g. inhalation of particles of decaying animal manure that supports these amoebae. It usually attacks children and young adults who enjoy an active life.

These amoebae are specifically neurotropic and cerebral invasion occurs through the olfactory nerves; the amoebae have been demonstrated in nerve filaments. The

THE NON-PATHOGENIC INTESTINAL AMOEBAE

Life cycle

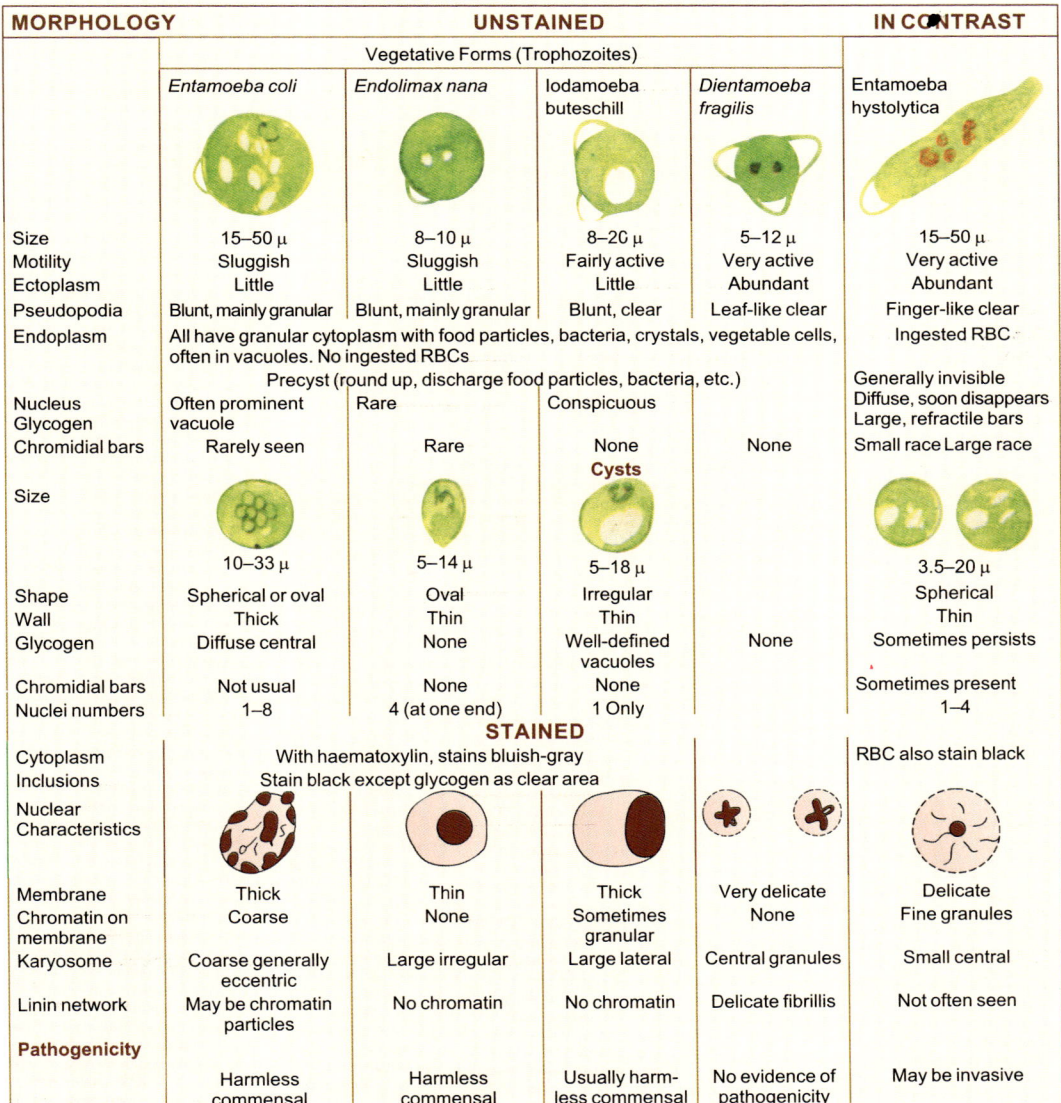

Cysts (Vegetative forms of *D. fragilis*) from environment

Excystation in small intestine

Encystation (except in *D. fragilis*) if dehydrated

Multiplication of vegetative forms in large intestine

Cysts (vegetative forms of *D. fragilis*) to environment in formed stools vegetative forms found in diarrhoea

MORPHOLOGY	UNSTAINED				IN CONTRAST
	Vegetative Forms (Trophozoites)				
	Entamoeba coli	*Endolimax nana*	Iodamoeba buteschill	*Dientamoeba fragilis*	Entamoeba hystolytica
Size	15–50 μ	8–10 μ	8–20 μ	5–12 μ	15–50 μ
Motility	Sluggish	Sluggish	Fairly active	Very active	Very active
Ectoplasm	Little	Little	Little	Abundant	Abundant
Pseudopodia	Blunt, mainly granular	Blunt, mainly granular	Blunt, clear	Leaf-like clear	Finger-like clear
Endoplasm	All have granular cytoplasm with food particles, bacteria, crystals, vegetable cells, often in vacuoles. No ingested RBCs				Ingested RBC
	Precyst (round up, discharge food particles, bacteria, etc.)				Generally invisible
Nucleus	Often prominent vacuole	Rare	Conspicuous		Diffuse, soon disappears
Glycogen					Large, refractile bars
Chromidial bars	Rarely seen	Rare	None	None	Small race Large race
			Cysts		
Size	10–33 μ	5–14 μ	5–18 μ		3.5–20 μ
Shape	Spherical or oval	Oval	Irregular		Spherical
Wall	Thick	Thin	Thin		Thin
Glycogen	Diffuse central	None	Well-defined vacuoles	None	Sometimes persists
Chromidial bars	Not usual	None	None		Sometimes present
Nuclei numbers	1–8	4 (at one end)	1 Only		1–4
	STAINED				
Cytoplasm	With haematoxylin, stains bluish-gray				RBC also stain black
Inclusions	Stain black except glycogen as clear area				
Nuclear Characteristics					
Membrane	Thick	Thin	Thick	Very delicate	Delicate
Chromatin on membrane	Coarse	None	Sometimes granular	None	Fine granules
Karyosome	Coarse generally eccentric	Large irregular	Large lateral	Central granules	Small central
Linin network	May be chromatin particles	No chromatin	No chromatin	Delicate fibrilis	Not often seen
Pathogenicity	Harmless commensal	Harmless commensal	Usually harmless commensal	No evidence of pathogenicity	May be invasive

subarachnoid basal cistern shows inflammatory exudate and it consists of neutrophils and macrophages (in equal proportions) along with amoebae. Sugar and protein levels of CSF are higher than those seen with bacterial infections. Fresh unstained preparations are essential to identify these amoebae. The possibility of this disease entity should be considered in every case of acute meningitis. If left untreated, it takes a fatal course. The incubation period is about 7 days and the treatment of choice is sulphadiazine along with the antifungal antibiotic amphotericin-B.

INTESTINAL, ORAL AND GENITAL FLAGELLATES

Flagellates inhabiting the intestine form the major group. Trichomonas tenax is found in the oral cavity, whereas *Trichomonas vaginalis* (genitalis) is found in the genital tracts (vagina, urinary tract and prostate). *Trichomonas hominis* is found in the ileo-caecal region. *Giardia intestinalis* (lamblia) lives in the duodenum.

GIARDIA LAMBLIA

Synonyn: *Giardia intestinalis, Lamblia intestinalis.* First seen by Leeuwenhoek (1681) while examining his own stool.

Geographical distribution: Worldwide.

Habitat: Duodenum and upper part of jejunum of man.

Morphology

Cultivation: A method for their cultivation was described in 1962 by Karapetyan by growing these with an yeast *Candida guillermondi*; it grew well on a medium of chick embryo extract, human serum, Hottinger's digest (tryptic meat digest) and Hank's solution.

Life cycle: Trophozoites multiply in the intestine by binary fission. When duodenal environment becomes unfavourable, encystment occurs, usually in the large intestine. During encystment, a thick resistant wall is secreted by the parasite and the cell then divides into two within the cysts. The cysts are ingested by a new host and within half an hour 2 trophozoites hatch out which multiply rapidly and colonise in the duodenum. To escape from the acidic environment of the duodenum, Giardia often localises in the biliary tract (gallbladder).

Pathogenicity: The sucking disc of the parasite attaches to the convex surface of the epithelial cells—leading to malabsorption. The patient may complain of persistently loose bowels, and mild steatorrhoea (passage of yellowish greasy stools—have excess of fat). The parasite can harm by producing allergic (toxic), traumatic, irritative and spoilative effects (diverting the nutriments).

   Clinically:
  1. It may not produce any symptom
  2. May cause chronic duodenitis, enteritis or acute enterocolitis
  3. General malaise, fever, anaemia (macrocytic) and allergic manifestations
  4. Chronic cholecystopathy.

Laboratory Diagnosis

  1. Microscopic examination of freshly passed stool for demonstration of giardia trophozoites and cysts (former are seen in diarrhoeic stools or after using a purgative).

2. Giardia trophozoites may be recovered both in bile A (aspirated from duodenum) and B (removed from bile duct) drawn by duodenal intubation.

Treatment

Same as for amoebiasis.

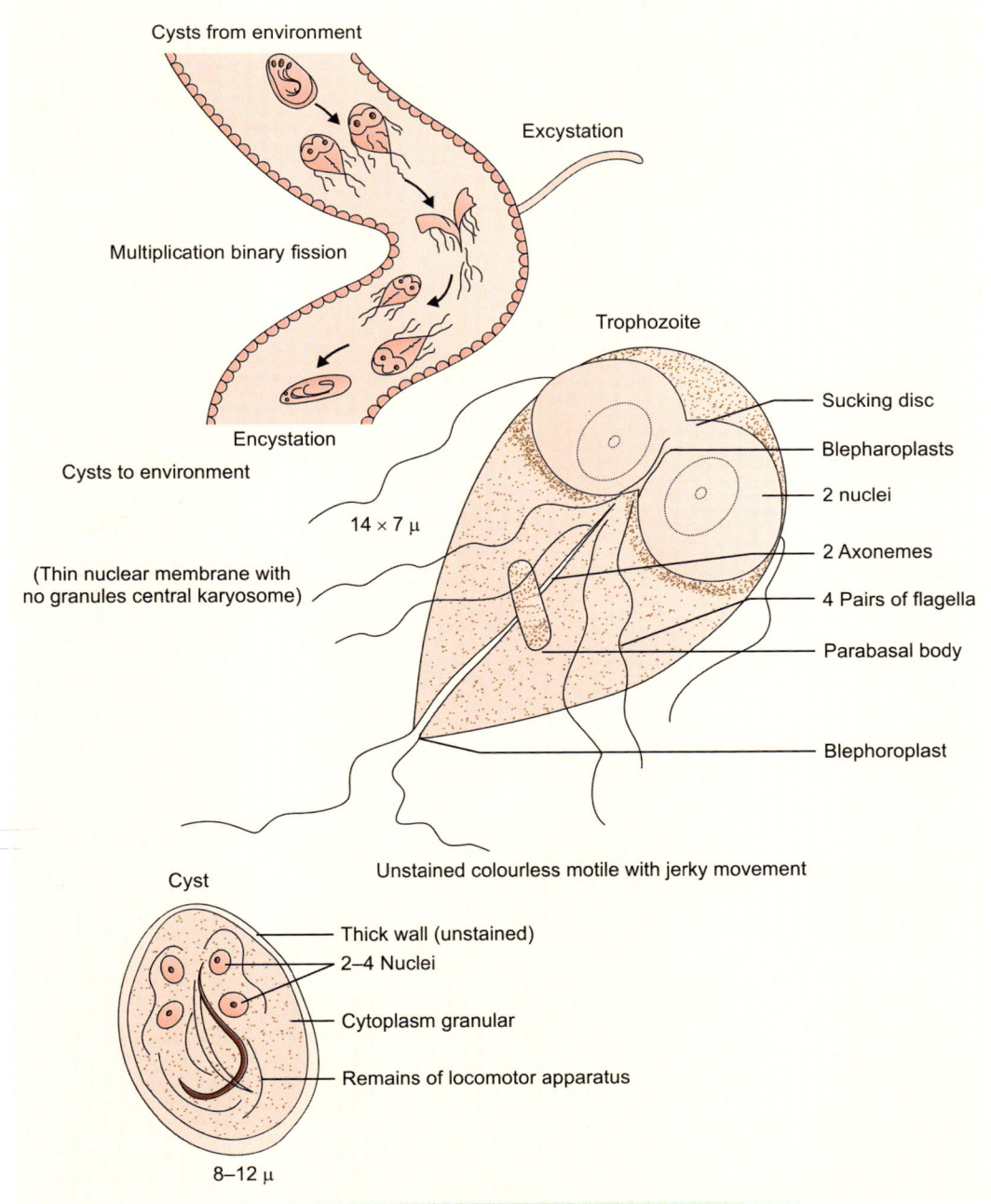

Cysts from environment

Excystation

Multiplication binary fission

Trophozoite

Encystation

Cysts to environment

Sucking disc

Blepharoplasts

2 nuclei

14 × 7 μ

2 Axonemes

(Thin nuclear membrane with no granules central karyosome)

4 Pairs of flagella

Parabasal body

Blephoroplast

Unstained colourless motile with jerky movement

Cyst

Thick wall (unstained)

2–4 Nuclei

Cytoplasm granular

Remains of locomotor apparatus

8–12 μ

Fig. 2.8: *Giardia lambila* (Morphology and life cycle)

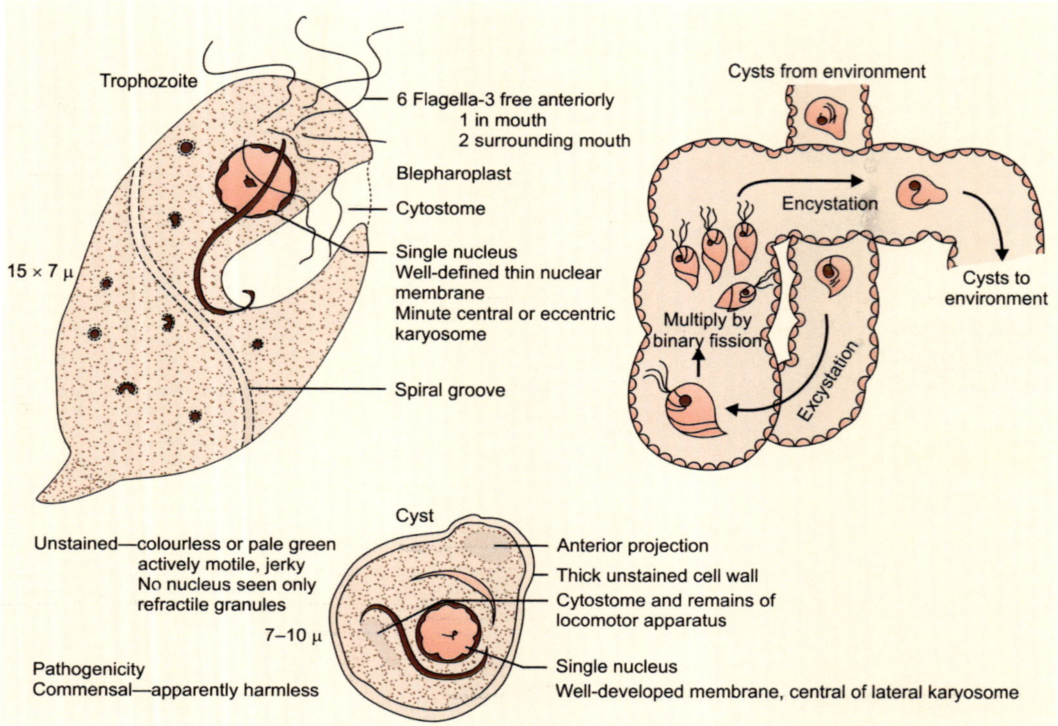

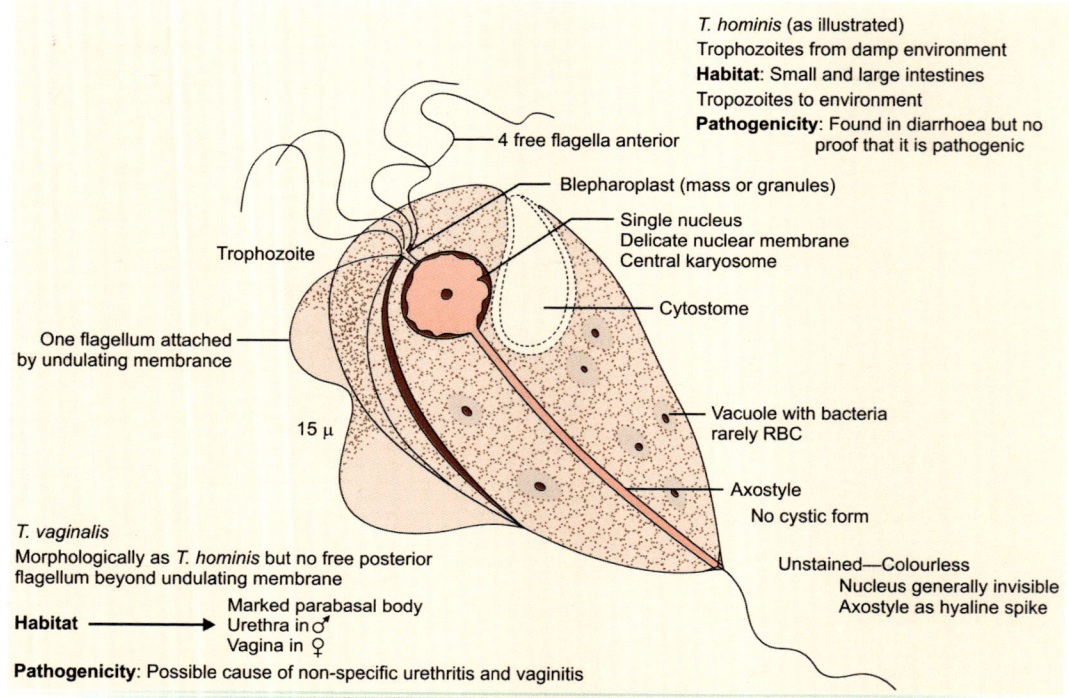

Trophozoite

6 Flagella-3 free anteriorly
1 in mouth
2 surrounding mouth

Blepharoplast

Cytostome

Single nucleus
Well-defined thin nuclear
membrane
Minute central or eccentric
karyosome

15 × 7 μ

Spiral groove

Cysts from environment

Encystation

Cysts to
environment

Multiply by
binary fission

Excystation

Cyst

Anterior projection
Thick unstained cell wall
Cytostome and remains of
locomotor apparatus

Single nucleus
Well-developed membrane, central of lateral karyosome

Unstained—colourless or pale green
actively motile, jerky
No nucleus seen only
refractile granules

7–10 μ

Pathogenicity
Commensal—apparently harmless

Fig. 2.9: *Chilomastix mesnili* morphology and llife cycle

T. hominis (as illustrated)
Trophozoites from damp environment
Habitat: Small and large intestines
Tropozoites to environment
Pathogenicity: Found in diarrhoea but no
                 proof that it is pathogenic

4 free flagella anterior

Blepharoplast (mass or granules)

Single nucleus
Delicate nuclear membrane
Central karyosome

Trophozoite

Cytostome

One flagellum attached
by undulating membrane

15 μ

Vacuole with bacteria
rarely RBC

Axostyle
No cystic form

T. vaginalis
Morphologically as T. hominis but no free posterior
flagellum beyond undulating membrane

Marked parabasal body

Habitat ⟶ Urethra in ♂
            Vagina in ♀

Unstained—Colourless
         Nucleus generally invisible
         Axostyle as hyaline spike

Pathogenicity: Possible cause of non-specific urethritis and vaginitis

Fig. 2.10: Morphology of Trichomonas

BLOOD AND TISSUE FLAGELLATES

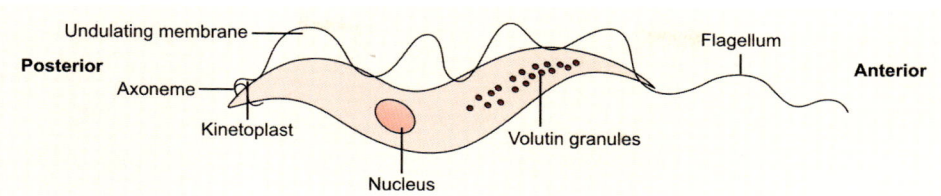

Undulating membrane — Flagellum
Posterior **Anterior**
Axoneme —
Kinetoplast
Volutin granules
Nucleus

MORPHOLOGICAL STAGES OF TRYPANOSOMATIDAE; GENERA AND SPECIES AFFECTING MAN

Trypanosoma cruzi			
Amastigote (Leishmanial)	Promastigote (Leptomonad)	Epimastigote (Crithidial)	Trypomastigote (Trypanosomal)
Intracellular in macrophages of man	In midgut then proboscis of sandfly		
	Transfer stage to man		
Leishmania donovani (Also in culture) *Leishmania tropica* *Leishmania braziliensis*		In salivary glands of tsetse fly.	In midgut, salivary glands and proboscis of tsetse fly Transfer stage to man In blood stream, lymph nodes and later CNS of man
			Trypanosoma rhodesiense *Trypanosoma gambiense*
		In midgut of bug	In midgut of bug In faeces of bug
Intracellular in macrophages and tissue cells of man.	Transitional stage only		Transfer stage to man In blood and tissue spaces of man

LEISHMANIASIS

Species	L. donovani	L. tropica	L. braziliensis
Disease	Visceral (Kala-azar)	Cutaneous (Oriental sore)	Mucocutaneous (Espundia)

Generic Character

Ross created the genus Leishmania in 1903, to include the parasite of Indian kala-azar, *Leishmania donovani*. Morphologically the flagellates belonging to the genus Leishmania are identical to those of the genus Leptomonas. Both genera have an amastigote and a promastigote stage, but they differ in the following respects:

	Genus Leptomonas	*Genus Leishmania*
Life cycle	Only in insect host No vertebrate host	Both in vertebrate and an insect host
Transmission	Ingestion of cyst	By intermediate host

Clinical Classification of Leishmaniasis

1. Visceral leishmaniasis or kala-azar: Caused by *L. donovani*. It is further subdivided depending upon the type of reservoir:
   (a) Rodent reservoir: African kala-azar (Sudan and East Africa)
   (b) Canine reservoir: Mediterranean kala-azar/infantile kala-azar/Chinese/Russian/South American kala-azar
   (c) Human reservoir: Indian kala-azar.
2. Cutaneous leishmaniasis (no visceral manifestations):
   (a) Oriental sore—caused by *L. tropica*
   (b) Espundia or mucocutaneous leishmaniasis—caused by *L. braziliensis*
   (c) Dermal leishmanoid or postkala-azar dermal leishmaniasis, a late complication of visceral form. Caused by *L. donovani*.

LEISHMANIA DONOVANI

(Causes visceral leishmaniasis or kala-azar)

Discovered by Leishman (in London, May 1903) and Donovan (Madras, 1903) simultaneously.

Geographical Distribution

Endemic in many places in India, China, Africa, Southern Europe, South America and Russia. In India, it is common in Assam, Bengal, Bihar along the coasts of Ganges and the Brahmaputra. It is also endemically seen in Orissa, Madras and Eastern UP as far as Lucknow.

Habitat

Inside the vertebrate host (man) the parasite is always intracellular, occurring in the amastigote form. Basically it is a parasite of the reticuloendothelial (RE) system.

Morphology: The parasite exists in two forms:
1. Amastigote (Leishmanial) form occurring in man
2. Promastigote (leptomanad) form occurring in the gut of the vector (sandly) and in cultures.

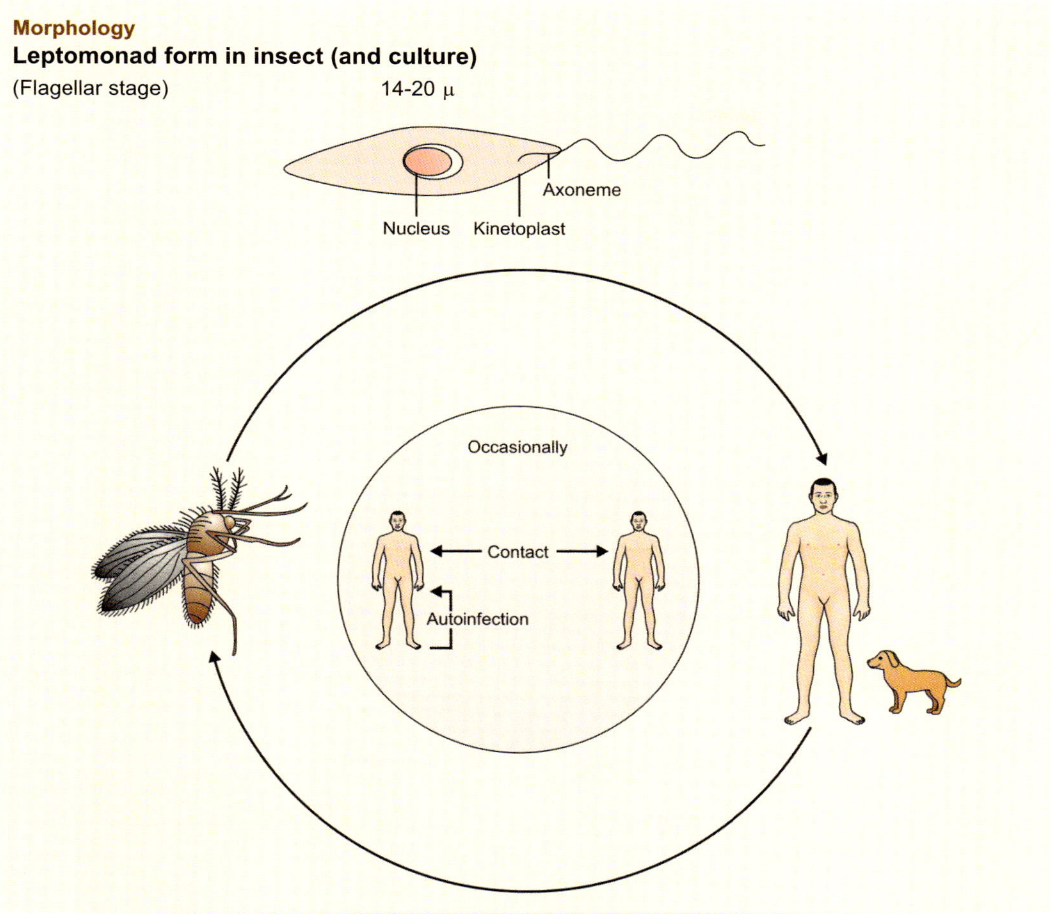

Morphology

Leptomonad form in insect (and culture)

(Flagellar stage)   14-20 μ

Axoneme

Nucleus   Kinetoplast

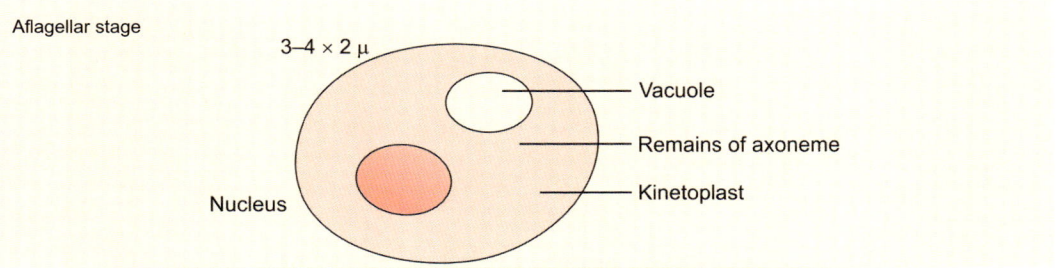

Occasionally

← Contact →

Autoinfection

Fig. 2.11: Life cycle and morphology of leishmania (similar in all three species)

Aflagellar stage

3–4 × 2 μ

Vacuole

Remains of axoneme

Kinetoplast

Nucleus

Fig. 2.12: Leishmanial form in reticuloendothelial cells of man

Amastigote stage (Aflagellar stage)

At this stage the parasite resides in the cells of the reticuloendothelial system of verte-brate hosts (man, dog and hamster).

Shape and size: Round or oval, 2–4 μm lengthwise

Cell membrane: Delicate, seen in fresh specimens only

Nucleus: Measures less than 1 μm, is round or oval and usually situated in the middle of the cells or along the side of the cell wall.

Kinetoplast: Lies tangentially or at right angle to the nucleus. It consists of a DNA containing body and a mitochondrial structure.

Axoneme (Rhizoplast) is a delicate filament extending from the kinetoplast to the margin of the body. It represents the root of the flagellum.

Vacuole is a clear unstained space lying alongside the axoneme.

Promastigote stage (Flagellar stage)

Seen only in cultures and insect vectors

Shape and size: Young forms—2–3 × 5–10 μm, short oval or pear-shaped. Maturer form—long, slender spindle-shaped, 1–2 × 15–20 μm.

Nucleus: Central

Kinetoplast: At the anterior end lies transversely.

Eosinophilic vacuole: Pale staining area lying in front of kinetoplast over which the root of the flagellum runs.

Flagellum: Equal to or longer than body length and projecting from the front. There is no undulating membrane as the flagellum does not curve round the body. Using Leishman's stain, the cytoplasm appears blue, nucleus pink or violet and kinetoplast bright red.

Cultivation: *L. donovani* can be cultured in a medium composed of two parts of salt agar and one part of defibrinated rabbit's blood. This medium was first introduced by Novy and MacNeal and later modified by Nicolle and is commonly referred to as NNN medium. The material for culture is inoculated into the water of condensation of the medium and incubated at 22–24° C. Bacterial contamination should not occur or else it would cause degeneration and death of *L. donovani*. The presence of haematin and ascorbic acid favour the growth of the parasite. In NNN medium the amastigote form changes into the promastigote form which then multiplies actively by longitudinal fission to produce numerous flagellates. By subculturing every 2–3 weeks, the strain can be preserved in the laboratory. The intracellular growth of *L. donovani* can be maintained in tissue culture at 37°C for up to 32 days.

Susceptible animals: In the Mediterranean region dogs are naturally infected with *L. donovani.* Common laboratory animals, such as mice, rats and guinea pigs are not suitable for transmission of infection. Some varieties of hamsters, however, can be infected.

Methods of infection: Reservoirs have been outlined earlier. However, the natural transmission of *L. donovani* from man to man is carried by a certain species of sandfly of the genera Phlebotomus and Lutzomiya. Undermentioned are the species involved.
  (a) Indian vector—*Phlebotomus argentipes*
  (b) Mediterranean vectors
      Phlebotomus perniciosus (Italy and Sicily)
      Phlebotomus major (Crete)
      Phlebotomus pernicious var. langeroni (Sudan)

Life Cycle

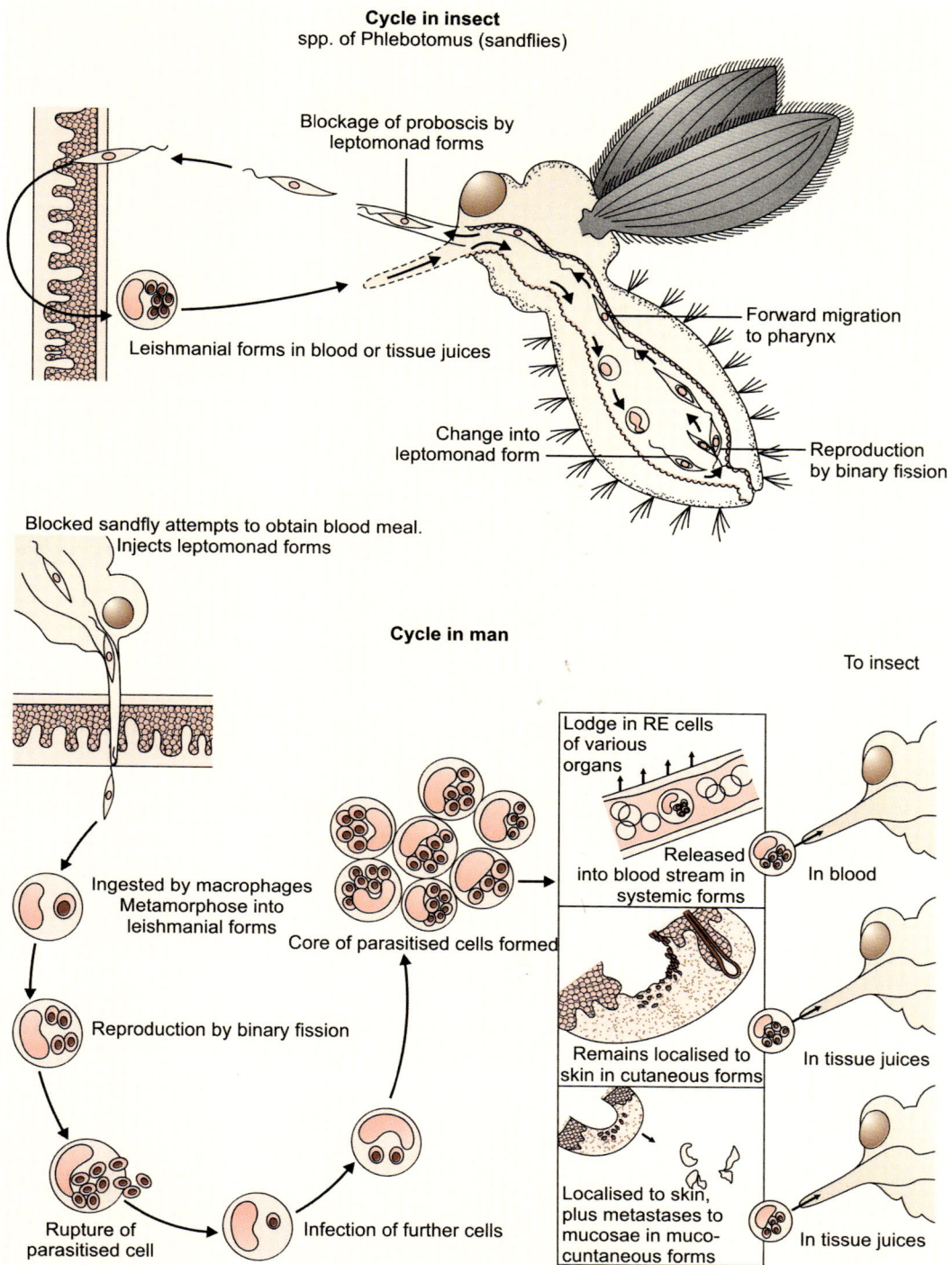

Cycle in insect
spp. of Phlebotomus (sandflies)

Blockage of proboscis by leptomonad forms

Leishmanial forms in blood or tissue juices

Forward migration to pharynx

Change into leptomonad form

Reproduction by binary fission

Blocked sandfly attempts to obtain blood meal. Injects leptomonad forms

Cycle in man

To insect

Lodge in RE cells of various organs

Released into blood stream in systemic forms

In blood

Ingested by macrophages Metamorphose into leishmanial forms

Core of parasitised cells formed

Remains localised to skin in cutaneous forms

In tissue juices

Reproduction by binary fission

Rupture of parasitised cell

Infection of further cells

Localised to skin, plus metastases to mucosae in muco-cuntaneous forms

In tissue juices

Fig. 2.13: Life cycle in insect

(c) Chinese vectors
  Phlebotomus chinensis and *Phlebotomus sergenti* var. mongolensis
(d) Sudanese vector
  Phlebotomus orientalis (Sudan)
  Phlebotomus martini (East Africa—Kenya)
(e) Brazilian vector
  Lutzomiya longipalpis
(f) Russian vector
  Phlebotomus arpaklensis

Other Methods of Transmission

1. Congenital infection of a child *in-utero*
2. Transmission by blood transfusion
3. Transmission by inoculation of cultures of *L. donovani*
4. Probable transmission during coitus.

Pathogenicity of *Leishmania donovani*

Incubation period: Usually about 3–6 months. May exceed 1–2 years.

Clinical features: Kala-azar or visceral leishmaniasis presents with:
1. **Pyrexia:** Early symptom, may be continuous or remittent type becoming intermittent later. About one-fifth of cases have double peaking in 24 hours. Intervening afebrile periods may stretch between febrile waves.
2. **Splenomegaly:** Gradually spleen increases markedly in size, may fill up the entire abdomen subsequently.
3. **Hepatomegaly:** Liver enlarges but not as much as spleen.
4. **Lymphadenopathy:** May be seen in Chinese and African forms.
5. **General features:** Not much malaise or apathy may be associated with pyrexia. The patient retains a good appetite and a clean moist tongue. Epistaxis may be a presenting feature. In a full blown case emaciation and anaemia may be significant.
6. **Skin:** Skin over the entire body is dry, rough and harsh and is often pigmented. Hair tend to be brittle and fall off. Watery eruptions on skin and a mucocutaneous lesion may be seen in African kala-azar.

Untreated, most patients would die within 2 years. Death occurs due to some complications, e.g. bacillary or amoebic dysentery, pneumonia, pulmonary Koch, cancrum oris (with severe neutropenia) and other suppurative infections. The immunosuppressive effect brings with it severe infections.

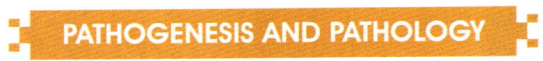

PATHOGENESIS AND PATHOLOGY

PATHOGENIC LESIONS

SPLEEN

Gross Features

1. Massively enlarged
2. Thickened capsule due to perisplenitis
3. Organ is soft in consistency and cuts easily

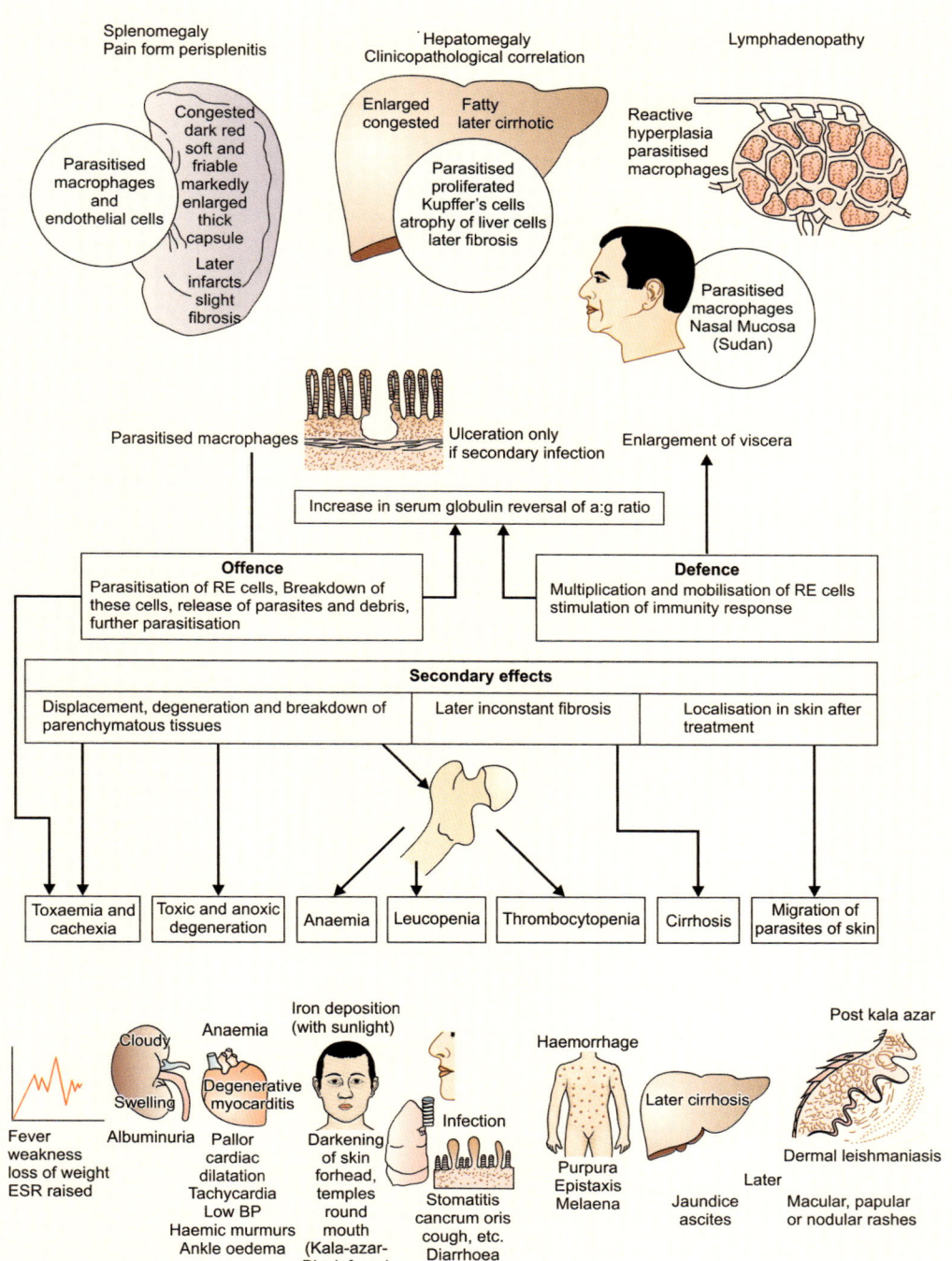

Fig. 2.14: Pathogenesis and pathology

4. Cut surface reveals marked congestion with a dull red or chocolate colour. In fresh splenectomy specimens alternating raised and depressed areas are seen. Spleen is markedly friable (lack of fibrosis).

Microscopic features

1. Vascular spaces widely dilated and engorged with blood.
2. The reticular cells of Billroth cords are markedly increased and are packed with amastigote forms of *L. donovani;* the sinus lining cells (littoral cells) do not exhibit any parasites.
3. There is no evidence of fibrosis in the parenchyma but there may be a slight increase in reticular fibrils that support the proliferating cells.
4. Trabeculae are thin and atrophic.
5. The malpighian corpuscles disappear almost because of pressure of the hyperplastic pulp tissue.
6. There is an increase in plasma cells.

LIVER

The organ is enlarged and congested. Cut surface may show a nutmeg appearance. Microscopically one finds:

1. Kupffer cells hyperplasia with the Kupffer cells being loaded with amastigote forms.
2. Sinusoidal capillaries are dilated and engorged with blood.
3. Hepatocytes are not parasitised. They may undergo thinning and atrophy because of pressure effect of dilated sinusoidal capillaries. A degree of fatty change may be present.
4. Slight increase in reticulin fibres may also occur.

Jaundice: Does not occur unless liver is greatly damaged.

BONE MARROW

Peripheral blood shows leucopenia. Whereas bone marrow exhibits a considerable replacement of the haematogenous tissues by the proliferated and parasitised macrophages and an increase in number of plasma cells. Demonstration of amastigote forms is an essential part of diagnosis of kala-azar.

ANAEMIA

Various causes put forward are:
(a) Hypoplasia of marrow.
(b) Haemolysis of RBC's (immune-based).

LYMPH NODES

Inconsistent changes. Parasites not seen in Indian kala-azar cases. Chinese and Mediterranean forms may show parasites in lymph nodes.

INTESTINES

Ulcers seen in intestine are because of secondary infections but not due to primary pathology caused by *L. donovani.*

IMMUNOLOGY

Amastigotes transformed from promastigotes excite a cellular reaction comprising histiocytic proliferation followed by invasion of mononuclear cells—lymphocytes and plasma cells. Histiocytes harbor the parasites where they multiply too. Lymphocytes help by providing cell-mediated immunity (CMI) through sensitised lymphocytes that destroy the Leishmania-filled macrophages. In *L. donovani* owing to lack of host response due to immunosuppressive effect, the CMI and delayed hypersensitivity reaction of the skin to Leishmanin antigen (a positive intradermal test—Leishmanin or Montenegro reaction) do not develop until the visceral infection has been cured. Therefore, the cells of the RE system of the organs involved proliferate and get massively parasitised, accompanied by an increase in the IgG fraction of the serum gamma globulin (hypergammaglobulinemia) which is in no way protective but is responsible for formol gel reaction (A/G ratio gets reversed).

Specific antibodies that form, can be used in complement fixation, haemagglutination, fluorescent or ELISA test for diagnostic purposes. NAT/ PCR techniques are available. They are highly sensitive and specific too.

Diagnosis of Leishmaniasis

Visceral

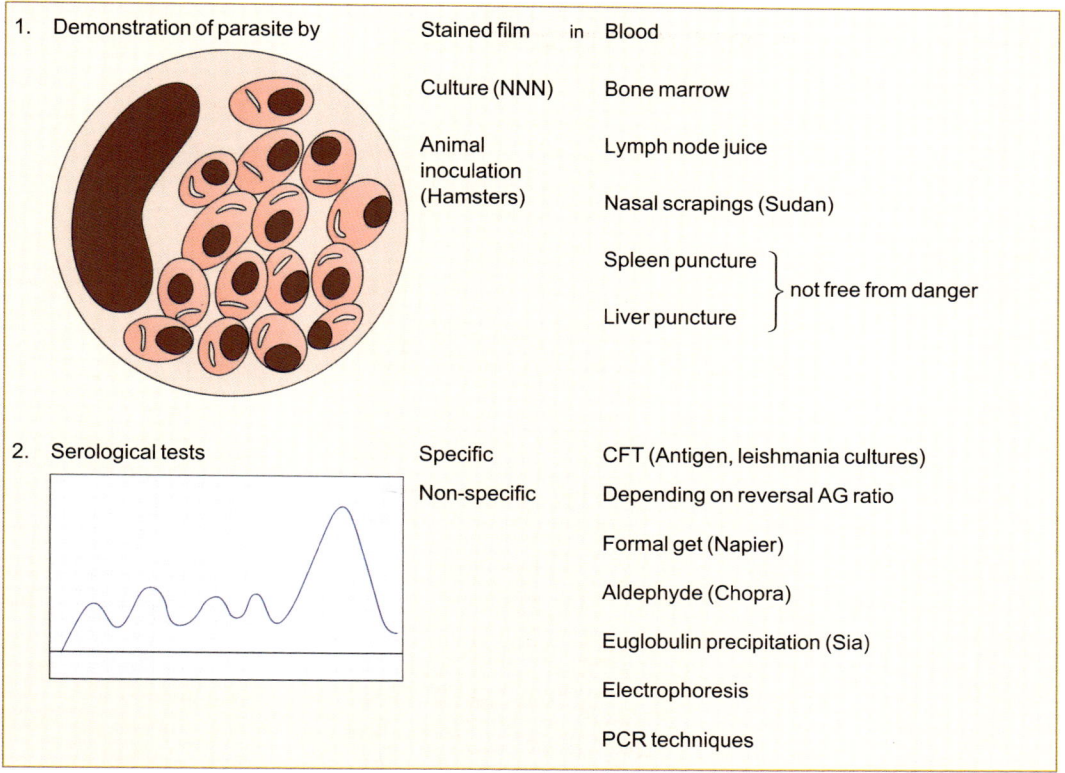

1. Demonstration of parasite by	Stained film	in	Blood
	Culture (NNN)		Bone marrow
	Animal inoculation (Hamsters)		Lymph node juice
			Nasal scrapings (Sudan)
			Spleen puncture ⎫ not free from danger
			Liver puncture ⎭
2. Serological tests	Specific		CFT (Antigen, leishmania cultures)
	Non-specific		Depending on reversal AG ratio
			Formal get (Napier)
			Aldephyde (Chopra)
			Euglobulin precipitation (Sia)
			Electrophoresis
			PCR techniques

Diagnosis can be made through direct/indirect evidences

Direct evidences

1. Peripheral blood (thick film method). Amastigote form.
2. Blood culture in NNN medium. Promastigote form
3. Biopsy material
   - Lymph node (in Chinese/Mediterranean forms but rarely needed in Indian kala-azar)
   - Sternal or iliac crest puncture (marrow)
   - Spleen puncture.

Indirect evidences

1. Progressive leucopenia
2. Serum tests
   - Aldehyde test (+ after 3 months)
   - Antimony test (less reliable)
   - Complement fixation tests (with WKK antigen)
   - ELISA tests (more reliable)
   - PCR/NAT techniques

Leishmanin test: A killed culture (0.1 to 0.2 ml volume and containing a suspension of 6 to 10 million promastigotes/ml) is injected intradermally. A positive reaction (an area of induration seen after 72 hours) is found in cured kala-azar cases 6–8 weeks after recovery and represents a delayed hypersensitivity reaction accompanied by cell-mediated immunity. The test is positive in African kala-azar but not in Indian and Mediterranean types. It is also negative in untreated kala-azar and postkala-azar dermal leishmaniasis.

Adler's test: The development of the promastigote forms of Leishmania in Locke's serum agar can be inhibited by specific immune serum but can occur in heterologous serum. The three species of Leishmania, can be differentiated serologically to a certain extent, although morphologically, culturally or by animal inoculation they are indistinguishable.

Direct evidences

Seeing is believing—demonstration of the parasite is the most conclusive evidence. This may be done by microscopic examination of a stained film and by culture.

Materials that can be Examined

(a) **Blood:** Blood film and blood culture.
(b) **Marrow:** Can be obtained by sternal/iliac crest puncture.
(c) **Splenic pulp tissue:** Biopsy material obtained by splenic puncture.

Blood: Stained blood film may show amastigote forms (often difficult to demonstrate). However, the chances of finding *L. donovani* can be enhanced by using any of the following methods:

(i) By examining a thick blood film, as for malarial parasites.
(ii) By producing a straight leucocytic edge while making a thin blood film and before the blood is exhausted, the spreading slide is abruptly lifted off. This produces a straight edge that contains a large number of WBCs. This region should be examined for the presence of amastigote forms of *L. donovani*.

(iii) By centrifuging citrated blood—the sediment at the bottom is sucked by means of a capillary pipette, smears prepared, stained and studied.

Blood culture: It is a slow, time consuming method (takes a month). 1–2 ml aseptically withdrawn blood is diluted with 10 ml of citrated saline solution (0.85% normal saline containing 2% sodium citrate). The cells are either permitted to settle in a cool incubator (22°C) overnight or centrifuged. The cellular deposit is then inoculated into the water of condensation of NNN medium and incubated at 22°C for 7 to 30 days. At the end of each week a drop of condensation fluid is examined for promastigote forms.

Splenic puncture: When splenomegaly occurs, this method is very useful for establishing a diagnosis. The amastigote forms are found in stained films or promastigote forms in culture. Haemorrhage from puncture site (can be fatal) is an important complication, however, the same can be avoided by ruling out haemorrhagic diathesis and leukaemia.

Bone marrow biopsy: From the sternum or iliac crest. In early cases, when splenomegaly has not yet occurred, this method is of utmost importance. It is safer than splenic puncture but is more painful. Another disadvantage is that when parasites are scanty, the amastigote forms may not be readily visible leading to a negative result. Material aspirated may be cultured in NNN medium and may then reveal the promastigote forms.

Indirect evidences

Evidences other than direct visualisation of the parasite:
 (i) Changes in the blood picture—blood counts.
 (ii) Changes in serum resulting from:
   (a) Rise in gamma globulin—detected by aldehyde and antimony tests.
   (b) Development of specific immune bodies detectable by complement fixation and ELISA techniques, etc.
   (c) Detecting parasite DNA through PCR techniques. Discussed towards the end of the book under New Diagnostic Protocols and Tools

Blood count: There is leucopenia (neutropenia) with relative lymphocytosis and monocytosis. Eosinophils are particularly absent. The TLC ranges around 3,000 cells/cu. mm and as the disease progresses it may fall to 1000 cells/cu. mm. There is reduction in numbers of erythrocytes also. The normal ratio of leucocytes: erythrocytes in 1:750 and this may be altered to about 1:1000 or 1:2000.

Serological tests:
(a) *Aldehyde (formol gel) test (Napier):* Depends upon hypergammaglobulinemia. To 1 to 2 ml of patients serum a drop or two of 40% formaline are added-jellification or milky white opacity implies a positive test. If the jellification occurs in 2 to 20 minutes, the test is said to be strongly positive. This test does not become positive till at least the disease is of 3 months duration. The test is found positive in other cases of hypergammaglobulinemias also, e.g. in infections with *S. japonicum* and *T. brucei*; it is also found to be positive in multiple myeloma and cirrhosis of liver.
(b) *Antimony test (Chopra et al):* This too detects raised gamma globulins. A positive test is indicated by the formation of a dense flocculent precipitate when a 4% urea

stibamine solution in distilled water comes in contact with whole serum or a serum diluted 1 in 10 from a kala-azar patient. It is, however, less sensitive.

(c) *Complement fixation test with WKK Antigen:* The antigen used is prepared from human tubercle bacillus (first prepared by Witebsky, Klingenstein and Kuhn and hence the name WKK). The test becomes positive within 3 weeks of acquiring the kala-azar infection. The test is also found to be positive in tuberculosis, leprosy and pulmonary tropical eosinophilia. Now Kedrowskey's AFB antigen is used.

Other serological tests: Immunofluorescent technique, indirect haemagglutination and Elisa techniques are more specific and sensitive. NAT/PCR techniques are fast overtaking other diagnostic platforms.

Diagnosis of acute kala-azar: Leucopenia. CFT with WKK antigen (after 3 weeks) and demonstration of parasites by thick blood film and by blood culture. Bone marrow aspiration/biopsy for direct examination or culture, spleen by this time is not enlarged enough for puncture.

Treatment

The specific chemotherapeutic drugs include:

1. **Antimony compounds:** Pentavalent antimony compounds are now the drugs of choice and include urea stibamine, aminostiburea, neostibosan, neostam, solustibosan and sodium-antimony-gluconate.
2. **Synthetic nonmetallic compound:** Pentamidine isethionate.

Prophylaxis

1. **Attack on parasite** is useful in India, i.e. measures for treatment. In China and Mediterranean the campaign should be directed against dogs serving as reservoirs of infections.
2. **Attack on the vector:** Consist of measures directed against the sandfly—the transmitting agent.
3. **Personal prophylaxis:** Use of mosquito-net or screen (22 meshes at least to the square inch), periodic fumigation and avoiding the ground floor for sleeping purposes.

POSTKALA-AZAR DERMAL LEISHMANIASIS (Dermal Leishmanoid) (PKDL)

This is a non-ulcerative cutaneous lesion seen in endemic areas of kala-azar in India. Mainly seen in Bihar and West Bengal and less so in Madras and least in Assam. About 10% of kala-azar cases develop these lesions after one or two years of antimonial treatment for the visceral kala-azar. Spontaneously cured cases may also develop PKDL. Sometimes seen in Africa but is rare in China. Mediterranean cases do not show PKDL.

Clinically: Three types of dermal lesions are seen:

(i) **Depigmented macules:** Earliest lesions that are distributed on the trunk and extremities, less common on the face. Pigment loss not as much as seen in tuberculoid leprosy.
(ii) **Erythematous patches:** Also early lesions that appear on the nose, cheeks and chin (after having symmetrical or 'butterfly erythema'). They are photosensitive and become prominent towards mid-day.

(iii) **Yellowish-pink nodules:** They replace the initial lesions but occasionally may appear at onset too. Nodules are found on the skin and rarely on the mucous membrane of the tongue and eyes. Usually seen on the face but may be seen elsewhere too. Nodules are soft, painless granulomatous growths of differing sizes. Absence of ulceration differentiates these lesions from Oriental sore and Espundia.

Diagnosis: Established by a microscopic examination of leishman-stained smear prepared from the biopsy material obtained from nodular lesions—shows amastigote forms. Direct smear examination from the depigmented macules does not generally reveal any parasite.

Treatment: Same as for visceral but in double the dosage. A subsequent course if needed should be administered after a gap of at least 2 months.

CUTANEOUS LEISHMANIASIS (Oriental sore, Chiclero's disease, Uta, etc.)

First demonstrated by Borovsky (1898) and Wright (1903), they described the morphology too, but Luhe (1906) named it *Leishmania tropica.*

Geographical distribution: The parasite is found along the coast of Mediterranean sea, Syria, Saudi Arabia, Iraq, Iran to Central Asia, the relatively drier parts of central and western India and in many places of Central Africa.

(*L. donovani* and *L. tropica* are not usually seen in the same locations. Iraq and Iran have endemic proportions of Oriental sore but do not have visceral leishmaniasis. Kala-azar is confined to moist/wet regions in India, whereas Oriental sore is observed in dry western regions of the country).

Habitat: Within the reticuloendothelial system cells of the skin (Clasmatocytes)

Morphology: Morphologically indistinguishable from *L. donovani.* Amastigote forms occur in man, while promastigote forms are seen in the sandflies and in culture.

Cultivation: Can be easily cultured in NNN medium. Cultures can be kept indefinitely by sub-inoculation.

Susceptible animals: Laboratory animals can be easily infected with *L. tropica.* In some animals intraperitoneal inoculation produces a visceral infection.

Immunology: In Oriental sore a well-defined cell-mediated immunity appears early in infection without any serum antibodies but accompanied by the development of a delayed hypersensitivity reaction with elimination of parasites. Therefore, a single attack of Oriental sore provides life-long immunity.

Life cycle and method of reproduction: Same as for *L. donovani,* except that the amastigote forms reside in the large mononuclear cells of the skin and not in the body viscera. The amastigote form in man and promastigote forms in sandflies, both divide by binary fission.

Reservoirs of infection: In endemic regions dogs serve as reservoirs, whereas in desert lands of central Asia Gerbils *(Rhombomys opimus,* a type of rodent) are the main source of infection.

Mode of transmission: Sandflies get infected by feeding upon Oriental sore cases. In 3 weeks' time the promastigote forms appear in the buccal cavity. Transmission to new host occurs by bite of the sandfly or by crushing of the infected sandflies into the punctured wound caused by the bite.

Pathology

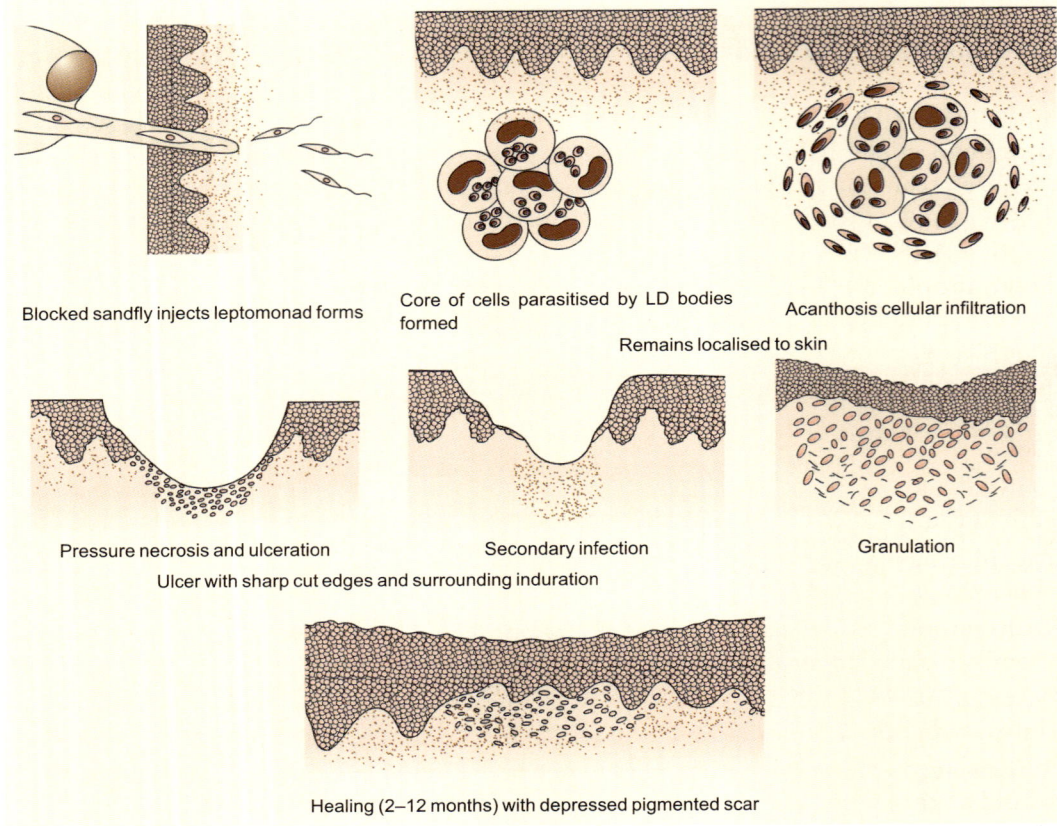

Blocked sandfly injects leptomonad forms

Core of cells parasitised by LD bodies formed

Acanthosis cellular infiltration

Remains localised to skin

Pressure necrosis and ulceration

Ulcer with sharp cut edges and surrounding induration

Secondary infection

Granulation

Healing (2–12 months) with depressed pigmented scar

The lesion of Oriental sore is a chronic infective granuloma with fibrosis. Initially, there is an aggregation of monocytes and macrophages with parasites within them; later round cell infiltration (lymphocytes and plasma cells) occurs with reduction in number of parasites and development of delayed hypersensitive skin reaction (*leishmanin reaction*).

Clinically

Incubation period is usually few weeks to 6 months and in a few cases may be up to one to two years. The lesion commences as a raised nodule about an inch in diameter. Mostly it ulcerates and shows a clean-cut margin with a raised indurated edge, surrounded by a red periphery. The parasites at this stage can be observed not in the floor of the ulcer but in the peripheral red areola. Slowly it heals spontaneously (takes 6 months or more). The ulcer gets filled by granulation tissue and leaves a depressed white scar. The sores are distributed on the exposed areas of the body, especially the face and extremities. Their number varies from 2 to 3 but sometimes there can be a single sore also. Blood picture shows a normal leucocytic count. As serum gamma globulins are normal, therefore, the aldehyde test is negative.

Laboratory diagnosis: Demonstration of parasites in the smear prepared from material obtained by a puncture of the indurated edge of the sore and stained by Leishman's/

Giemsa's stain. Amastigote forms are seen in large numbers within the macrophages. If smears are found negative, cultures should be done an NNN medium.

Skin test (Leishmanin reaction): Intradermal injection of Leishmanin (a suspension of promastigotes) of *L. tropica* gives a positive skin test in cases of Oriental sore.

Treatment: A pentavalent preparation of antimony is the drug of choice. Dehydro-emetine orally in 100 mg dosage given daily for 10–21 days gives satisfactory results.

Prophylaxis: Measures include:
- (i) Elimination of reservoir hosts.
- (ii) Control of sandflies.
- (iii) Individual protection from sandfly bites.
- (iv) Prophylactic immunisation with a culture of *L. tropica*.

ESPUNDIA (Muco-cutaneous Leishmaniasis caused by *Leishmania brasiliensis*)

First observed by Carini (1911) and described by Vianna (1911).

Geographical distribution: Confined to Central and South America.

Habitat: Occurs as an intracellular parasite (amastigote form) inside macrophoges of skin and mucous membrane of the nose and buccal cavity.

Morphology: *L. brasiliensis* resembles morphologically and culturally the other two species *L. donovani and L. tropica.*

Cultivation: Easily cultivable on NNN medium. Can also be grown on chorio-allantoic membrane of chick embryo.

Susceptible animals: Inoculation into Syrian hamsters causes a localised skin lesion only, intreperitoneal inoculation does not produce any visceral infection.

Life cycle: The insect host is a wild species of sandfly (Genus Lutzomyia) commonly found in regions where espundia occurs. Life cycle, reproduction methods resemble other types of leishmania.

Reservoir hosts: Small (forest) rodents.

Transmission: The South American Leishmaniasis is a zoonosis, affecting the skin of small forest rodents and is maintained by a variety of sandflies that feed on them. Man is infected by bite of these sandflies. The disease can spread from man to man; therefore, direct contact plays a significant role in the transmission of infections.

Immunity: In espundia with metastasis in the skin and mucous membrane the cell-mediated immunity (CMI) does not develop until metastasis takes place.

Pathology

The skin pathology in *L. tropica* and *L. bransiliensis* is identical. The initial lesion has a tendency to enlarge radially forming an ulcer with a clear-cut margin and oozing surface. Microscopically, the skin and the mucous membrane lesions show infiltration of lymphocytes, plasma cells and large mononuclear cells with necrotic tissue. The parasites are found (amastigote forms) in huge numbers within the macrophages and the monocytes at the periphery of the lesion.

Clinically: Incubation period exactly not known, may be from a few days to few weeks. One finds a specific ulcerative granuloma of the skin followed subsequently by involvement of the mucocutaneous regions.

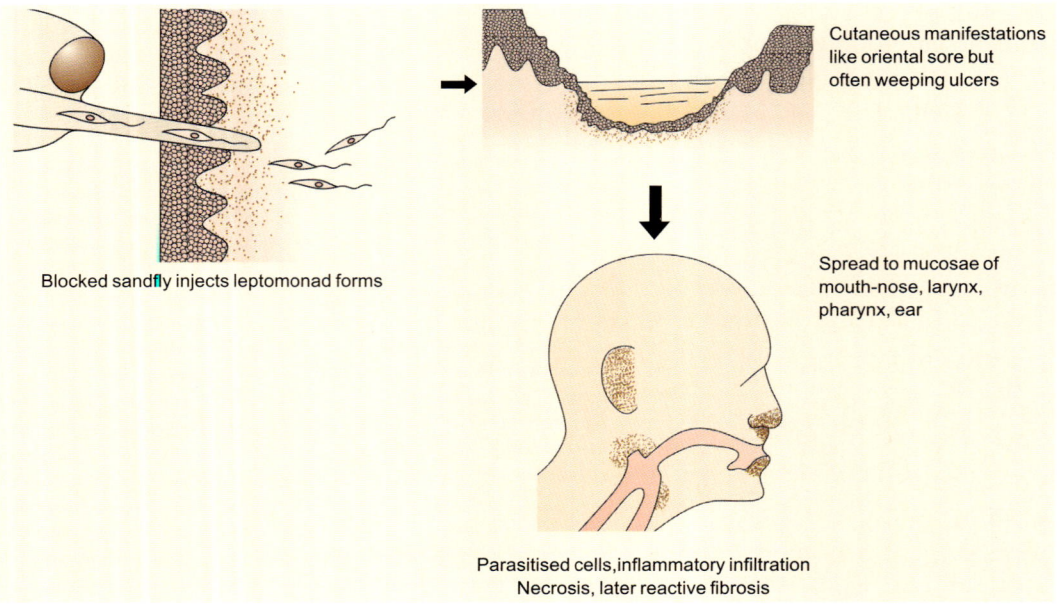

Blocked sandfly injects leptomonad forms

Cutaneous manifestations like oriental sore but often weeping ulcers

Spread to mucosae of mouth-nose, larynx, pharynx, ear

Parasitised cells, inflammatory infiltration
Necrosis, later reactive fibrosis

Secondary effects in loose mucosal tissues		
Oedema and capillary involvement Interference with local blood supply Necrosis: Extensive destruction	Secondary infection Deep erosion locally Spread of infection to lungs or elsewhere	Healing with fibrosis
Leading to Extensive disfiguring lesions	General constitutional upset (fever, pain, anaemia.)	Bronchopneumonia and septicaemia

Diagnosis: Confirmed by demonstration of the amastigote forms in skin and mucocu-taneous lesions in smear or biopsy. An intradermal skin test (delayed hypersensitivity reaction) can also be performed by using cultures of *L. brasiliensis.*

The leishmaniae are scanty in skin smears in cases of Chicle ulcer (Bay sore) and therefore, a biopsy of skin lesion becomes essential.

Treatment: A pentavalent antimonial preparation is the drug of choice. In resistant cases amphotericin-B or pyrimethamine can be used.

Prophylaxis: Being a zoonoses, it is difficult to control. Forest workers should take protective measures against sandfly bites.

BLOOD FLAGELLATES

CLASS ZOOMASTIGOPHOREA

FAMILY TRYPANOSOMATIDAE

Developmental Stages of Trypanosomatid Flagellates

Various developmental stages are named after the arrangement of the flagellum in the body, as determined by its starting point (in relation to the kinetoplast), its course and point of emergence. The root term is mastigote and various prefixes are used to name the various stages.

1. **Amastigote (leishmanial stage):** Represented by rounded stage without any external flagellum

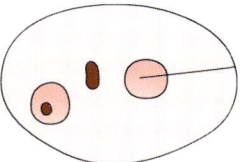

2. **Promastigote (leptomonad form):** It is the form where kinetoplast lies anterior to the nucleus; the flagellum arising near it emerges from the anterior end of the body.

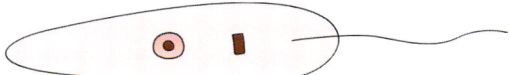

3. **Opithomastigote (trypanosome or trypanomorphic stage):** Here the kinetoplast lies posterior to the nucleus; the flagellum arises near it, then passes through the body and emerges from the anterior end (no undulating membrane present). This stage is not seen in flagellates that infect humans.

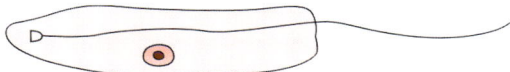

4. **Epimastigote (crithidial stage):** Here the kinetoplast lies anterior and close to the nucleus; the flagellum arising near it emerges from the side of the body to run along a short undulating membrane.

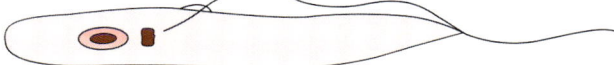

5. **Trypomastigote (true trypanosome stage):** Here the kinetoplast is posterior to the nucleus and is situated at the posterior end of the body; the flagellum arises near it and emerges from the side of the body to run along a long undulating membrane.

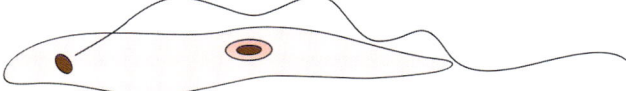

6. **Choanomastigote (barley-corn form):** Kinetoplast lies at the anterior end of the body; the flagellum arises near it and emerges at the anterior end of the body through a wide funnel-shaped reservoir.

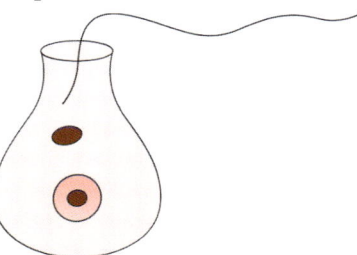

TRYPANOSOMA

Characteristics of the genus Trypanosoma: These exist as trypomastigotes in verte-brate hosts (man and animals), some, e.g. *T. cruzi,* assume amastigote forms. They need two hosts to complete their life cycle—vertebrate and insect. They pass through the stages of amastigote, promastigote, epimastigote and metacyclic form of trypo-mastigote. They can multiply and reproduce in any of the above-mentioned forms. Transmission from one vertebrate host to another is effected via blood-sucking insects. They need to develop in the insect vector too. Infectivity of an insect depends on the final development of metacyclic form of trypomastigotes.

Mainly two types of development are observed.

1. **Anterior station (Salivaria):** The trypomastigotes ingested develop in the mid-gut and they move towards the proventriculus, labial cavity and the salivary glands as seen in *T. brucei* subgroup. Transmission occurs through the bite of the insect.
2. **Posterior station (Stercovaria):** Ingested trypomastigotes develop in the intestine from where they proceed backwards to the hindgut, as seen in *T. cruzi* and *T. lewisi.* Transmission is effected by ingestion of faeces of the insect, or by rubbing the faecal matter into the wound caused by the bite of the insect, as in *T. cruzi.*

Morphology of Trypomastigotes

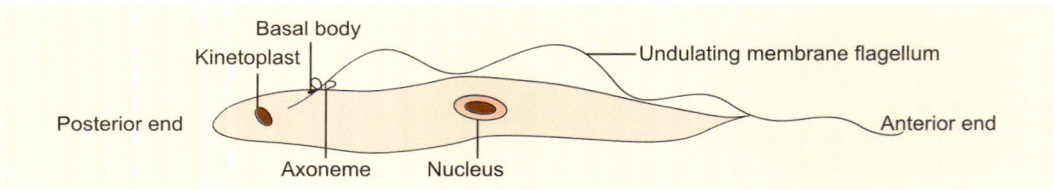

Method of Reproduction

Reproduction occurs by binary longitudinal fission. It commences by division of the kinetoplast and the basal body, followed later by that of the nucleus. The flagellum with the undulating membrane stays with one of the daughter cells while the other one develops them afresh. At the end, the cytoplasmic body splits longitudinally from the anterior end.

Classification: Those infective to man are:

1. *T. brucei* subgroup (human strain)—causes African trypanosomiasis (Gambian, Rhodesian and Zambezi forms of sleeping sickness)
2. *T. brucei*—Causes South American trypansomiasis
3. *T. rangeli*—A non-pathogenic trypanosome found in the blood of man in some of the Latin American countries (Venezuela and Colombia)

ANIMAL TRYPANOSOMES

Non-pathogenic: *T. lewisi* in rat; transmitted by rat fleas.

Pathogenic: *T. brucei* (animal strain)—wildgame and domestic animals in tropical Africa, causes Nagana.

T. evansi—in horses and mules in India, mechanical transmission.

T. equiperdum—a venereal disease in horses and asses in Europe, America, North Africa and India. Transmitted sexually.

T. *equinum*—causes 'mal de caderas' amongst horses in South America. Mechanical transmission, has no kinetoplast and no insect cycle.

T. *vivax* and T. *congolese*—cause disease in cattle transmitted by tsetse flies.

Trypanosoma brucei

Causes African trypanosomias is in man and Nagana in domestic animals.

Discovered by David Bruce in 1890, suggested it to be causative agent of 'nagana' in cattle in Zululand. The trypanosome causing disease in man was first discovered by Forde and Dutton in Gambia in 1902 and in Rhodesia by Stephens and Fantham in 1909.

T. *brucei subgroup*

It is realised that T. *brucei* subgroup comprises a single species containing strains or subspecies of varying host-specificity and virulence. It includes:

(a) Animal strain—spread through the tsetse belt of Africa. It does not infect man.
(b) Human strains—on clinico-epidemiological pattern basis, the undermentioned forms are recognised
    (i) 'Rhodesian' sleeping sickness, acute form.
    (ii) 'Gambian' sleeping sickness, chronic form.
    (iii) 'Zambezi' sleeping sickness, although chronic, is more like the acute 'Rhodesian' form.

Strict classification on above basis should not be done. Hoare in 1970 suggested that the brucei-rhodesiense-gambiense complex should be considered as subspecies of T. *brucei* and may be termed:

T. *brucei brucei*, T. *brucei gambiense*, T. *rhodesiense* as a virulent nosodeme of T. *gambiense*. Morphologically these strains are indistinguishable from each other, they can only be differentiated by their behaviour in man (can be tested directly by infecting human volunteers).

Blood incubation infectivity test to identify whether a strain, isolated from a tsetse fly or a domestic or a game animal, is an animal strain (T. *brucei*) or a human infectivity strain (T. *rhodesiense*).

The strain to be tested is at first inoculated into rats or mice and on establishment of parasitaemia, cardiac blood is withdrawn. About 0.25 ml of this blood is taken in each of 2 Bijou bottles. To one bottle 2 ml of human blood and an anticoagulant (0.25 mg of 2% potassium oxalate with glucose added to a strength of 3 mg/ml of blood) is taken. This constitues the test sample.

In the other bottles instead of the human blood, 2 ml of phosphate-buffered saline (pH = 7.4) is added. This represents the control sample.

Both the samples are mixed gently and are incubated in a water bath at 37°C for 5 hours. Each of the mixtures is then tested separately by inoculating into a rat. If a later development of persistent parasitaemia occurs in both the rats, the result is interpreted as positive, i.e. the strain is human infective form and the infectivity to rats having remained unimpaired. If the parasitaemia occurs only in the rat inoculated with the control sample, the test is interpreted to be negative, i.e. the strain is of animal origin and inoculation with the human blood having rendered it non-infective to the rat.

Habitat: T. *brucei* is basically a parasite of connective tissues, where it divides readily. It consumes a large amount of glucose.

It reaches the draining lymph nodes and also reaches the blood circulation causing parasitaemia. Ultimately it localises in the brain. The African sleeping sickness is a disease of the central nervous system.

Prevalence of *T. brucei*: The animal strains occur throughout the tsetse belt of Africa but the human strains are less widespread. The chronic 'gambiense' strain is found mainly in West Africa (from Gambia to Congo), Central Africa (Zambia and surrounding countries) and scattered regions in East Africa, especially Uganda.

The chronic 'Zambezi' strain (pathology similar to 'gambiense') is found in Botswana, Zimbabwe, and Zambia. The acute 'Zambezi' strain (resembling 'rhodesiense') is found in Tanzania, Uganda and Kenya.

Morphology: In vertebrates, *T. brucei* exists in trypomastigote form. These are elongated rather flattened spindle-shaped organisms with a blunted posterior end and an acutely pointed anterior end. The centrally placed nucleus is large and oval. The small kineto-plast is placed at the posterior end. The flagellum originates from the posterior end near the kinetoplast, it curves around the body in the form of an undulating membrane and then continues beyond the anterior end as a free flagellum. The undulating membrane is thrown into folds (usually 3 or 4 depending upon the length of the parasite). The flagellum assists the parasite in rapid motility.

Polymorphism: The parasites differ in size and shape during different stages of their development. Two main forms are recognised:

1. Short, thick stumpy form (10 × 5 μ) with no or a very small flagellum.
2. Long slender (20 × 3 μ) with a conspicuously long flagellum.

Forms between the two forms described above may be seen. Initially, the long form is seen but as the infection establishes the short, stumpy form with inter-mediate forms appear. Antigenic *variants* appear at 3–4 days' intervals, possibly by selection of mutants. As host's defence gets activated, variants develop and finally some variant multiplies. Each parasitaemia wave is accompanied by fever and followed by leucocytosis (monocytosis). Another feature is that the antibodies develop to a series of immunologically distinct type variant in the serum of hosts. Each antibody titre rise coincides with the disappearance of the homologous variant and when this has been eliminated, a new antigenic type immediately appears. The outer proteinaceous coat protects the parasite from the hosts' defence mechanisms.

Demonstration of parasites: Peripheral blood taken during parasitaemia can be stained with Leishman's/Giemsa's stain—here the cytoplasm and the undulating membrane appear pale blue; the nucleus reddish purple or red; the kinetoplast and flagellum dark red.

Cultivation: NNN is not suitable. It can be cultivated. It has been cultivated in a medium of Ringer's solution with sodium chloride, Tyrode's solution and citrated human blood. Long slender forms of trypomastigote, similar to midgut forms of tsetse fly are encountered in culture.

Animal inoculation: Laboratory animals, like mice, rats and guinea pigs can be inocu-lated if peripheral blood smear examination does not show the trypomastigotes. In laboratory animals it causes marked parasitaemia and kills the animal in a few days. *T. brucei* in rabbits (syringe inoculated infection) causes a chronic infection lasting a few weeks and most die in about 4–5 weeks.

Immunology: Non-specific IgM immunoglobulins in large quantities are produced by the host. These antibodies, however, do not offer any significant effect. On the contrary African trypanosamiasis is associated with profound immunosuppressive effect especially the humoral component.

Life cycle: *T. brucei* passes its life cycle in two different hosts. The vertebrate hosts are man, game and domestic animals, while the insect hosts comprise various species of tsetse fly (glossina) which include *G. palpalis, G. tachinoides, G. pallidipes, G. swynnertoni* and *G. moristans.*

Development in man (Vertebrate host): Infected glossina bites and deposits the metacyclic trypanosomal forms and these divide by binary fission at the inoculation site. They become shorter and stumpy later parasitaemia ensues. These short stumpy forms are taken up by tsetse fly with its blood-meal and undergo further developmental changes inside it.

Development in tsetse fly: First change in midgut is transformation to long slender forms (with kinetoplast lying midway between posterior end and the nucleus), these then pass to the posterior end of the extra-peritrophic space (space between the peritrophic membrane and the epithelial cells), where also they multiply for some time. Around 15th day anterior end of the space is reached and the parasites enter the lumen of the proventriculus. Subsequently, they migrate to the buccal cavity pass onto the hypopharynx and ultimately reach the salivary glands through the opening of the salivary ducts. Once here, they again change their morphology, first becoming the epimastogote and then tansferring into the metacyclic (short stumpy trypomastigote) form which is infective to man. The cycle within the fly takes about 20 days time and thereafter these flies stay infective for the rest of their lives that may extend up to 185 days. The flies cannot transmit the disease to their offsprings (about 6–12 larvae are produced during its life span).

Vectors and Reservoirs of Infection

T. brucei animal strain is transmitted by *Glossina morsitans* amongst wild and domestic animals.

T. brucei gambiense strain is transmitted by *G. palpalis, G. pallidipes* and *G. tachinoides.*

G. palpalis sucks blood from birds, reptiles and man. *G. tachinoides* feeds on blood of mammals (especially antelopes) other than man. These are shade and moisture-loving flies and are found in shrubs and shady trees near water (called riverine species). Animal reservoirs of infection for this strain are not yet identified. So far as the 'gambiense' strain is concerned man himself is the reservoir of infection. The site where bites take place is near the water supply of the village.

The transmitting agents for *T. brucei rhodesiense* strain are *G. morsitans, G. swynnertoni* and *G. pallidipes.* These flies feed on other wild animals too but important amongst these is bushbuck. Wild animal to man transmission is responsible for sporadic spread while endemic spread occurs from man-fly-man transmission.

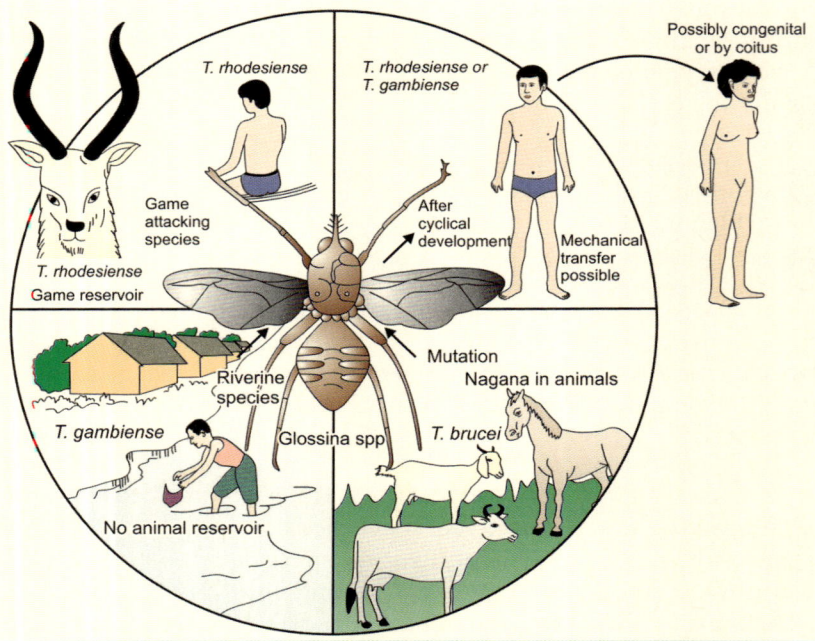

Fig. 2.15: Life cycle: General

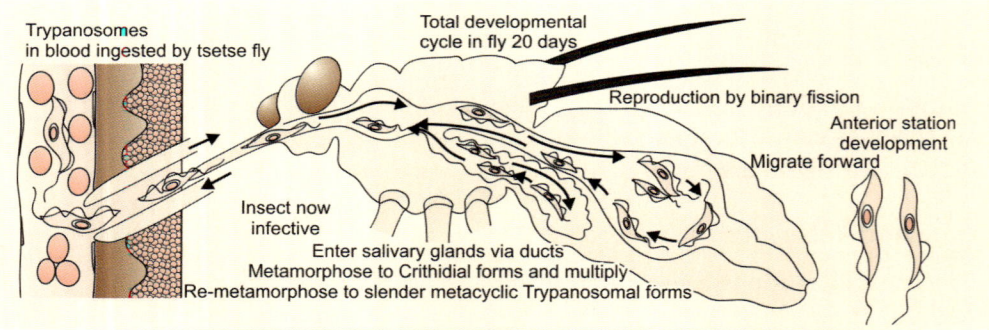

Fig. 2.16: Life cycle in insect

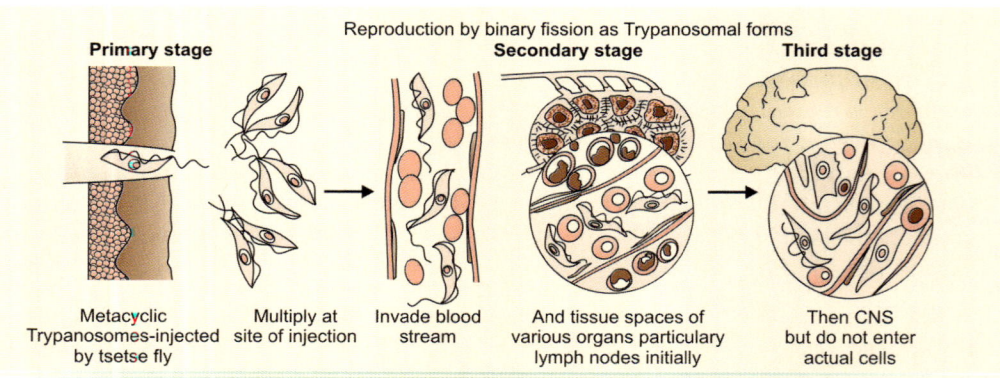

Fig. 2.17: Life cycle in man

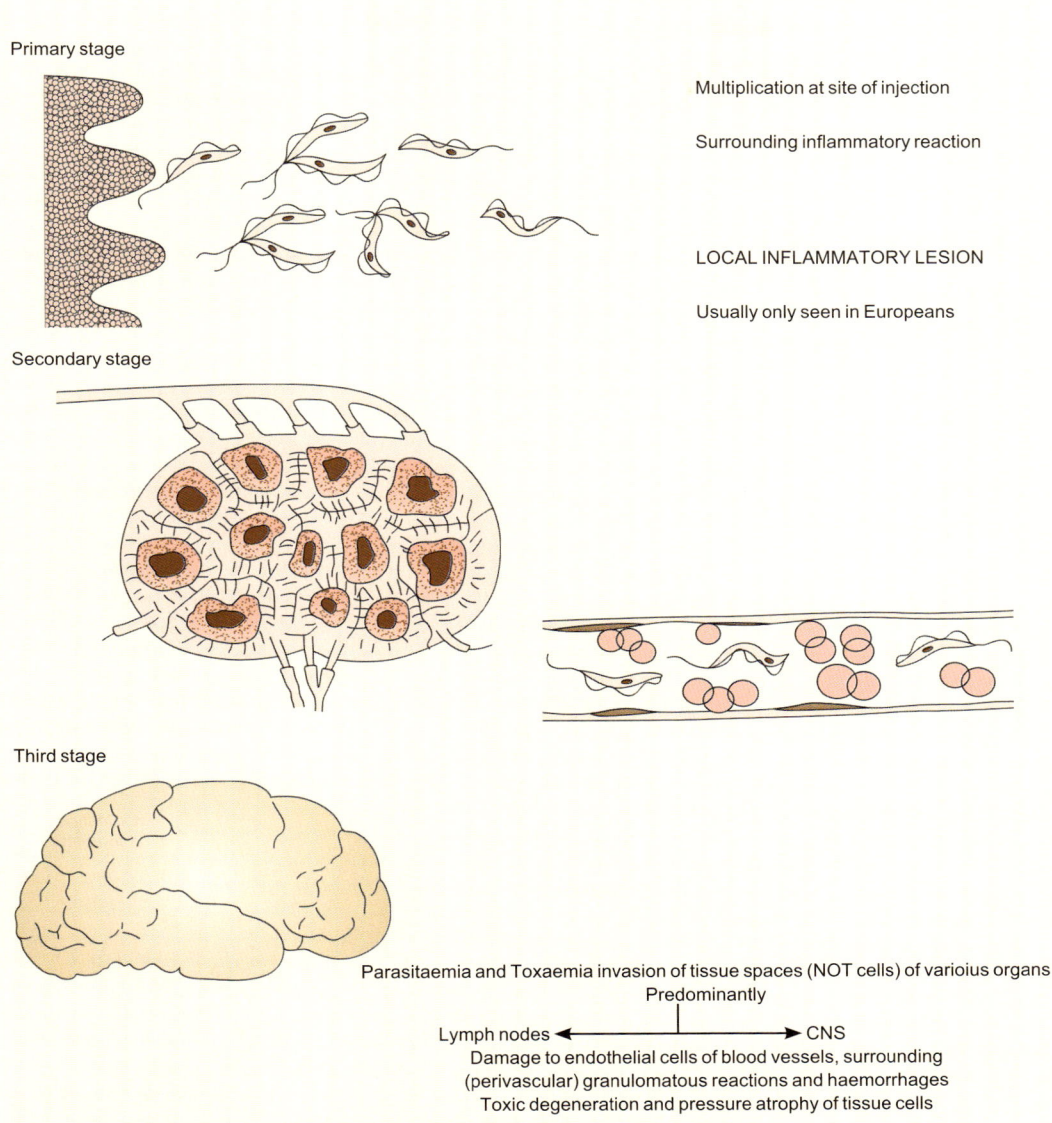

Primary stage

Multiplication at site of injection

Surrounding inflammatory reaction

LOCAL INFLAMMATORY LESION

Usually only seen in Europeans

Secondary stage

Third stage

Parasitaemia and Toxaemia invasion of tissue spaces (NOT cells) of varioius organs
Predominantly

Lymph nodes ← | → CNS
Damage to endothelial cells of blood vessels, surrounding
(perivascular) granulomatous reactions and haemorrhages
Toxic degeneration and pressure atrophy of tissue cells

Fig. 2.18: Pathogenesis and pathology

PATHOGENESIS

Mode of infection: By bite. Both male and female flies can transmit and bite by daylight—usually early morning and evening. The trypomastigotes get entangled in the tissue spaces and some enter the blood stream. In tissue spaces the organisms evade the action of antibodies.

Initially parasitaemia is mild. It has been suggested that the connective tissue damage caused may be on account of exaggerated immune response (autoimmune reaction or extensive kinin release) rather than any direct effect (mechanical damage due to their movement) of this relatively non-toxic organism. The trypomastigotes in the connective tissue induce reaction by two ways:

1. By producing exessive amounts of non-specific immunoglobulins (not useful to the patient), these are produced in response to the secretion of an exo-antigen of the trypomastigote.
2. By heavy infiltration of the site by macrophages, the microphages (neutrophils) exhibit no interest. CMI plays a dominant role.

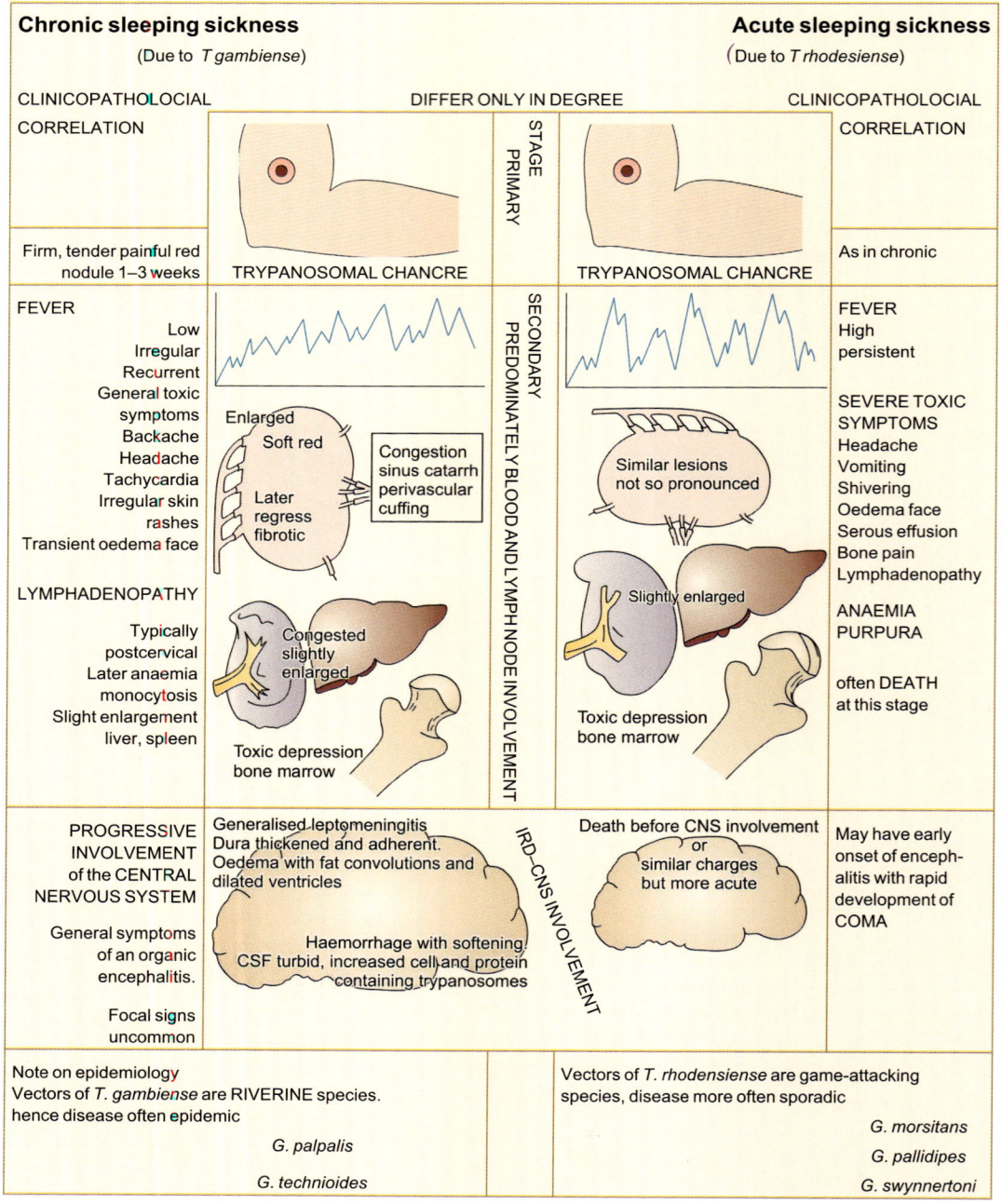

Chronic sleeping sickness
(Due to *T gambiense*)

Acute sleeping sickness
(Due to *T rhodesiense*)

CLINICOPATHOLOCIAL CORRELATION — DIFFER ONLY IN DEGREE — CLINICOPATHOLOCIAL CORRELATION

STAGE PRIMARY

TRYPANOSOMAL CHANCRE — Firm, tender painful red nodule 1–3 weeks / TRYPANOSOMAL CHANCRE — As in chronic

SECONDARY PREDOMINATELY BLOOD AND LYMPH NODE INVOLVEMENT

FEVER — Low, Irregular, Recurrent — General toxic symptoms, Backache, Headache, Tachycardia, Irregular skin rashes, Transient oedema face

Enlarged Soft red — Congestion sinus catarrh perivascular cuffing — Later regress fibrotic

LYMPHADENOPATHY — Typically postcervical — Later anaemia monocytosis — Slight enlargement liver, spleen

Congested slightly enlarged

Toxic depression bone marrow

Similar lesions not so pronounced

Slightly enlarged

Toxic depression bone marrow

FEVER — High, persistent

SEVERE TOXIC SYMPTOMS — Headache, Vomiting, Shivering, Oedema face, Serous effusion, Bone pain, Lymphadenopathy

ANAEMIA PURPURA

often DEATH at this stage

IRD–CNS INVOLVEMENT

PROGRESSIVE INVOLVEMENT of the CENTRAL NERVOUS SYSTEM — General symptoms of an organic encephalitis. Focal signs uncommon

Generalised leptomeningitis. Dura thickened and adherent. Oedema with fat convolutions and dilated ventricles. Haemorrhage with softening. CSF turbid, increased cell and protein containing trypanosomes

Death before CNS involvement or similar charges but more acute

May have early onset of encephalitis with rapid development of COMA

Note on epidemiology
Vectors of *T. gambiense* are RIVERINE species. hence disease often epidemic

G. palpalis

G. technioides

Vectors of *T. rhodensiense* are game-attacking species, disease more often sporadic

G. morsitans
G. pallidipes
G. swynnertoni

Pathogenic lesions: There is massive damage of the perivascular connective tissue. The collagen bundles are disrupted and fibroblasts destroyed. Chiefly, the lesions are seen in the lymph nodes and central nervous system (CNS).

In CNS an increase in glial cells occurs diffusely. The cerebral perivascular spaces are 'cuffed' with mononuclear cells (perivascular cuffing). Cerebral softening may result from thrombosis of these cuffed blood vessels. The choroid plexus is markedly congested and infiltrated with monocytes with many filled with parasites. There is massive cellular infiltration in the leptomeninges but slight infiltration in the brain substance.

The lymph nodes in initial stages show congestion, haemorrhages and profound proliferation of macrophages; later they undergo degenerative changes with extensive fibrosis.

Blood and CSF

Blood shows leucocytosis (monocytosis) and anaemia. ESR rises due to hypergammaglobulinemia and for the same reason serum aldehyde test becomes positive; it also causes RBC auto-agglutination. CSF has raised pressure and cell count (50–100 cells/cu mm) and elevated protein levels (100–150 mg%). The rise in globulin contents gives a 'tabetic' type of colloidal gold curve. The parasites may be seen in CSF.

Clinically

A history of tsetse fly bite is often elicited. A trypanosomal chancre may develop at the site of bite (is often unnoticed or passed of as a normal tsetse bite). It is a hard painful nodule and fluid withdrawn from it reveals actively dividing trypomastigotes; it subsides in about 2 weeks without suppurating.

In 'rhodesian' form the symptoms appear about 2 weeks after the bite, while in 'zambezi' and 'gambian' forms symptoms may be delayed for up to a year.

It is characterised with parasitaemia, lymphadenopathy (first regional and later generalised) and eventually involvement of the CNS. The initial symptoms are fever (high and fluctuating in rhodesian form), severe headache, loss of nocturnal sleep rhythm and a feeling of general debility and ill feeling. A fleeting circinate erythematous rash may appear on chest and shoulders (not so easy to detect on black skin). Lymph node enlargement especially of the posterior triangle of the neck, is a feature of 'gambian' form while in 'rhodesian' form CNS invasion is rapid. As it advances, meningoencephalitis develops with appearance of classical sleeping sickness. Later, patient becomes emaceated with signs of malnutrition. In 'rhodesian' form patients die earlier (if left untreated) but with 'gambian' and 'zambezi' forms the patient may survive longer (up to several years). In the 'zambezi' form the patient may spontaneously overcome infection and become a healthy carrier.

Laboratory diagnosis

1. *Demonstration of the parasite*

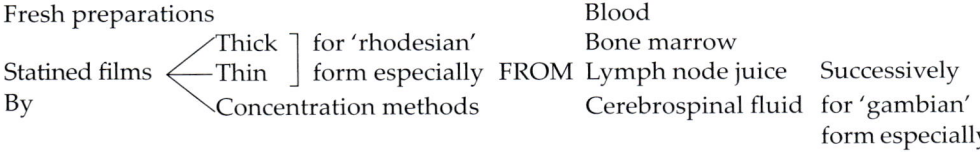

2. *Serological methods*
   - Indirect fluorescent antibody test,
   - A complement fixation test for *T. gambiense* now available
   - Formol gel test (as for Leishmaniasis) may be positive
   - Note: Paul-Bunnell test (for heterophile antibodies) may be positive.

   Parasite DNA detection by NAT-PCR techniques

Treatment

Suramin and pentamidine are drugs of choice for early acute infections. These drugs cannot cross the blood–brain barrier (BBB), therefore, they are not usable in CNS involved cases—in these cases an arsenical is needed, e.g. tryparsamide, melarsen, melarsoprol (Mel-B) and trimelarsen. Nitrofurazone may be used in arsenical resistant cases.

Prophylaxis includes:
   (i) Destroying vectors' habitat, supplemented by use of pesticides.
   (ii) Game destruction to eliminate the reservoirs.
   (iii) Staying away from regions known to harbor the infective/infectable game and treatment of all infected human beings.
   (iv) Chemoprophylaxis—Pentamidine is effective against 'gambian' form. A single 4 mg/kg body weight injection given intramuscularly provides chemoprophylaxis for 6 months against the 'gambian' form.

SOUTH AMERICAN TRYPANOSOMIASIS

CHAGAS' DISEASE

Trypanosoma cruzi

Geographical distribution: South and Central America

Habitat: Resides in nervous and muscular tissues and also in the RE system existing in the amastigote form. Trypomastigote forms appear in the peripheral blood from time to time.

Two main morphological forms are found in human beings *Trypomastigote forms.* The parasite appears as a C- or U-shaped organism in the peripheral blood. Measure 20 μ in length, has a large central ucleus, an oval posteriorly placed kinetoplast. Two forms are identified in the peripheral blood:
   1. A slender long form.
   2. A short and broad form.

The parasite does not multiply in peripheral blood. These trypomastigotes may be taken up by the insect vector or enter the tissue cells to live as amastigote forms.

Amastigote forms: Especially seen inside skeletal muscle cells (cardiac and skeletal), neuroglial cells in the CNS and cells of RE system. The amastigote forms are round to oval, 2–4 μ in diameter and possess a nucleus and a kinetoplast. On full development numerous amastigotes may be found enclosed in a cystic cavity. Parasitic multiplication occurs at this stage only.

Staining: By any of the Romanowsky stains.

Cultivation: Easily cultivated in NNN medium or its modifications.

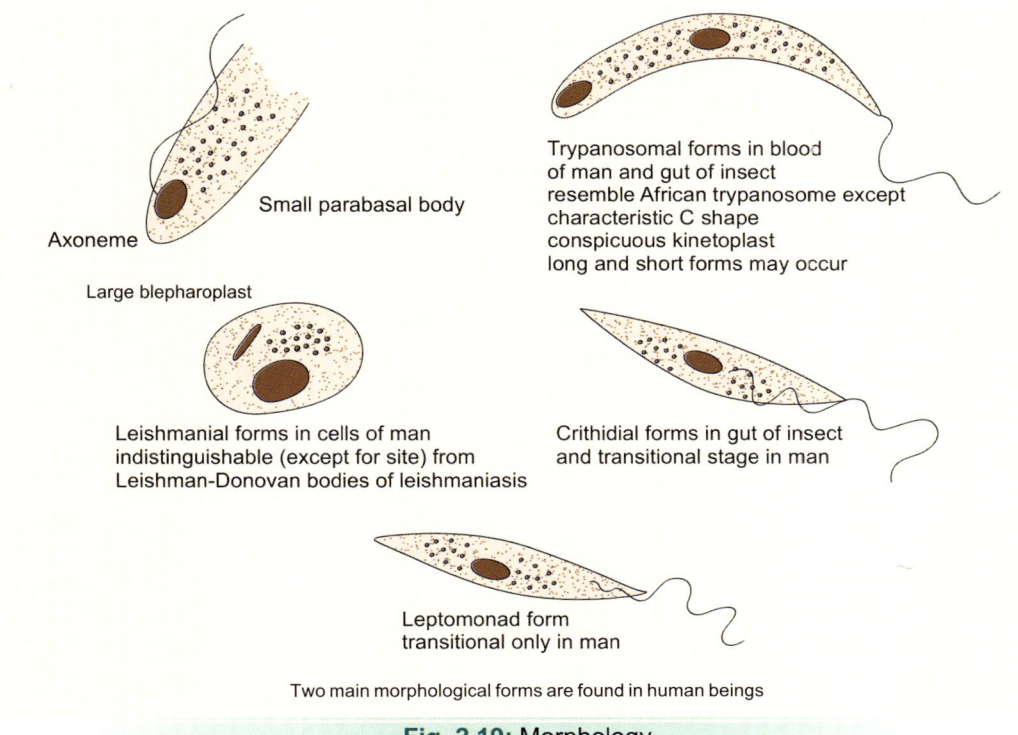

Axoneme

Small parabasal body

Large blepharoplast

Trypanosomal forms in blood
of man and gut of insect
resemble African trypanosome except
characteristic C shape
conspicuous kinetoplast
long and short forms may occur

Leishmanial forms in cells of man
indistinguishable (except for site) from
Leishman-Donovan bodies of leishmaniasis

Crithidial forms in gut of insect
and transitional stage in man

Leptomonad form
transitional only in man

Two main morphological forms are found in human beings

Fig. 2.19: Morphology

Immunology: Serum antibodies develop in Chagas' disease but the parasites being intracellular are not exposed to them.

Life cycle: *T. cruzi* passes its life cycle in two hosts: One in man or the reservoir host; the other in the transmitting insect, the reduviid big *(Panstrongylus megistus, Triatoma infestans and Rhodnius prolixus).*

Development in Reduviid Bug

The trypomastigotes taken up by the bug are transformed into amastigote forms and multiply by binary fission. Later transformed into epimastigote forms they pass backwards to the hindgut and multiply by longitudinal fission. In one week to 10 days time the metacyclic trypomastigote forms appear that are excreted with the faeces.

Development in Man

Man gets infected either by faecal matter of the bug that is rubbed into the bite wound or by a likely contamination of the conjunctivae and other exposed mucous membranes with fingers. The metacyclic forms in the human host are converted into amastigotes which multiply by binary fission and after passing through promastigote and epimastigote forms they are transformed into trypomastigotes that cause parasitaemia.

Reservoir Hosts

These are armadillos and opossums. Man being a secondary host. Other animals that can get infected are bats, rats and cats.

Domestic animals
Possibly congenital by coitus
Triatoma spp. (Cone bug)
Cyclical development
Possibly
Wild animals man and reservoirs
Bed bug
Tick
New host

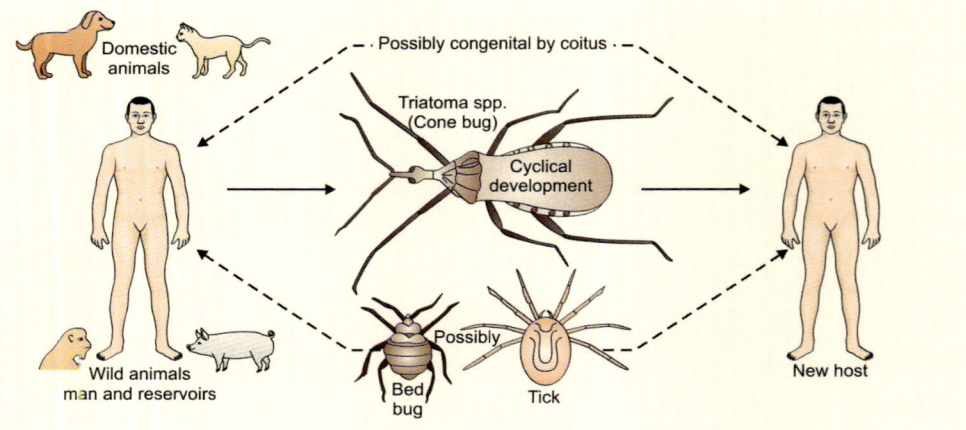

Fig. 2.20: Life cycle: General

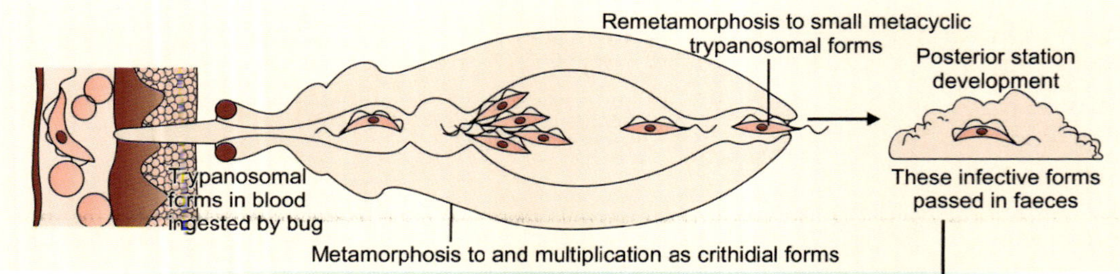

Remetamorphosis to small metacyclic trypanosomal forms
Posterior station development
Trypanosomal forms in blood ingested by bug
These infective forms passed in faeces
Metamorphosis to and multiplication as crithidial forms

Fig. 2.21: Life cycle in insect

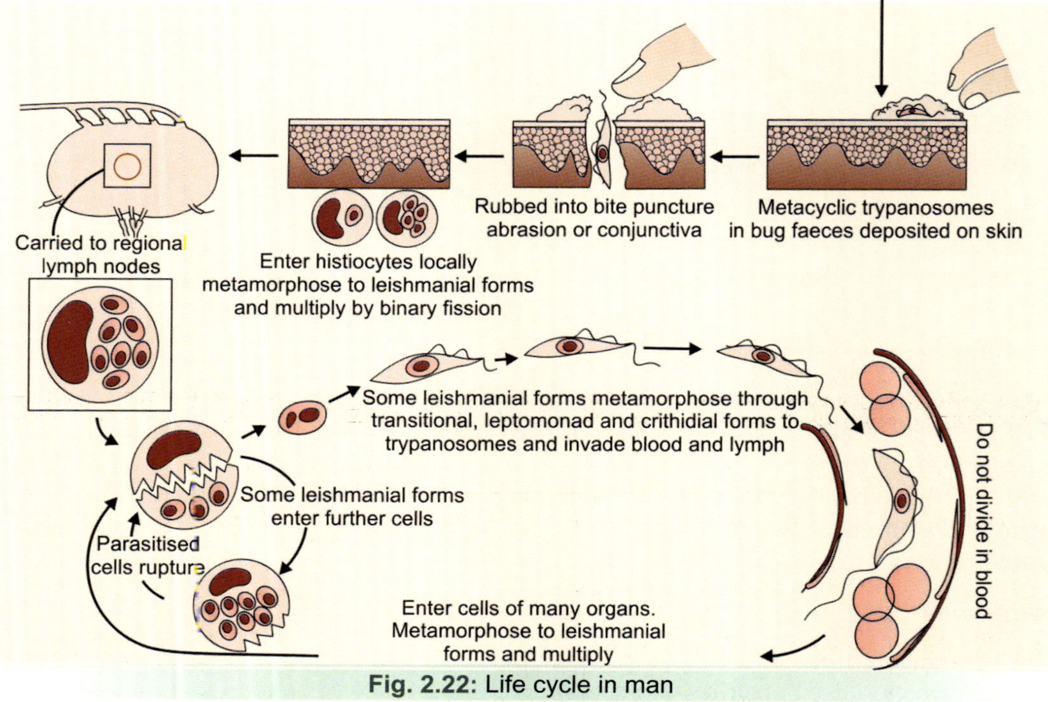

Carried to regional lymph nodes
Enter histiocytes locally metamorphose to leishmanial forms and multiply by binary fission
Rubbed into bite puncture abrasion or conjunctiva
Metacyclic trypanosomes in bug faeces deposited on skin
Some leishmanial forms metamorphose through transitional, leptomonad and crithidial forms to trypanosomes and invade blood and lymph
Some leishmanial forms enter further cells
Parasitised cells rupture
Do not divide in blood
Enter cells of many organs. Metamorphose to leishmanial forms and multiply

Fig. 2.22: Life cycle in man

Pathogenesis (Fig. 2.23)

Mode of infection: By contamination through the Reduviid bug. Portal of entry being skin or conjunctiva. The swelling that occurs in the skin is called 'Chagoma', whereas, the oedematous swelling in the conjunctival entry site is designated as 'Romana's sign'. Transmission can also occur transplacentally to newborns and otherwise by blood transfusion of infected blood.

Lesions: The parasites invade heart, skeletal muscle, nervous system (and thyroid in certain regions) cells. The RE system cells are especially involved. The parasites multiply in the amastigote stage only and the pathogenic lesions are due to amastigotes themselves which ultimately destroy the cell they infect.

Clinically

Incubation period: One to two weeks and assumes acute or chronic forms of Chagas' disease.

Acute form: It is seen in infants and children. It is characterised by fever, conjunctivitis, asymmetric or unilateral facial oedema, lymphadenopathy, splenomegaly, anaemia and lymphocytosis. Left untreated it terminates fatally with symptoms of meningo-encephalitis or cardiomyopathy (cardiac failure).

Chronic form: It is observed in adolescents and adults. It brings about cardiac arrythmias (cardiac block, Adams Stokes syndrome) and nervous system abnormalities (spastic aparalysis and psychotic changes). This period may last for a period of 12 years.

By causing degeneration of entramural autonomic nerve plexuses, it leads to dilatation of the tubular organs—megaoesophagus and megacolon. Cardiomyopathy may also occur. As a result of myopathy, ventricular apical aneurysm may occur and at autopsy these are often found to be filled with thrombus.

Laboratory Diagnosis

1. **Demonstration of the parasite:**

Fresh preparations	Blood (Trypanosomal forms)	
Stained films	Lymph node juice	*(Trypanosomal forms)*
	(Leishmanial forms)	
Animal inoculation	Blood inoculation into a guinea pig	
By Culture	*From* Lymph node juice	
	Blood (clean bred triatomid bugs fed on patient or his blood develop Trypanosomes in gut in 2 weeks time)	
Histological	Biopsy material (lymph node, calf/deltoid muscle)	
techniques	Postmortem material	

2. **Serological methods:** Specific complement fixation test available (Machado-Guerretro test). Antigen obtained from culture of *T. cruzi.*
   Also available NAT-PCR techniques or sensitive and specific diagnosis.

Intradermal test: A delayed hypersensitivity reaction is obtained by using an extract 'cruzin' prepared from culture of *T. cruzi.*

Treatment

Nitrofurazone tablet can be given spread over 3–4 weeks time. Benznidazole has also been tried with some success in acute case.

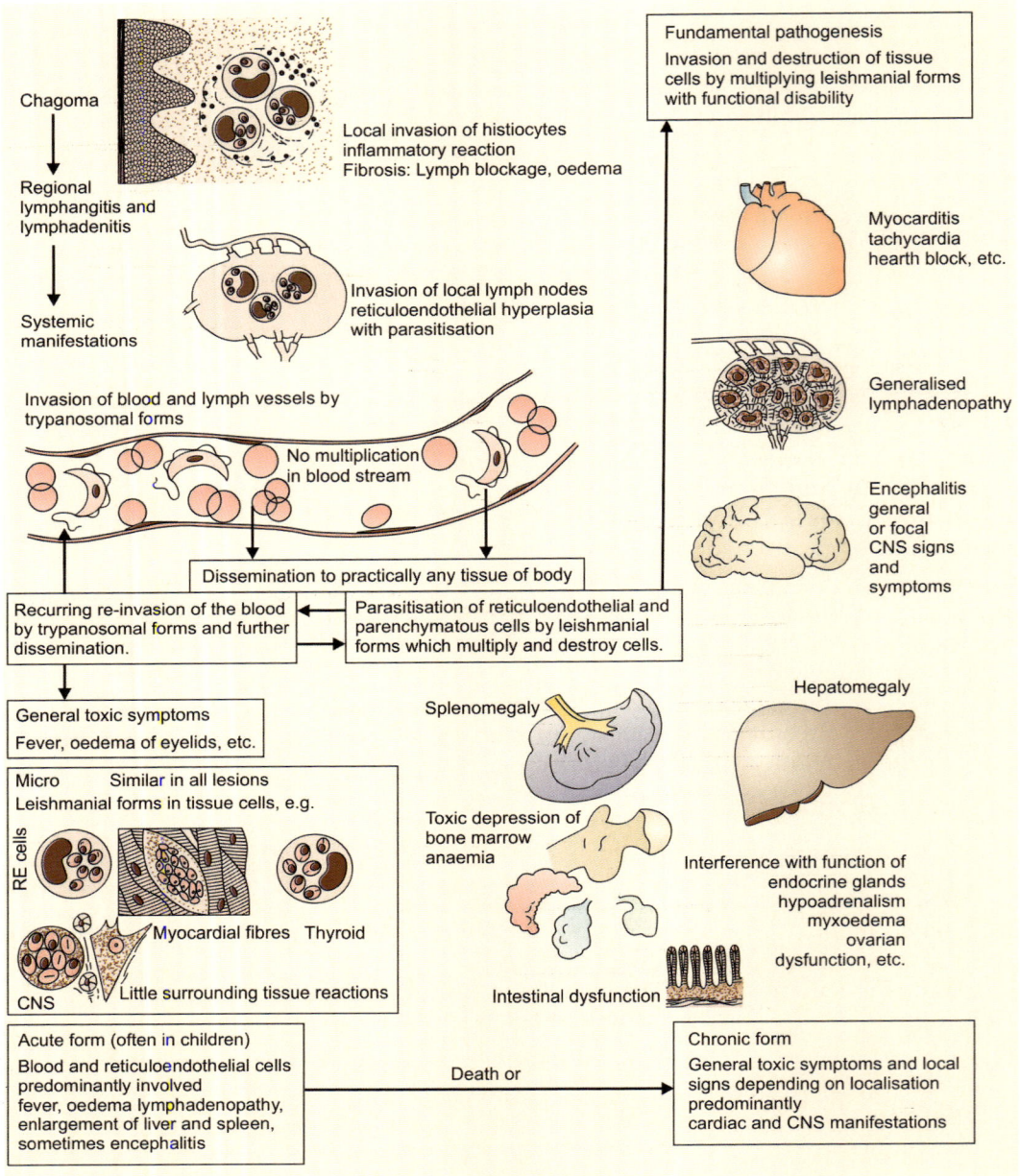

Fig. 2.23: Pathogenesis and pathology

Prophylaxis

(i) Attack on parasite—treatment with a drug

(ii) Attack on vector—using insecticides or using building material that repels the bug.

(iii) Personal prophylaxis—using mosquito nets, etc., i.e. avoiding the bites.

Table 2.2: The essential differences between African trypanosomiasis, South American trypanosomiasis and visceral leishmaniasis

	African trypanosomiasis (Sleeping sickness)	South American trypanosomiasis (Chagas' disease)	Visceral Leishmaniasis (Kala azar)
CAUSED BY	*Trypanosoma gambiense* or *Trypanosoma rhodesiense*	*Trypanosoma cruzi*	Leishmania donovani
VECTOR	Glossina spp. (tsetse flies)	Triatonida spp. (cone-nosed bugs)	Phlebotumus spp. (sand files)
CYCLE IN VECTOR			
	Anterior station development	Posterior station development	Anterior station development
Stage ingested	Trypanosomal	Trypanosomal	Leishmanial
		Metamorphose to Crithidia	
Then	Multiply and move forward Enter salivary glands via duct	Multiply	Metamorphose to Leptomonad, Multiply
	Metamorphose to Crithidla Multiply	Move backward	Move forward
	Metamorphose to metacylic Trypanosomes	Metamorphose to metacyclic Trypanosomes	Block proboscis
	INFECTIVE: INJECTED IN SALIVA	INFECTIVE: PASSED IN BUG FAECES	INFECTIVE: INJECTED FROM PROBOSCIS
CYCLE IN MAN Form injected	Metacyclic Trypanosome	Metacyclic Trypanosome	Leptomonad
Metamorphosis	NONE—remain as Trypanosomes	Enter histiocytes locally and become Leishmanial	Enter histiocytes locally and become Leishmanial
Multiplication (all by binary fision)	as TRYPANOSOMES in BLOOD and tissue spaces	As Leishmanial forms in cells	As Leishmanial forms in macrophage cells
Then	Remain in blood stream as Trypanosomes	Carried to regional nodes: some	Further dissemination as Leishmanial forms ONLY
		Leishmanial forms infect further histiocytes: Some metamorphose through transitional Leptomonad and Crithidial forms to gain blood as Trypanosomes. Do not multiply as such but disseminated, enter further tissue cells, metamorphose to Leishmanial forms and multiply	
Pathogenesis	Circulating, multiplying Trypanosomes cause Parasitaemia and Toxaemia, damaging tissues	Parasitisation and destruction of all types of tissue cells. Circulating Trypanosomes produce toxaemia	Parasitisation and destruction of RE cells
Pathological effects	Mainly general toxaemia Lymphadenopathy CNS involvement	General toxaemia Local functional disability of whichever tissues invaded, especially lymph nodes, heart, CNS	General toxaemia from breakdown of RE cells Proliferation of RE cells (mainly spleen, liver, bone marrow, lymph nodes) No CNS involvement
Clinico-pathological correlation	Acute (*T. rhodesiense*) Fever and severe toxaemia	Fever Enlarged nodes, spleen and liver Protean manifestations depending on localisation in tissues especially Cardiac	Fever Anaemia Enlarged liver and spleen
	Chronic (*T.gambiense*) Fever, lymphadenopathy, encephalitis	CNS syndromes	

DISTINCTION BETWEEN HUMAN AND ANIMAL TRYPANOSOMES

In epidemological surveys of infection rates of trypanosomes in vectors (e.g. Glossina spp.) domestic animals or game reservoirs (e.g. Antelopes), certain animal or reptilian trypanosomes may be found and require differentiation from human trypanosomes.

Table 2.3: Groups, subgroups and species

	Brucei—Evansi	Vivax	Congolense	Lewisi
Size	18–42 μ	12–20 or 20–26 μ	9–18 or 12–24 μ	Varies 20–90 μ
Shape	POLYMORPHIC (various forms encountered)	MONOMORPHIC (all one form)	MONOMORPHIC or POLYMORPHIC	MONOMORPHIC for spp.
Posterior end	Blunt (except in slender forms)	Blunt	Blunt	Pointed
Kinetoplast	SMALL (none in T. equinum) typically SUBTERMINAL	LARGE, generally TERMINAL	MEDIUM, typically MARGINAL	VERY LARGE TERMINAL or SUBTERMINAL
Undulating membrane	CONSPICUOUS	INCONSPICUOUS	CONSPICUOUS INCONSPICUOUS	INCONSPICUOUS (except in T. grayi and T. theieri)
Free flagellum	PRESENT (except in slumpy forms)	PRESENT	ABSENT or VERY SHORT	PRESENT
Nucleus	Central (except in post-nucleate forms)	CENTRAL	CENTRAL	CENTRAL (anterior in T. lewisi)
Forms	**Evansi** — Always Polymorphic slender and stumpy forms plus others. *T. gambiense* in man and Tsetse flies; *T. rhodesiense* in man. Tsetse flies and game; *T. brucei* in cattle. Tsetse flies and game. **Brucei** — Polymorphism INCONSTANT always slender forms, stumpy rare. *T. evansi* in domestic animals; *T. equinum*, *T. equiperdum* in horses. (slender 29–42 μ; stumpy average 18 μ; intermediate average 23 μ; post-nucleate)	SPP. *T. uniforme* 12–20 μ; *T. vivax* 20–26 μ. *T. vivax* — In domestic animals; *T. uniforme* — Tsetse flies and game	SPP and FORMS. Monomorphic — *T. congolense* 9–24 μ; Polymorphic — slender, short, stout — *T. simiae* 12–24 μ. *T. congolense.* In domestic animals and game; *T. simiae* in pigs, sometimes in tsetse flies	SPP. *T. cruzi* 20 μ; *T. lewisi* 25 μ; *T. grayi* 90 μ; *T. theilleri* 70 μ. *T. cruzi* In man, animals and bugs; *T. grayi* In crocodiles and tsetse flies; *T. lewisi* In rats; *T. theileri* In cattle and game

3

Ciliates

Subphylum - Ciliophora
Class - Ciliatea
Order - Heterotrichida

The parasite's body is covered with hair-like process (cilia). They are binucleate organisms and the shape of the body is defined by a distinct cell membrane

BALANTIDIASIS

Class   **PROTOZOA**
|
Ciliata
Move by cilia
Generally have mouth (cytosome)
Oesophagus and anal opening
|
Genus   **Balantidium**
Ovoid
Coarse cilia
Contractile vacuoles
Horseshoe or kidney-shaped macronucleus
Reproduce by binary fission

Balantidium coli

Causes dysentry in man (ciliate dysentry or balantidiasis)

Geographical distribution: Worldwide.

Habitat: Largest protozoal parasite inhabiting the gut of man. Also seen in pigs and monkeys. In pigs they are nonpathogenic.

Morphology

Classification

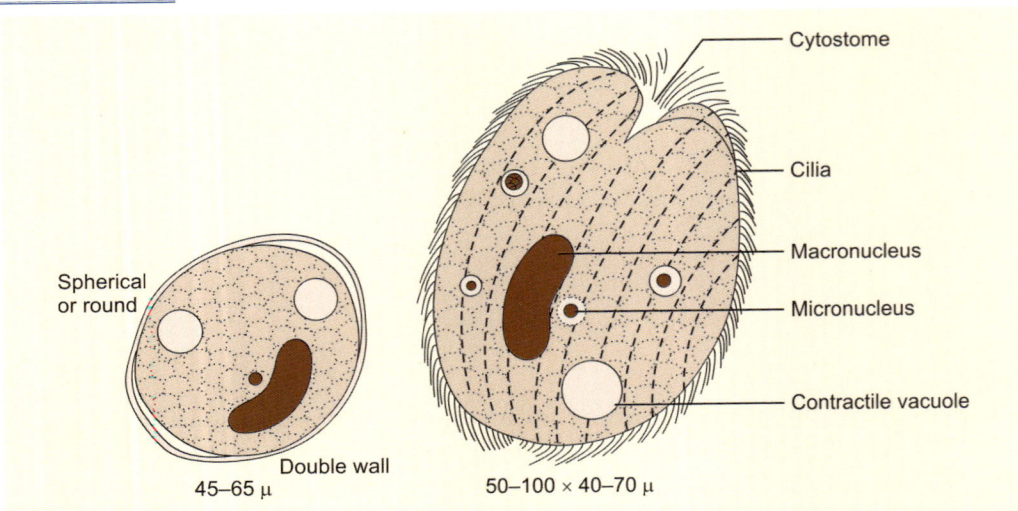

Cytostome

Cilia

Macronucleus

Micronucleus

Contractile vacuole

Spherical or round

Double wall
45–65 μ

50–100 × 40–70 μ

Cyst

Vegetative

The parasite exists in two forms. Cysts (found in chronic cases and carriers). Trophozoites are observed in dysenteric stools.

Trophozoite

Oval-shaped with variable size 40–50 × 60–70 μ. Body covered with delicate pellicle exhibiting longitudinal striations. Short delicate uniformly long cilia cover the body except near the mouth called "adoral cilia" are longer. Beneath the pellicle is a thin layer of clear ectoplasm. Body is chiefly composed of granular endoplasm. The anterior end shows a groove (peristome) that leads to the mouth (cytostome). The cytostome terminates into a short funnel-shaped gullet (cytopharynx) extending up to one-third of the body length. There is no intervening intestine while the posterior end reveals a fixed anus (cytopyge).

The internal structures are:
  (i) *Two nuclei:* A large bean-shaped macronucleus at the middle of the body. The concavity of the larger nucleus shows a micronucleus.
 (ii) *Two contractile vacuoles:* One in the middle and the other at the posterior end.
(iii) Multiple food vacuoles consisting of debris from the host's gut-content and sometimes tissue debris, erythrocytes and leukocytes.

Cyst

Smaller than trophozoite, measuring 50–60 μ in diameter. The granular cytoplasm contains a macro and a micro nucleus plus a refractile body. During encystment the contractile vacuoles are active for some time. Exteriorly the cyst is surrounded by a thick transparent bi-layered wall.

Cultivation: B. coli cultivation characteristics are like those of *E. histolytica*.

Life cycle consists of two stages but in the same host. While pig happens to be the main host, man gets infected only rarely. Cyst is the infective stage and is ingested by man.

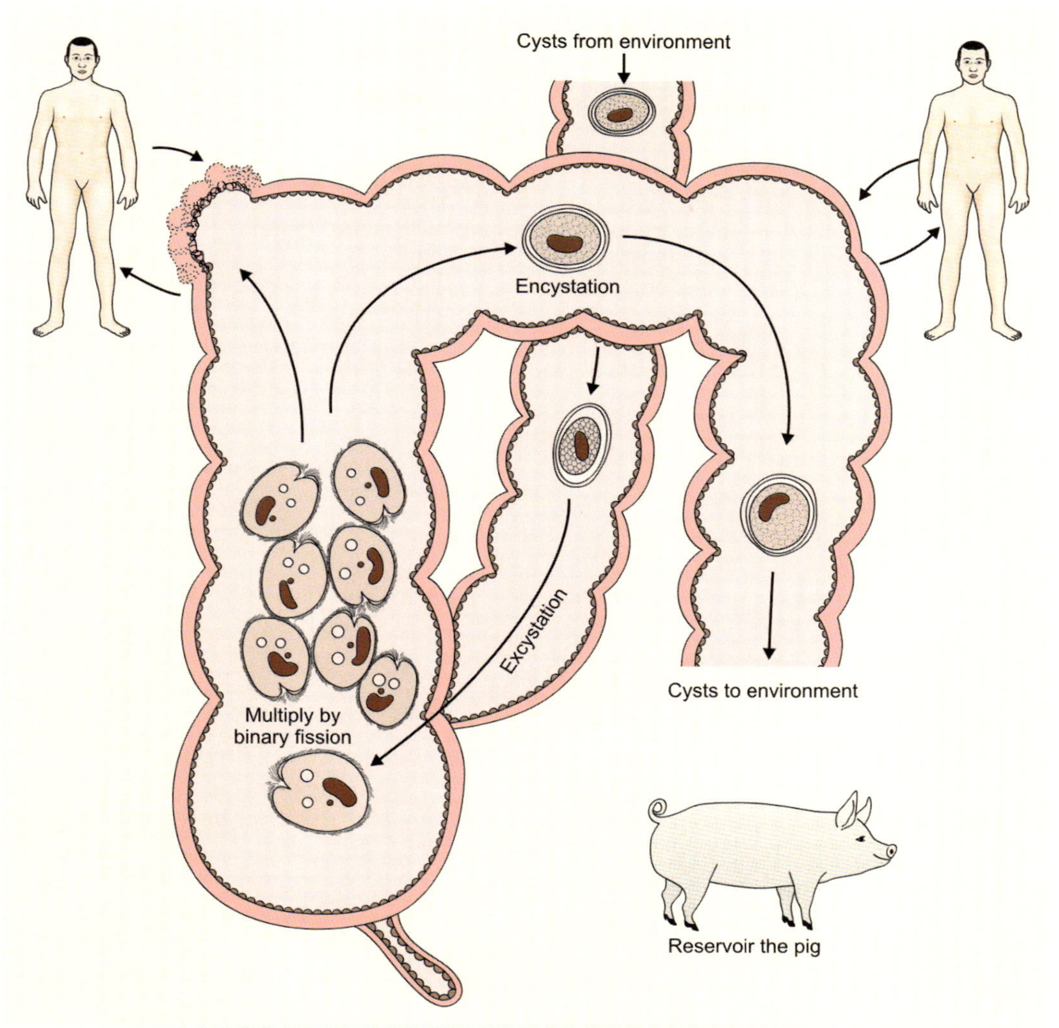

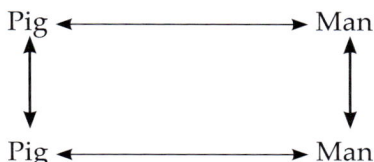

Fig. 3.1: Life cycle and reproduction

Transmission: Occurs from pig to pig, pig to man and man to man.

Pig ⟷ Man

Pig ⟷ Man

Each ingested cyst liberates a single trophozoite. The trophozoites may remain in the lumen or enter into the sumucous coat of colon, growing and multiplying there. Each division forms two trophozoites leading to colony formation. Division starts with micronucleus, then the macronucleus and finally the body by a transverse fission (consequently the daughter-individual that gets the cytostome develops the anus and vice versa). After some time of growth and multiplication or when environment gets hostile—encystment occurs. During conjugation two trophozoites get encysted, exhange nuclear materials and separate.

Invade like *E. Histolytica* by $\left\{\begin{array}{l}\text{Motility} \\ \text{Cytolytic ferment}\end{array}\right.$

Ulcers wider-mouthed than in amoebic dysentery
Secondary infection frequent so cellular infitration around
Localised to intestine. No extra-intestinal spread
Complications—perforation

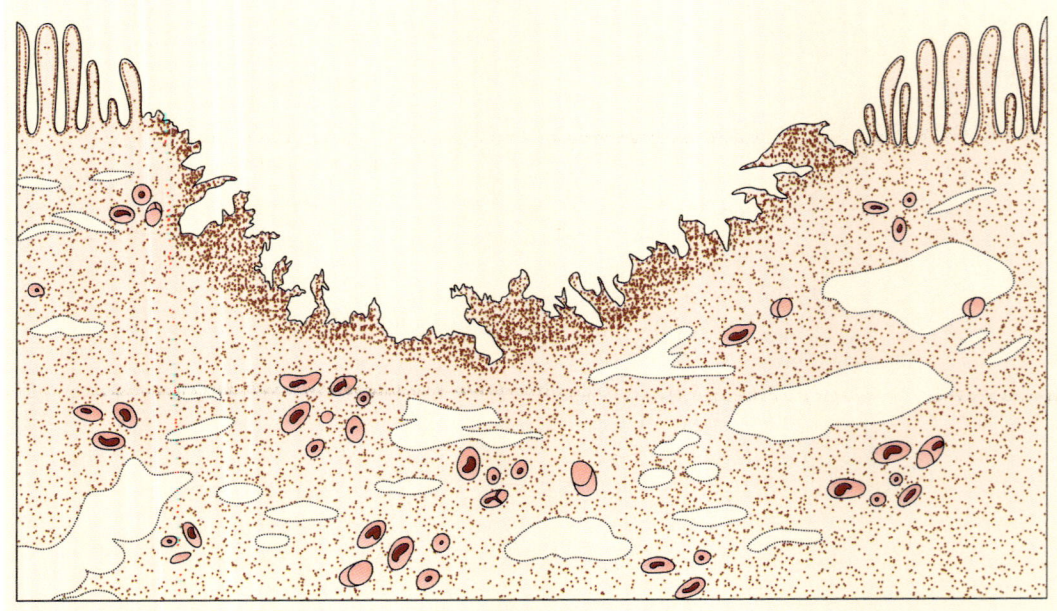

Fig. 3.2: Pathology

People running piggeries often contract the infection. Cyst-contaminated food is ingested, scarcity of starchy food in humans makes it invade the intestinal epithelial cells (pigs consume abundant starchy food and therefore *B. coli* do not invade their tissues but derive the food from the luminal starches). Less of starchy food also explains the rarity of balantidiasis in man.

Lesion: Consists of colonic ulceration. Diagnosis is established by demonstrating the parasite in the tissues. The necrosis may extend to the muscle coat. Hepatic invasion does not occur.

Clinically: No fever. Passage of blood and mucous in stool.

Diagnosis: By demonstration of trophozoites in the stool sample

Treatment: Drugs effective are arsenicals (carbarsone), diiodohydroxyquinoline (diiodoquin) and oxytetracycline. Emetine has no role here.

Prophylaxis: Protection of food and drink from getting contaminated with faeces of pig or an infected man.

Sporozoa (Subphylum)

CLASSIFICATION

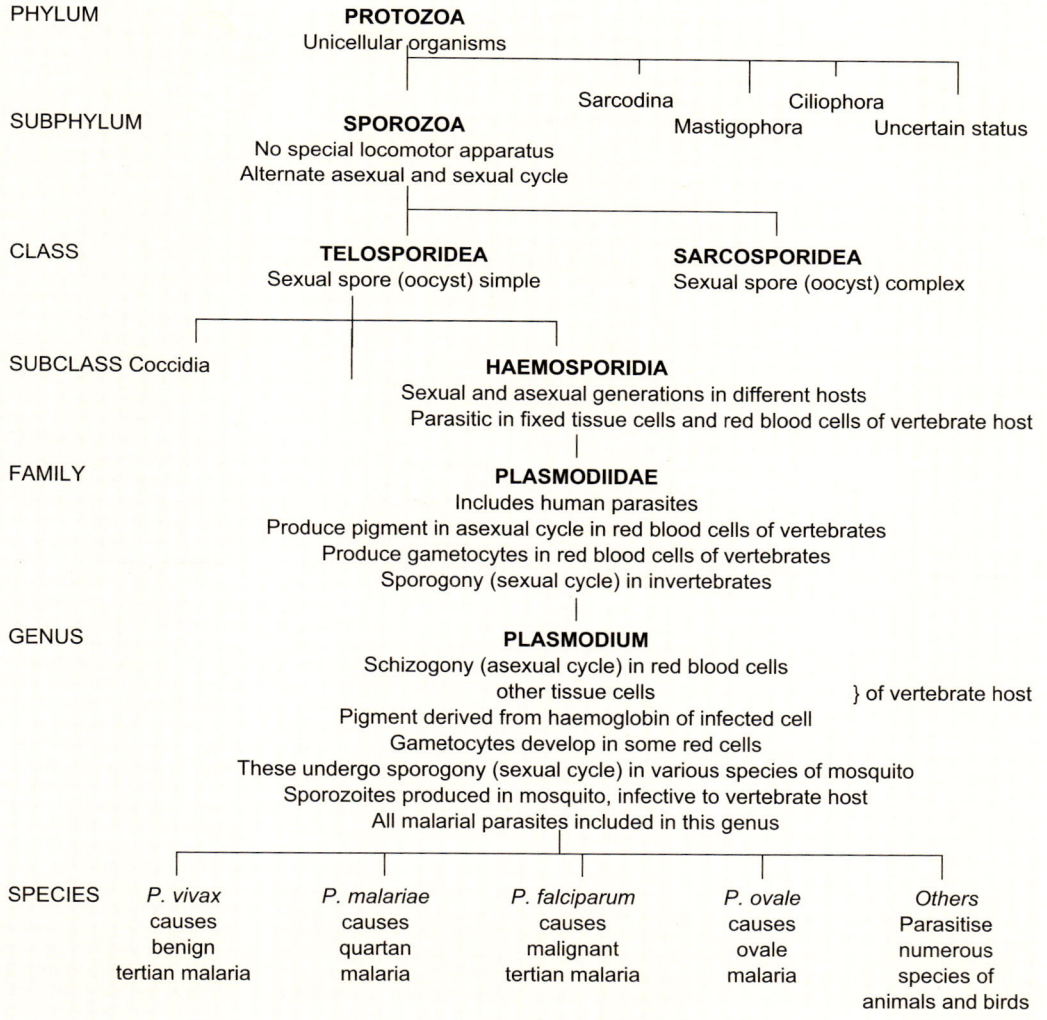

PHYLUM	**PROTOZOA** Unicellular organisms				
SUBPHYLUM	**SPOROZOA** No special locomotor apparatus Alternate asexual and sexual cycle	Sarcodina Mastigophora	Ciliophora Uncertain status		
CLASS	**TELOSPORIDEA** Sexual spore (oocyst) simple	**SARCOSPORIDEA** Sexual spore (oocyst) complex			

SUBCLASS Coccidia

HAEMOSPORIDIA
Sexual and asexual generations in different hosts
Parasitic in fixed tissue cells and red blood cells of vertebrate host

FAMILY

PLASMODIIDAE
Includes human parasites
Produce pigment in asexual cycle in red blood cells of vertebrates
Produce gametocytes in red blood cells of vertebrates
Sporogony (sexual cycle) in invertebrates

GENUS

PLASMODIUM
Schizogony (asexual cycle) in red blood cells
other tissue cells } of vertebrate host
Pigment derived from haemoglobin of infected cell
Gametocytes develop in some red cells
These undergo sporogony (sexual cycle) in various species of mosquito
Sporozoites produced in mosquito, infective to vertebrate host
All malarial parasites included in this genus

SPECIES

P. vivax causes benign tertian malaria	*P. malariae* causes quartan malaria	*P. falciparum* causes malignant tertian malaria	*P. ovale* causes ovale malaria	*Others* Parasitise numerous species of animals and birds

PLASMODIUM

(Genus)

Generic characters: Parasites of this genus exhibit alternation of generation accompanied by an alternation of host. Asexual cycle (schizogony) occurs inside RBCs of the vertebrate host and sexual cycle (sporogony) occurs within the invertebrate host. Schizogony produces merozoites, whereas sporogony produces sporozoites. Gametogony (formation of gametocytes) actually commences within erythrocytes and completes in various species of blood-sucking mosquitoes with production of sporozoites (these are infective to the vertebrate host).

Species Parasitising Man

1. *Plasmodium vivax* (Grassi and Feletti, 1890)
2. *Plasmodium falciparum* (Welch, 1897)
3. *Plasmodium malariae* (Laveran, 1881; Grassi and Feletti, 1890)
4. *Plasmodium ovale* (Stephens, 1922)

Primate Malarial Parasites that can Infect Man

1. Benign tertian type   *P. cynomolgi* (Mayer, 1907)
                                P. cynomolgi bostianelli (Garnham, 1959)
2. Ovale tertian type   *P. simium* (Fonseca, 1951)
3. Quartan type   *P. inui* (Halberstadter and Von Prowazek, 1907)
                                P. brasilianum (Gonder and von Berenberg-Gossler, 1908)
                                P. shortii (Bray, 1963)
4. Quotidian type   *P. knowlesi* (Sinton and Mulligan, 1932), has been used to develop antimalarial vaccine

Animal malarial parasites: Large number of species parasitise monkeys, birds, rodents, bats and cold-blooded animals like lizards. Anopheline mosquitoes transmit malarial parasites of man and monkeys while avian parasites are transmitted by culicine mosquitoes.

Evolution of Knowledge Regarding Malarial Parasites (MP)

Year	Discovery/remarks
1753	Disease named malaria
	Treatment of malaria came first, much before the malarial parasite was identified
1847	Muckel ⎫
	⎬ disovered presence of pigment in organs in malarial infections.
1849	Virchow ⎭
1880	Laveran discovered MP in unstained blood preparations.
1883	Machafava employed methylene blue to stain MP.
1885	Golgi established erythrocytic schizogony of quartan MP.
1886	Golgi demonstrated erythrocytic schigony of benign tertian MP.
1891	Romanowsky introduced staining method for MP.
1897	Ross in India (Secunderabad) found oocysts in the gastric wall of an anopheline mosquito which had earlier fed on a malaria patient

1898	Ross in Calcutta described the mosquito cycle with avain MP. Bignami et al., showed the same with human MP.
1900	Patrick Manson proved beyond doubt the theory of mosquito transmission
1934	Tissue phase of MP showed in avian malaria.
1948	Shortt and others worked out the pre-erythrocytic schizogony of MP in hepatic parenchymal cells (first with cynomolgi and then with vivax malaria)
1949	Shortt and others explained pre-erythrocytic schizogony of *P. falciparium.*
1954	Garnham and associates discovered the pre-erythrocytic schizogony of *P. ovale.*

HUMAN MALARIAL PARASITES

(Plasmodium—vivax/lfalciparum/malariae/ovale)

Geographical distribution: All nations falling between 40° S and 60° N. The tropical zone shows the endemic infections. *P. malariae* is a subtropical parasite while *P. vivax* prevails in the temperate climates. *P. ovale* has been chiefly reported from East Africa, West Africa (especially Nigeria), and Philippines.

Habitat: After been through the phase in hepatic parenchymal cells, the cells then reside within the RBCs and are carried by the circulating blood to various organs.

Life cycle: MP needs two different hosts
1. **In man:** The parasites in the liver cells and RBCs multiply asexually (schizogony). Man, therefore, represents the intermediate host of the malarial parasite.
2. **In female anopheline mosquitoe:** The sexual forms male and female gametocytes develop in the human host. The mosquito sucks them up where they are transformed into sporozoites which are infective to humans. On account of occurrence of sexual reproduction in the mosquito, it is the definitive host of the malarial parasite.

HUMAN CYCLE

Mosquito introduces sporozoites via the bite. It later undergoes through the undermentioned stages.
   A. **Pre-erythrocytic schizogony:** Sporozoites do not directly enter the RBCs to commence erythrocytic schizogony but undergo developmental phase in other human tissues. This phase is designated as pre-erythrocytic schizogony and consists of only a single generation of pre-erythrocytic schizont. This cycle lasts for about 8 days in *P. vivax, 6* days in *P. falciparum* and 9 days in *P. ovale.* This pre-erythrocytic schizogony occurs within hepatic parenchymal cells. The liberated merozoites are called cryptozoites. The larger (macro-merozoites) ones re-enter liver cells but the smaller (micro-merozoites) enter the blood stream. [Sporozoites are minute thread-like curved organisms with tapering ends. Measuring 9–12 µ in length with a central elongated nucleus while the cytoplasm reveals no pigment as seen with a light microscope]. No pathological changes or any symptoms appear while the parasite multiplies within hepatocytes. During this phase there is no parasitaemia.
   B. **Erythrocytic schizogony:** Parasite lives within the red blood cells and passes through the stages of trophozoite, schizont and merozoite. These asexual

forms of parasites can be demonstrated in thick/thin smears of the peripheral blood about 3–4 days after the completion of pre-erythrocytic schizogony i.e. roughly 12 days in *P. vivax* and 9 days in *P. falciparum*, after exposure. Each erythrocytic schizogony cycle lasts for 48 to 72 hours in *P. vivax/ovale*, it is 48 hours in *P. falciparum*, while in *P. malariae* it is 72 hours. The symptoms of hyperpyrexia occur during the erythrocytic phase. This cycle may last for considerable time, but in due course of time the infection tends to die out either due to exhaustion of the asexual reproductive capacity or due to spontaneous killing of the parasites.

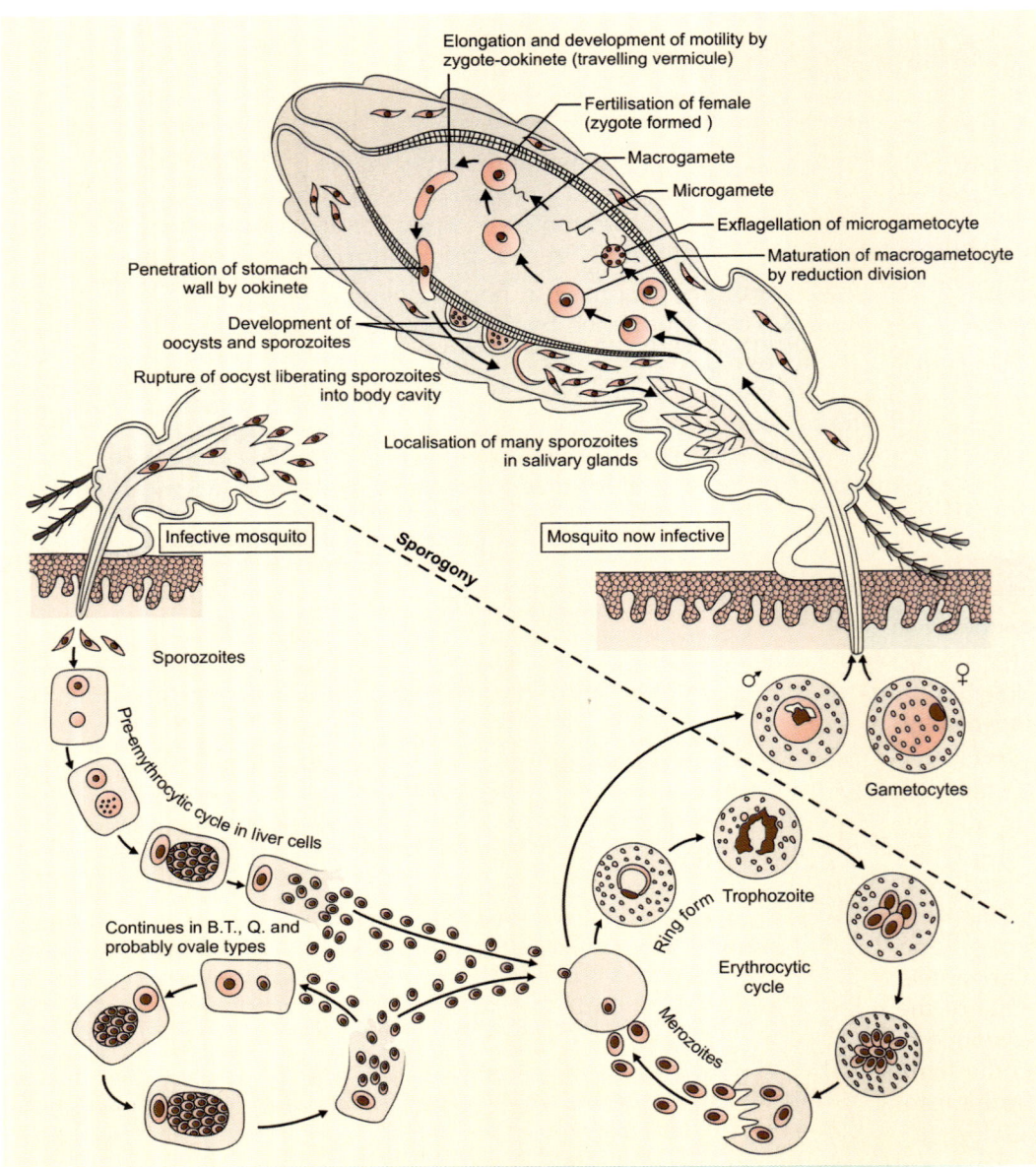

Fig. 4.1: Life cycle of malarial parasites

C. **Gametogony:** Having undergone erythrocytic schizogony for sometime (varies with different species), some of the merozoites, instead of developing into trophozoites and schizonts, give rise to gametocytes which develop in the RBCs of the capillaries of internal organs (e.g. spleen and bone marrow). Peripheral blood reveals only the mature gametocytes. Maturation time is 96 hours or 4 days. No febrile reaction occurs in the host during gametogony. A person who harbors the gametocytes is referred to as a carrier.

D. **Exo-erythrocytic schizogony:** After parasitaemia occurs the initial tissue phase (pre-erythrocytic phase) disappears completely in *P. falciparum,* whereas in *P. vivax/ovale/malariae* it carries on in the form of a local hepatic cycle. This phase is designated as exo-erythrocytic schizogony. The exo-erythrocytic forms never originate from asexual parasites of erythrocytic schizogony and are now thought to be responsible for relapses of vivax, ovale and quartan malaria. In the absence of fresh infection this forms the source of asexual parasites. The micro and macro-merozoites liberated from the exoerythrocytic schizogony are together called phanerozoites.

It can be summarized that there are two phases of development within the human host

  I. In liver (tissue or exo-erythrocytic phase) (no pigment)
    (a) Pre-erythrocytic (primary exo-erythrocytic) schizogony
      No symptoms, signs or any pathological destruction.
    (b) Exo-erythrocytic (secondary exo-erythrocytic) schizogony. Responsible for relapse.

  II. In RBCs (erythrocytic phase) (pigmentation seen)
    (a) Erythrocytic schizogony—causes symptoms
    (b) Gametogony—infects mosquito

MOSQUITO CYCLE

(Sexual Cycle)

Female anopheles sucks up gametocyte containing blood from an infected host. Both, sexual and asexual forms are ingested but only the mature sexual forms develop and the rest die. At least 12 gametocytes per cubic millimetre of blood are thought essential to be able to infect the mosquito (female gametocytes should be more than the male gametocytes).

In the gut, from one microgametocyte, 5 to 8 filamentous (thin-thread-like) micro-gametes are formed. From one macrogametocyte only one macrogamete is evolved, maturation involves condensation of nucleus and extrusion of polar bodies. The *P. falciparum* crescents get rounded, rest of the process is common with other species. Once ready, chemotactically, the microgametes are attracted towards the macrogametes.

One of the male gametes attaches to the periphery of the female gamete at the site of a small protrusion and penetrates inside the body. Fusion occurs between the male and the female pronuclei and zygote is formed. The zygote is formed in 20 minutes to 120 minutes after the blood meal. In the next 24 hours, the zygote lengthens into an ookinete.

Ookinete comes to lie in contact with the peritrophic membrane. Having crossed this barrier they push aside the brush border of the mucosal cell and their anterior end comes in close contact to the host cell membrane. By secretion of a proteolytic substance the cell membrane is lysed and it enters the cell to ultimately rest against the external border of the cell basement membrane, where it develops into an oocyst.

Oocysts are spherical (6–12 µ in diameter) and surrounded by a structureless capsule. They contain a single vesicular nucleus and the pigment granules of the macrogamete. As it matures it enlarges up to 60 µ in diameter and divides meiotically and mitotically to form a large number of haploid sporozoites (hundreds to thousands). Number of oocysts in the stomach wall may vary from a few to over a hundred. Around the tenth day of infection the oocyst ruptures, releasing sporozoites in the body cavity (haemocele) of the mosquito. These sporozoites are then distributed through the circulating fluid into various organs and tissues of the mosquito excepting the ovaries. These sporozoites have a special predilection for the salivary glands and attain maximum concentration in its ducts. At this stage the mosquito becomes infective and a single bite does the job.

Different species of the malarial parasites can develop in the same mosquito, such a mosquito can transmit mixed infection commonest being *P. vivax* and *P. falciparum*.

MORPHOLOGY OF MALARIAL PARASITES (STAINED BY LEISHMAN OR GIEMSA)

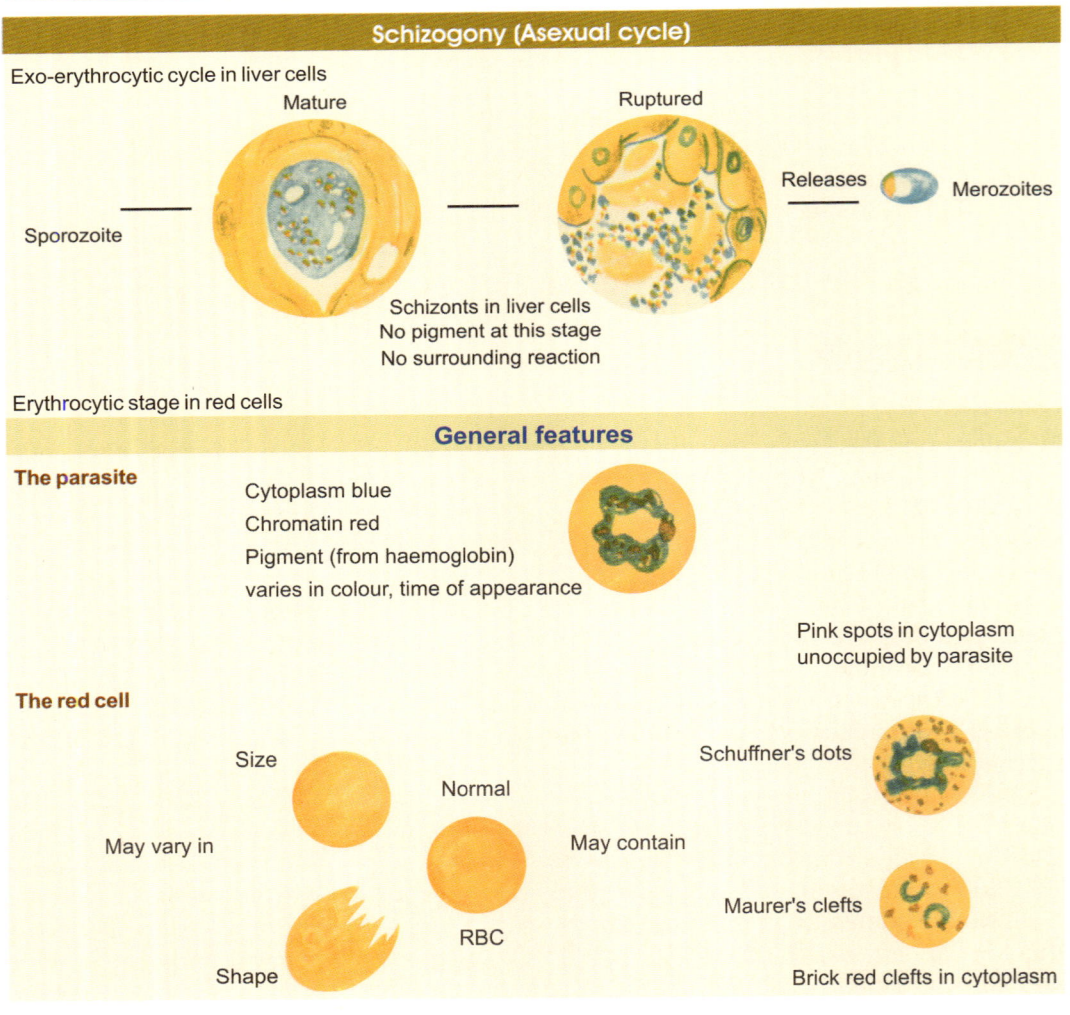

	P. vivax	P. malariae	P. falciparum	P. ovale
Size	Enlarged	Not enlarged	Not enlarged	Slightly enlarged
Colour	Pale	Normal	Normal	Pale
Shape	Round	Round	Round	Oval
			May be crenated	May be fimbriated
Schuffner's dots	Present	None	None	Conspicuous
Maurer's clefts	None	None	May be present	None

Stages in thin films

P. vivax   P. malariae   P. falciparum   P. ovale

RING FORMS (EARLY TROPHOZOITES)

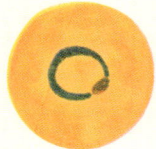 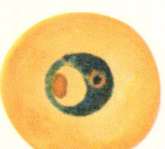 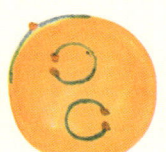 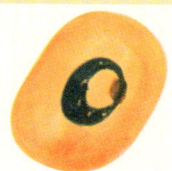

Size	1/3 Red cell	Up to 1/3	1/5 red cell	1/3 red cell
Shape	Delicate ring	Compact ring	Very delicate ring	Dense ring

 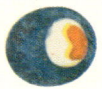 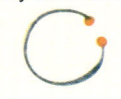

Chromatin	Fine dot Sometimes two	One mass often inside ring	Fine dots Frequently two	Dense, well-defined mass
Accole forms	Sometimes	None	Frequent	None
Pigment	None at this stage	May be present	None at this stage	None at this stage

DEVELOPING TROPHOZOITES

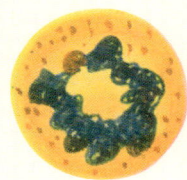 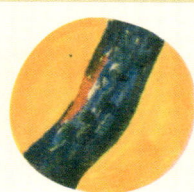  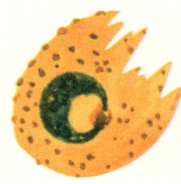

(Rarely seen in peripheral blood)

Size	Large	Small	Small	Small
Shape	Very irregular	Compact, often band forms	Compact	Compact
Vacuole	Prominent	Inconspicuous	Inconspicuous	Inconspicuous
Chromatin	Dots or threads	Dots or thread	Dots or thread	Large irregular clumps
Pigment				
Texture	Fine	Coarse	Coarse	Coarse
Colour	Yellow brown	Dark brown	Black	Dark yellow brown
Quantity	Medium	Abundant	Medium	Medium
Distribution	Scattered fine particles	Scattered clumps and rods	Aggregated in two clumps	Scattered coarse particles

Contd.

Stages in thin films *(Contd.)*

P. vivax	P. malariae	P. falciparum	P. ovale

IMMATURE SCHIZONTS

Rarely seen in peripheral blood

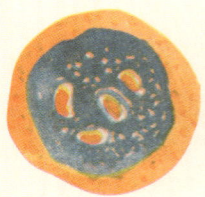 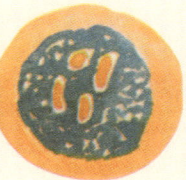 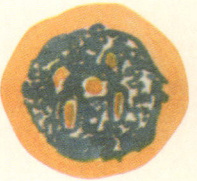 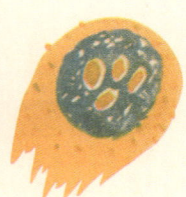

	P. vivax	P. malariae	P. falciparum	P. ovale
Size	Almost fills red cell	Almost fills red cell	Almost fills red cell	Almost fills red cell
Shape	Somewhat amoeboid	Compact	Compact	Compact
Chromatin	Numerous irregular masses	Few irregular masses	Numerous irregular masses	Few irregular masses
Pigment	Scattered	Scattered	Scattered	Scattered

MATURE SCHIZONTS

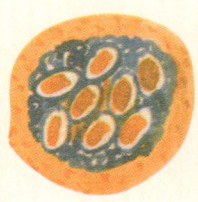 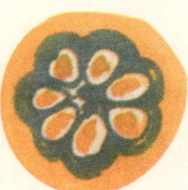 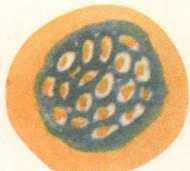 

Rarely seen in peripheral blood

	P. vivax	P. malariae	P. falciparum	P. ovale
Size	Fills red cell	Nearly fills red cell	Nearly fills red cell	Fills of red cell
Shape	Segmented	Segmented daisy head-like	Segmented	Segmented
Chromatin				
Range	14–24	6–12	8–32	6–12
Mean	16	8	24	8
Size	Medium	Large	Small	Large
Pigment	Aggregated in centre (yellow brown)	Aggregated in centre (dark brown)	Aggregated in centre (black)	Aggregated in centre (dark yellow brown)

Contd.

Stages in thin films *(Contd.)*

MICROGAMETOCYTES

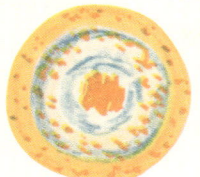 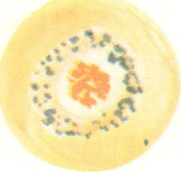 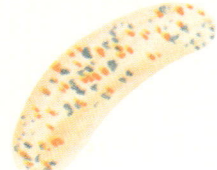 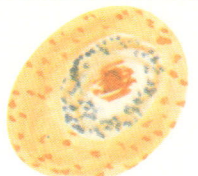

Time of appearance	3–5 days	7–14 days	7–12 days	12–14 days
Number in blood stream	Many	Scanty	Many	Scanty
Size	Fills enlarged red cells	Smaller than red cell	Larger than red cell	Size of red cell
Shape	Round or oval compact	Round compact	Kidney shaped bluntly round ends	Round compact
Cytoplasm	Pale blue	Pale blue	Reddish blue	Pale blue
Chromatin	Fibrils in skin with surrounding unstained area	As for *P. vivax*	Fine granules scattered throughout	As for *P. vivax*
Pigment	Abundant brown granules throughout	As for *P. vivax*	Dark granules throughout	As for *P. vivax*

MACROGAMETOCYTES

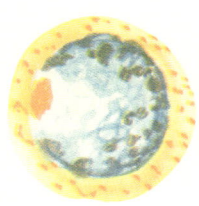 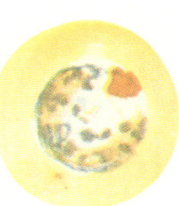 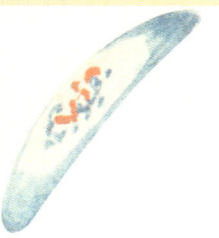 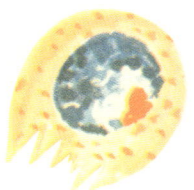

Time of appearance	3–5 days	7–14 days	7–12 days	12–14 days
Number in blood stream	Many	Scanty	Many	Scanty
Size	Fills enlarged red cell	Smaller than red cell	Larger than red cell	Size of red cell
Shape	Round or oval compact	Round compact	Crescentic-sharply rounded or pointed ends	Round compact
Cytoplasm	Dark blue	Dark blue	Dark blue	Dark blue
Chromatin	Compact peripheral mass	As for *P. vivax*	Compact masses near centre	As for *P. vivax*
Pigment	Small masses round periphery	As for *P. vivax*	Black granules round nucleus	As for *P. vivax*

MORPHOLOGY IN STAINED THICK FILMS

GENERAL

Parasites not flattened so are smaller than in thin film

Red cells haemolysed in processing so no guide to: Size | Shape | Colour } of red blood cell

Schüffner's dots indefinite   No Maurer's clefts

PARTICULAR

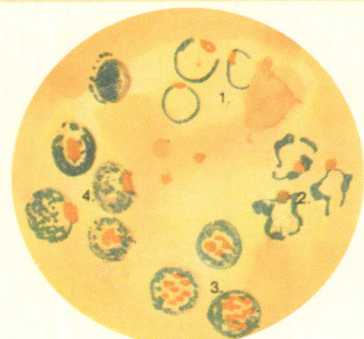

P. vivax

1. Ring forms, small, fine rings often broken
2. Trophozoites, markedly irregular cytoplasm
3. Schizonts, many (average 16) small merozoites
4. Gametocytes compact parasites with features of ♂ and ♀ as described
5. White blood cell

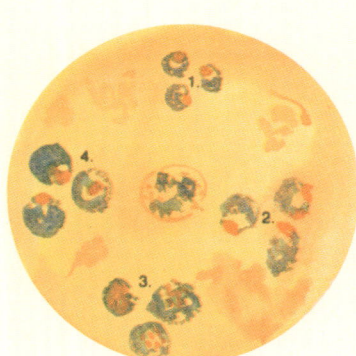

P. malariae
P. ovale } Almost identical but Schuffner's dots may be visible in later

1. Ring forms. Compact rings
2. Trophozoites. Solid regular cytoplasm
3. Schizonts. Few (average 8) large merozoites
4. Gametocytes. Very difficult to distinguish from *P. vivax*
5. White blood cell

P. falciparum

1. Ring forms very small, fine rings usually unbroken

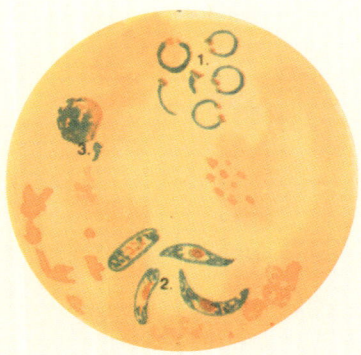

Trophozoites
Schizonts } Not seen in peripheral blood usually

2. Gametocytes, characteristic crescentic ♂ and ♀ forms
3. White blood cell

Species identification in the mosquito—pigment in oocysts				
Oocysts	P. vivax	P. malariae	P. falciparum	P. ovale
Length of cycle in days	9	15–21	10	15
Size in μ	10–46	5–44	8–60	9–37
Pigment Colour	Greenish brown	Dark brown or nearly black	Blackish	Dark brown or nearly black
Texture	Fine	Medium coarse	Very coarse	Medium coarse
Number of grains	50–100	30	10–20	50–60
Pattern				

Pattern — Days

Days	P. vivax	P. malariae	P. falciparum	P. ovale
3	None	Distributed, some clumping		
4				
5	Typical Prince of Wales feather design		Concentrated at periphery in double row often	Concentrated at periphery in semi-circles or dotted lines
6				
7				
8	Obscured by nuclei	Increased clumping	Mainly obscured	Most clearly defined, dotted lines often crossed
9				
10				
After 10		If visible, clumped at periphery	Seldom visible	Mainly obscured

Recapitulation of distinctive features	Prince of Wales feather design	Distributed then clumped	Peripheral in rows	Semicircular or crossed line design

Comparison of course of natural infection of *P. vivax* and *P. falciparum* in man		
Stage	*P. vivax*	*P. falciparum*
Pre-erythrocytic schizogony	Consists of a single cycle, lasts 8 days. Number of merozoites produced by each schizont = 12,000 approximately.	Consists of a single cycle, lasts 6 days. Each schizont produces about 40,000 merozoites.
Erythrocytic schizogony	Each cycle lasts 48 hours In thick smears the parasites appear by 12th day. First temperature peak by 16th day of infection Primary attack lasts 3 to 4 weeks.	Each cycle lasts for 36 to 48 hours In thick smears the parasites appear by 10th day. First fever peak occurs by 12th day. Primary attack lasts 10 to 14 days.
Gemetogony	Gametocytes appear in peripheral blood on 16th day of infection (1st day of fever: 4 days after the appearance of asexual forms in peripheral blood).	Gametocytes in peripheral blood seen on 21st day of infection (after 9 days of fever: about 10 days after appearance of asexual forms in peripheral blood).
Exo-erythrocytic schizogony	Present, can continue for up to 3 years. Relapses often occur.	Absent. Relapses do not occur.
A single infection	Can last up to 3 years.	Lasts up to a month to a maximum of one year.

Appearance of parasites: Microscopic density of about 10 parasites per cubic millimeter of blood.

Fever peak: Pyogenic density (fever threshold) About 50 parasites per cubic millimeter of blood are necessary for pyrexia peak.

Cultivation: Cultivation of malarial parasites has not been fully successful. Attempts are being made to cultivate them in human erythrocytes.

Animal inoculation: Human malarial parasites can be transferred to several primate species and vice versa.

Immunology: Immunity here implies tolerance to infection (cessation of symptoms in spite of existing parasitaemia) and this occurs as a result of active immunity (both CMI and humoral). The RE system cells (especially in liver and spleen) actively phagocytose the malarial parasites and therefore keep them at subclinical levels. So, it has been suggested that the immunity in malaria depends upon a persistent latent infection—designated as—infection immunity or premunition. It has also been shown that immunity in malaria may be complete and may on occasions persist for some time, even after elimination of parasites/parasitaemia.

It is now clear that plasmodial antigens derived from asexual erythrocytic phases of the parasite evoke production of specific antibodies, both protective and precipitating, that are present in the IgG and IgM fractions of gamma globulins. The antibodies bind to the parasites and make them more acceptable to macrophages. They have no effect on sporozoites, therefore, new infection is not prevented.

The CMI-humoral defence mechanisms are effective against asexual erythrocytic parasites only (mature schizonts and free merozoites). The gametocytes and exo-erythrocytic forms are free from the defence mechanisms' action. The merozoites released from the exo-erythrocytic source serve to infect the RBCs and may bring about a clinical attack of malaria, in the absence of re-infection. As long as immunity presists, the merozoites released by the liver are immediately destroyed and therefore, cannot invade RBCs; however, those that re-enter hepatocytes are not affected. Only when this immunity mechanism fails do the merozoites escaping from hepatic-schizonts succeed in infecting the RBCs and thereby produce a relapse.

The malarial antigens: These are soluble antigens present in sera of infected individuals and these can be detected by various immunological techniques. They can also be extracted from infected RBCs. *P. falciparum* antigens have been classified on the basis of their heat stability/lability.

The malarial antibodies: The protective malarial antibodies are IgG type but the precipitating antibodies exist in IgG and IgM forms. Antibodies can cross the placental barrier and appear in the sera of infants born to immune mothers. The protective antibodies persist for months or years and diminish in the absence of reinfection. Persistence of the immunity hence depends upon frequency of antigenic stimulation.

Malarial Infection: Immunological Consequences

1. **Protective immunity:** Neonates derive passive (congenital) immunity for up to 6 months from immune mothers via transplacental access or by passage of IgG antibodies via milk. In the older age groups the toxic products of the parasite are neutralised—this is called antitoxic immunity.
2. **Associated pathological states:**
   (a) Tropical splenomegaly syndrome (TSS)
   (b) Malarial nephrosis, especially in *P. malariae* infection
   (c) Auto-immune haemolytic anaemia seen in pregnant women with *P. falciparum* infection
   (d) Aberrant immunological responses
3. **Immunosuppression:** There is an immunosuppressive effect towards other antigenic stimuli, this explains the less frequent occurrence of autoimmune diseases in malarial infections (for instance tetanus toxoid fails to evoke an antitoxin response in children with malarial parasitaemia).

It is now increasingly asserted that Burkitt's lymphoma occurs due to synergic action between plasmodial and oncogenic viral infections. Perhaps the malarial infection is by immunosuppressive effect allows virus proliferation or interferes with immune reactions to neoplastic. cells.

Reservoirs of infection: Human malarial parasites are not harbored by other lower vertebrates. Primates/apes may sometimes act as reservoirs.

Mode of transmission: Female anopheline mosquitoes serve as intermediaries in transmitting infection to man. The infection is spread by bite/inoculation. The mosquito's proboscis pierces the skin and the salivary secretion (containing sporozoites) is injected into the bite wound.

Other Methods of Transmission

A. Experimentally injecting emulsion of salivary glands containing sporozoites can induce infection—called sporozoite-induced malaria.

B. Infusion/injection of blood containing asexual forms of erythrocytic schizogony can produce malaria—called trohozoite-induced malaria.
   (i) *Transfusion malaria:* Infected blood transfusion produces malaria in recipient.
   (ii) *Congenital malaria:* Defective placenta can help spread of malarial infection from mother to foetus. (A physiologically and structurally normal placenta presents an effective barrier.)
   (iii) *Malaria in drug addicts*—through the use of same syringe, when one of them is infected.

THERAPEUTIC MALARIA (Not used any more)

To produce hyperpyrexia for treating cases of neurosyphilis (general paralysis of insane). The methods employed were:
   (i) By inoculating blood of an infected donor
   (ii) By letting laboratory-bred infected mosquitoes to bite the patient
   (iii) By injecting emulsion of salivary glands containing sporozoites.
   Sporozoite and Trophozoite induced malaria are different in the following respects.

	Sporozoite-induced malaria	*Trophozoite-induced malaria*
Pre-erythrocytic schizogony	Present	Absent
Incubation period	Long	Short
Exo-erythrocytic schizogony	May be present	Absent
Relapses	May occur	Do not occur
Schizonticidal medicines	No radical cure, because of presence of exo-erythrocytic forms	Can be radically cured, because of absence of exo-erythrocytic forms

Spread of malaria: Factors responsible
   (i) Presence of a gametocyte carrier
   (ii) A suitable Anopheles vector to spread and
   (iii) A susceptible person

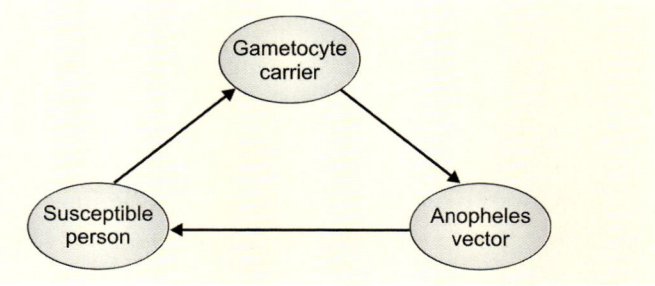

This cycle needs to be broken at any stage to prevent spread of malaria.

PATHOLOGY

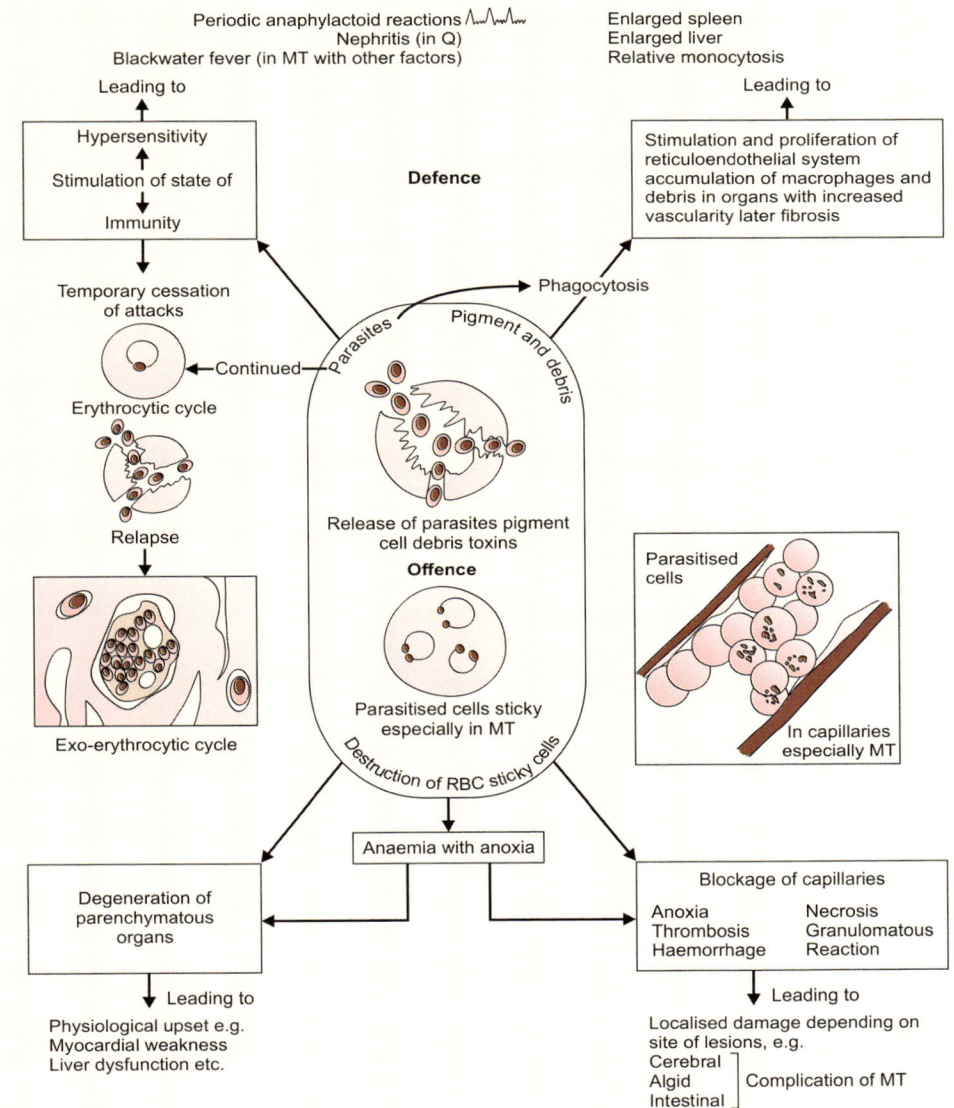

Periodic anaphylactoid reactions /\w/w/w
Nephritis (in Q)
Blackwater fever (in MT with other factors)

Leading to

Enlarged spleen
Enlarged liver
Relative monocytosis

Leading to

Hypersensitivity

Stimulation of state of

Immunity

Defence

Stimulation and proliferation of
reticuloendothelial system
accumulation of macrophages and
debris in organs with increased
vascularity later fibrosis

Temporary cessation
of attacks

Phagocytosis

Continued

Parasites

Pigment and debris

Erythrocytic cycle

Relapse

Release of parasites pigment
cell debris toxins

Offence

Parasitised
cells

Exo-erythrocytic cycle

Parasitised cells sticky
especially in MT

Destruction of RBC sticky cells

In capillaries
especially MT

Anaemia with anoxia

Degeneration of
parenchymatous
organs

Blockage of capillaries

Anoxia   Necrosis
Thrombosis   Granulomatous
Haemorrhage   Reaction

Leading to

Physiological upset e.g.
Myocardial weakness
Liver dysfunction etc.

Leading to

Localised damage depending on
site of lesions, e.g.
Cerebral ⎤
Algid   ⎟ Complication of MT
Intestinal ⎦

Incubation Period

In *P. vivax*, *P. ovale* and *P. falciparum* incubation period is 10–14 days. In *P. malariae* it
is about 18 days to 6 weeks. Clinical features: Main features are fever peaks followed
by anaemia and splenomegaly.

1. **Febrile paroxysms**
   P. vivax: Vivax malaria (benign tertian malaria)—has a 48-hour cycle.
   P. falciparum: Falciparum malaria (malignant tertian malaria, causes pernicious
   malaria and Blackwater fever. Also has 48-hour cycle.
   P. malariae: Quartan malaria (Malariae malaria). Has a 72-hour cycle.
   P. ovale: Ovale malaria.

The febrile paroxysm shows a succession of 3 stages:
(a) Cold stage—lasting 20 minutes to an hour
(b) Hot stage—lasting 1 to 4 hours and
(c) Sweating stage—lasting 2 to 3 hours.
Total duration varies from 6 to 10 hours
The fever proxysm coincides with erythrocytic schizogony of the malarial parasite
(a) With a 48-hour cycle fever recurs every third day, tertian malaria and
(b) With a 72-hour cycle fever recurs every fourth day, quartan fever
(c) Fever recurring at 24-hour periodicity, quotidian malaria has been observed in infections with *P vivax* and *P. malariae*. This is on account of maturation of two generations of tertian parasites on two successive days (tertiana duplex) or three generations of quartan parasites on three successive days (quartana triplex). When two generations of quartan parasites occurs on two successive days followed by an afebrile day (quartana duplex)
In *vivax malaria* (benign tertian malaria) the typical intermittent periodic fever establishes only in later stages, initially there may be continuous/quotidian/remittant fever. Initially two broods of parasites undergo schizogony on alternate days, thereby releasing two generations of merozoites with a febrile reaction each day. Later one brood drops out and then the febrile curve becomes tertian.
In *quartan malaria* the intermittent fever commences from the begining. *In falciparum malaria* the febrile paroxysm may not show the three successive cold, hot and sweating stages. The fever in these cases may be continuous or remittent instead of being intermittent. This occurs due to the fact that several generations of the parasite are multiplying at different intervals. After the first paroxysm there is no remission of fever and temperature may remain constant or may show a drop (remittent) towards the latter part and then merge on to the next paroxysm which comes on before the period of 48 hours has elapsed.

2. **Anaemia:** Occurs as a result of RBC's breakdown on account of their parasitisation.

3. **Splenomegaly:** Initially splenomegaly is mild or negligible but after some paroxysms and usually by the second week, palpable splenomegaly occurs.

PERNICIOUS MALARIA

Series of phenomena that occur during the course of an untreated *P. falciparum* infection (can be life-threatening) within 1 to 3 days is referred to as pernicious malaria.

Pathogenesis

There is diffuse capillary blockage leading to diminished effective circulation of blood (blockage of capillaries occurs due to agglutination of parasitised RBCs). Internal organs are involved—this is a special feature of *P. falciparum* where asexual parasites recede from peripheral circulation to the capillaries of internal organs for later stages of schizogony. Assisted by stickiness of infected erythrocytes (fibrin coated) and causing occlusion of capillaries. Stasis occurring as a result of vasoconstriction (sympathetic hyperactivity) is also thought to contribute to capillary obstruction. Pernicious manifestations usually occur when 5% more RBCs are parasitised. The peripheral smear shows heavy parasitaemia and schizonts as well as ring-forms are seen.

PATHOLOGY IN MALARIA

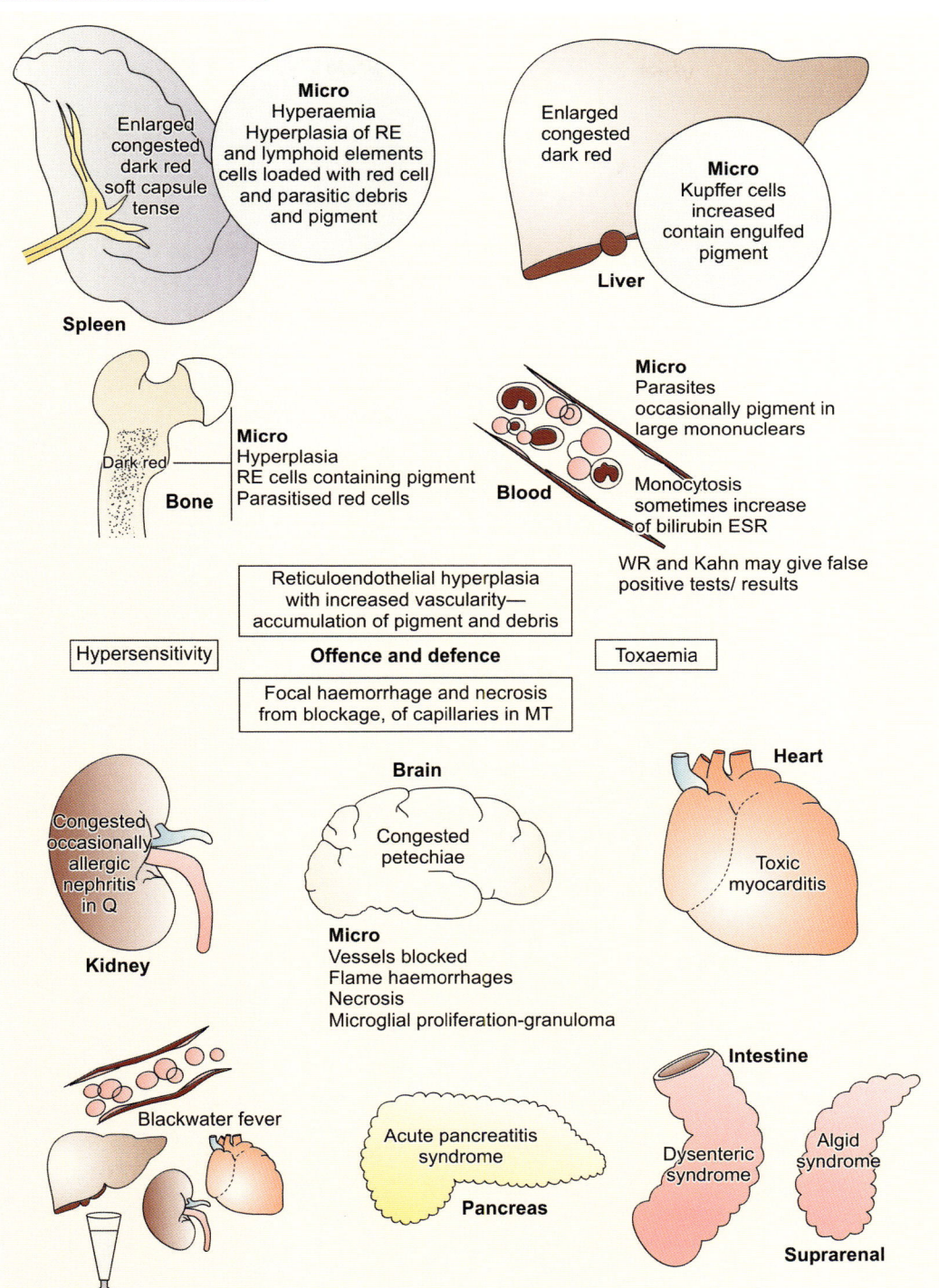

Spleen

Enlarged congested dark red soft capsule tense

Micro
Hyperaemia
Hyperplasia of RE and lymphoid elements cells loaded with red cell and parasitic debris and pigment

Liver

Enlarged congested dark red

Micro
Kupffer cells increased contain engulfed pigment

Bone

Dark red

Micro
Hyperplasia
RE cells containing pigment
Parasitised red cells

Blood

Micro
Parasites occasionally pigment in large mononuclears

Monocytosis sometimes increase of bilirubin ESR

WR and Kahn may give false positive tests/ results

Reticuloendothelial hyperplasia with increased vascularity— accumulation of pigment and debris

Hypersensitivity

Offence and defence

Toxaemia

Focal haemorrhage and necrosis from blockage, of capillaries in MT

Kidney

Congested occasionally allergic nephritis in Q

Brain

Congested petechiae

Micro
Vessels blocked
Flame haemorrhages
Necrosis
Microglial proliferation-granuloma

Heart

Toxic myocarditis

Blackwater fever

Acute pancreatitis syndrome

Pancreas

Intestine

Dysenteric syndrome

Algid syndrome

Suprarenal

Fig. 4.2: Acute phase

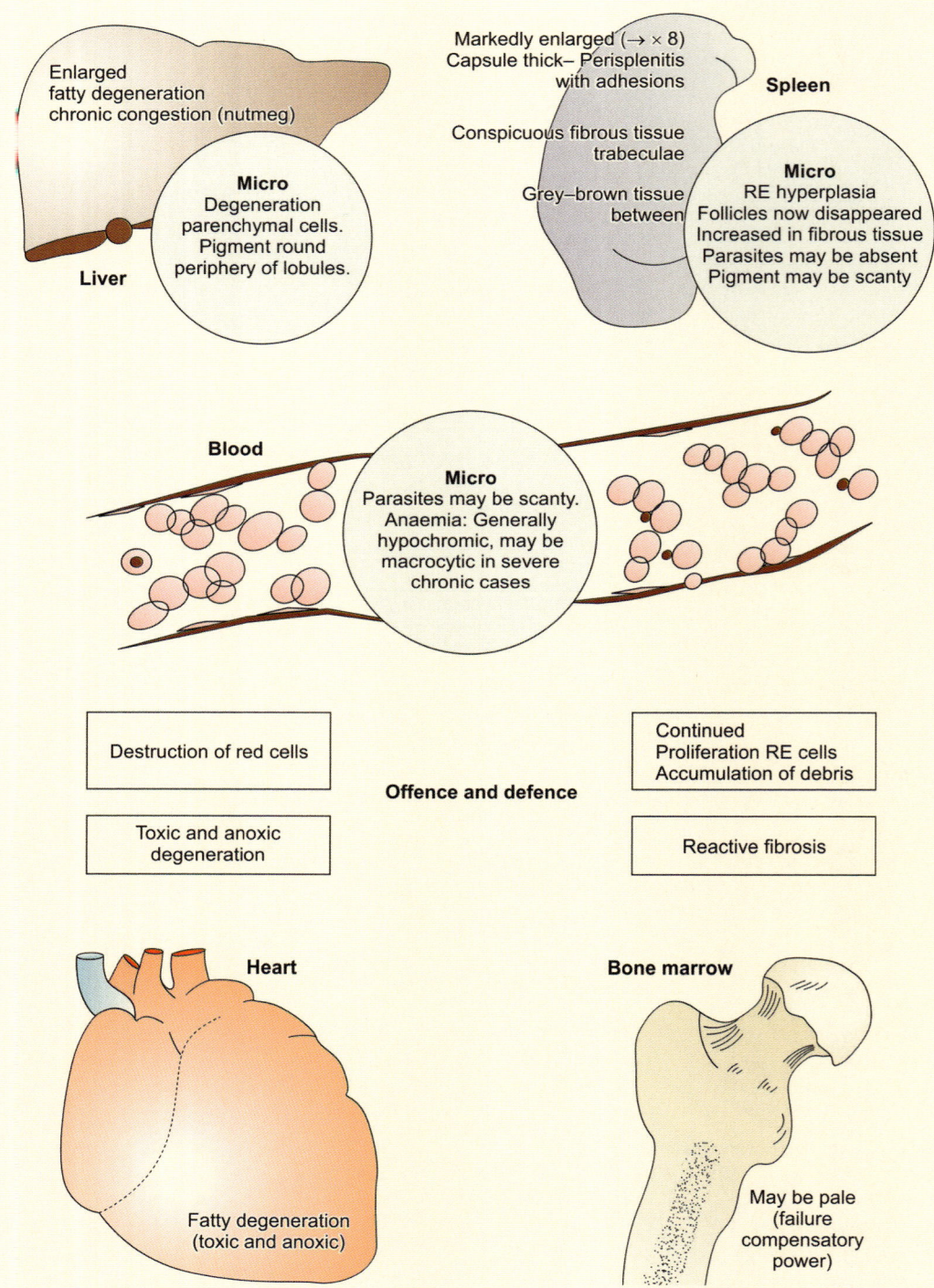

Liver
Enlarged
fatty degeneration
chronic congestion (nutmeg)

Micro
Degeneration
parenchymal cells.
Pigment round
periphery of lobules.

Spleen
Markedly enlarged (→ × 8)
Capsule thick– Perisplenitis
with adhesions

Conspicuous fibrous tissue
trabeculae

Grey–brown tissue
between

Micro
RE hyperplasia
Follicles now disappeared
Increased in fibrous tissue
Parasites may be absent
Pigment may be scanty

Blood

Micro
Parasites may be scanty.
Anaemia: Generally
hypochromic, may be
macrocytic in severe
chronic cases

Destruction of red cells

Offence and defence

Toxic and anoxic
degeneration

Continued
Proliferation RE cells
Accumulation of debris

Reactive fibrosis

Heart
Fatty degeneration
(toxic and anoxic)

Bone marrow
May be pale
(failure
compensatory
power)

Fig. 4.3: Chronic phase

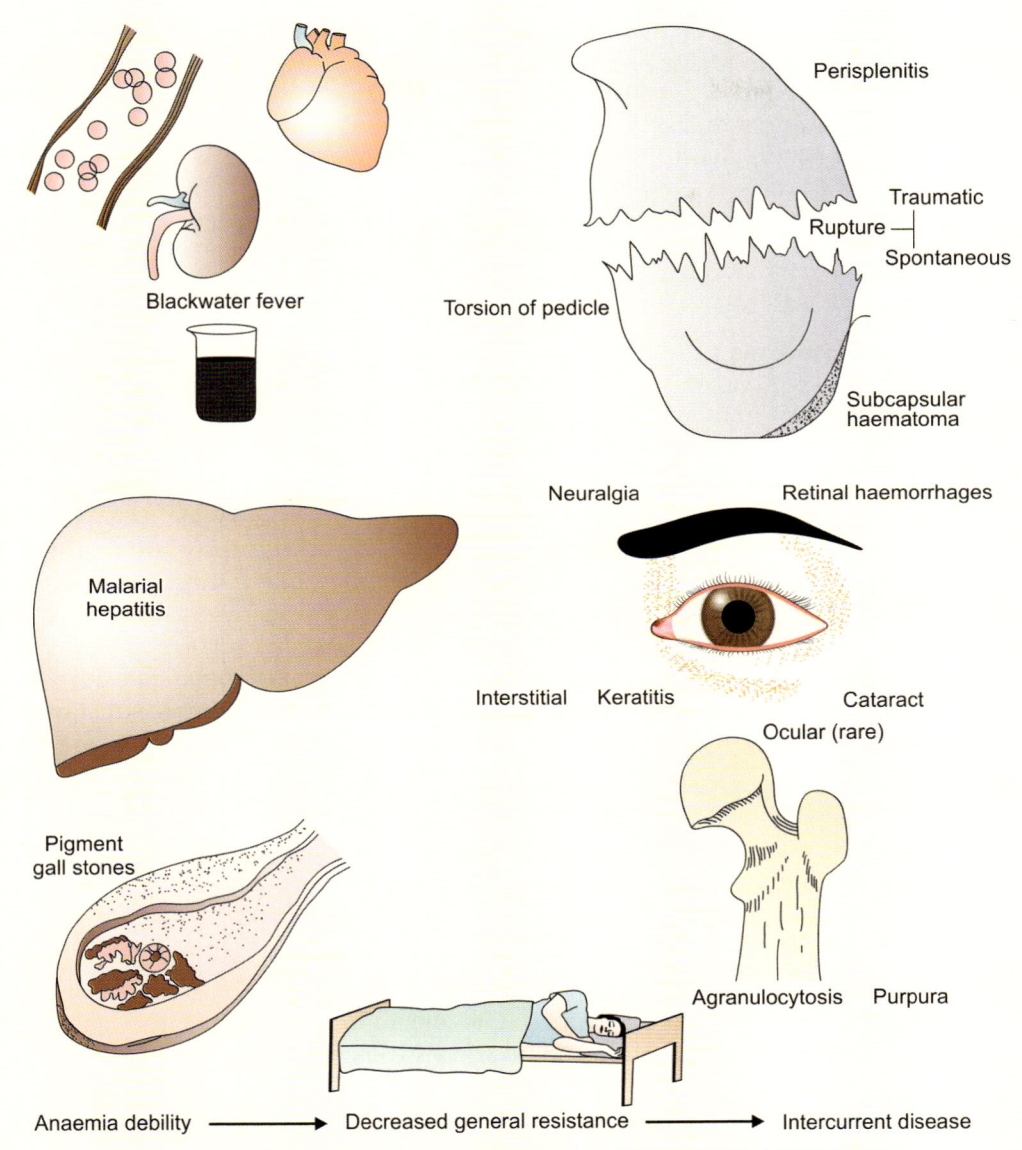

Perisplenitis

Traumatic

Rupture

Spontaneous

Blackwater fever

Torsion of pedicle

Subcapsular haematoma

Neuralgia

Retinal haemorrhages

Malarial hepatitis

Interstitial   Keratitis

Cataract

Ocular (rare)

Pigment gall stones

Agranulocytosis   Purpura

Anaemia debility ⟶ Decreased general resistance ⟶ Intercurrent disease

Fig. 4.4: Complications and sequelae

Significant Pathological Features

A. Organ pigmentation—slate grey or black discolouration. Malarial pigment is always found within the cells of RE system (pigment granules are physiologically inert).

B. RE system hyperplasia—the system proliferates to deal with plasmodia and their effete products, e.g. toxins, haematin, etc.

C. Parasitised RBCs filling the lumina of capillaries of internal organs (especially in *P. falciparum* malaria)

D. Vascular changes—congestion, engorgement and dilatation of sinusoidal vessels. Perivascular haemorrhages resulting from the damaged capillary endothelium occur in falciparum malaria.

E. Hypoxia occurring as a result of capillary obstruction leads to degenerative changes of parenchymal cells of internal organs (in falciparum malaria)

F. Fibrosis that occurs due to reparation of local damage is never so extensive as to cause organ-fibrosis.

G. Immunosuppression observed with malaria can bring secondary bacterial infections.

Specific Organ Changes

Spleen: Spleen functions as a filter for the removal of parasites and the products of their schizogony. All stages of development of the parasites are found in abundance in the spleen (more so in falciparum malaria).

The parasites and haematin pigment are actively phagocytosed by splenic macrophages.

Grossly: Spleen is *enlarged* (moderately). Splenomegaly as big as seen in kala-azar is never observed. Spleen turns *slate grey or black,* depending upon the amount of pigmentation. In acute cases the splenic capsule gets *thinned* but in chronic cases it gets *thickened* due to associated perisplenitis. The *consistency* of spleen *initially is soft* while in *chronic cases* it becomes *firm (ague cake consistency).* The cut surface appears as a homogeneous black area with scattered white fibrous bands (trabeculae). Occasionally one can detect haemorrhages in the subcapsular region and splenic substance in falciparum malaria (rarely spleen may rupture spontaneously).

Microscopically: Splenic sinusoids are congested. Significant amount of pigments, both haematin and haemosiderin are found scattered diffusely. The haematin pigment is present intracellularly within the macrophages which themselves are increased in number. The malpighian corpuscles (white pulp) are free from pigment and parasites. The parasites can be identified as blackish dots within RBCs in H and E stained sections. The reticulin fibrils may be increased in number.

Tropical splenomegaly syndrome (TSS): Seen in adults in hyperendemic malarial regions. Occurs due to abnormal immune response to plasmodial antigen (parasitaemia is usually absent). Continuous malaria chemoprophylaxis helps in reducing the spleen size.

Liver

Grossly: Uniformly enlarged due to vascular congestion and reticuloendothelial cells' proliferation. Colour varies from dark chocolate-red to slate-grey or even black, and depends upon the stage of congestion and the amount of haematin pigment. The cut surface reveals dilated lobular veins and where the fatty change is restricted to the central zone of the lobule, it stands out as a yellowish area against the brownish red background.

Microscopically: The central veins of lobules and the sinusoidal capillaries are dilated and engorged with RBCs (many of the red cells are parasitised). The Kupffer cells are hyperplastic and filled with haematin (malarial pigment) and parasitised RBCs. The parenchymal hepatocytes lying in the central zone show fatty degeneration, atrophy and necrosis (centrilobular necrosis). This has been attributed to hypoxia resulting from interference to escape of hepatic venous blood. Parasites in various stages of development within the RBCs may be seen lying in the sinusoidal lumina or phago-cytosed within the Kupffer cells.

Brain: Brain shows hyperaemia and discolouration. Cut surface may show petechial haemorrhages. Microscopically capillaries are found filled with parasitised red cells. There are ring haemorrhages around some capillaries. These later develop into "malarial granulomas" obstructed capillaries with proliferating glial cells around them.

Algid Malaria: Pathology

Gastrointestinal tract: Mucous membranes show slate-gray pigmentation. Occasion-ally there may be punctiform haemorrhages but ulcerations are not seen. The intes-tinal contents may be watery or darkbrown with little mucous. Microscopically, the mucosal and submucosal capillaries are found engorged with parasitised RBCs, however, the capillaries of the muscle and serous coats contain very few parasites.

Peripheral blood vessels: Peripheral circulatory failure (vascular collapse) occurs second-arily to adrenal damage or may arise independently—this accounts for the fatality in these cases. Heart does not show any significant damage in these cases at autopsy.

Adrenal glands: One finds necrosis of zona fasciculata and haemorrhages with conges-tion of zona reticulata. Parasitised RBC's and pigmented phagocytes are found in the sinusoidal capillaries of the adrenal glands.

Septicaemic Malaria: Pathology

Heart: Macroscopically normal. Microscopically it reveals markedly congested blood vessels filled with parasitised RBCs. Fatty degeneration and necrosis of cardiac muscle are also found.

Lungs: Pneumonic symptom cases exhibit small areas of haemorrhages with patches of oedema and collapse. Microscopically, alveolar capillaries are found to be congested with parasitised RBCs. The alveoli show extravasated RBCs and pigmented monocytes.

Blood: Marked parasitaemia is the hallmark in this form with both schizogony and gametogony seen in the peripheral smear and also within the capillaries of internal organs. Severe parasitaemia leads to profound anaemia quickly.

CLINICAL PATHOLOGY

Haematological changes: Anaemia occurs as a result of red blood cell destruction during each cycle of schizogony (haemolytic anaemia). Degree of anaemia is maximum in *P. falciparum* as the parasitaemia is heavier and both young and mature RBCs are invaded. Anaemia is of normocytic hypochromic type. During the period of rising temperature there is leucocytosis which returns to normal as temperature becomes normal. With recurring paroxysms there is leucopenia with neutropenia. Monocy-tosis occurs and both, the monocytes and neutrophils, may show ingested haematin pigment.

Biochemical Changes

(a) There is hypoalbuminaemia perhaps due to liver dysfunction. Globulins rise leading to a reversal in A/G ratio.

(b) Cholesterol rises with rigor but falls during a febrile period.

(c) Hyperglycaemia (raised blood sugar) is correlated to adrenal function. Hypoglycaemia is seen in falciparum malaria.

(d) The lysing red cells release potassium so there is hyperkalemia (raised serum potassium)

(e) ESR rises. Related to altered plasma proteins and increased stickiness of red blood cells.

(f) With increase in pyruvates and lactates there is fall of pH and loss of alkali reserve.

(g) Unconjugated or indirect bilirubin rises, as liver cannot cope with increased workload presented to it.

(h) Pathological haemoglobinemia and haemoglobinuria is unusual.

(i) Within the RBCs' there is raised sodium with proportional decrease in potassium.

Laboratory Diagnosis of Malaria

Malarial parasites in thin film of blood. Stained by Leishman and Giemsa

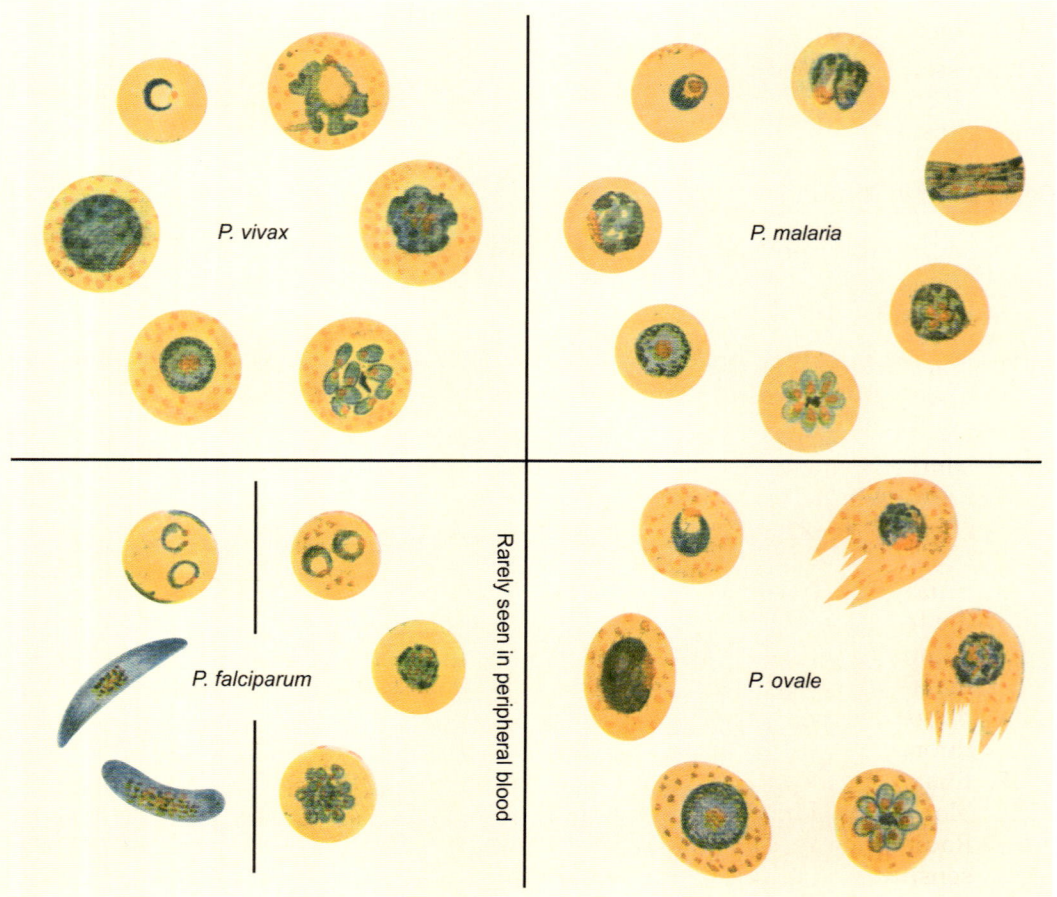

P. vivax

P. malaria

P. falciparum

Rarely seen in peripheral blood

P. ovale

Thick film of blood stained by field or giemsa
in thick or thin film of bone marrow

Concentration ⎫
Serological ⎬ Techniques academic rather than practical
Cultural ⎭

| Black water fever |

In addition to above

Spectroscopic examination of urine and faeces

Tests to exclude other causes of haemoglobinuria
(e.g. Donath-Landsteiner reaction for cold agglutinins)

The most important diagnostic tool is the microscopic examination of peripheral blood smear.

In most cases of symptomatic malaria (if no treatment has been given) a thin smear will usually reveal the parasite. However, both thin and thick smears may be taken. Attempt should be made to identify the species (difficult when only a few ring forms are seen).

Malarial parasites may not be seen when
(a) Smears are prepared after commencement of antimalarial therapy
(b) Blood films are made during afebrile periods
(c) Smears are made in the initial 2–3 days in primary infections

It is essential to remember (for diagnosing) that a malarial parasite must be inside a red cell and show a red coloured chromatin and a blue cytoplasm in Romanowsky stained smears.

Other Methods

1. **Cultural examination:** Not needed except in special circumstances when species identification is required.
2. **Observing pigment:** Presence in monocytes—signifies past or present malarial infection.
3. **Flocculation tests:** Nonspecific, imply hyperglobulinemia only.
4. **Serologic tests:** Irrelevant for acute infections but are used for studying immunologic aspects of populations living in highly endemic areas and for detecting latent malaria in blood donors.
5. **Complement fixation test:** It shows high positivity in children from hyperendemic areas (parasitaemia may or may not be positive) and also in parasitaemia positive adults.
6. **Immunofluorescence test (direct and indirect):** The fluorescent dye used in the test conjugates with the gamma globulin of the serum to be tested. If such a gamma globulin contains malarial antibody, it will adhere to the relevant malarial parasite and will be recognised as glistening particles under the fluorescent microscope. *Becton and Dickinson* (USA) have come out with the fluorescence test where parasite can be demonstrated alive in human blood.
7. **Elisa test:** It is the most specific test to detect malarial antigen in the peripheral blood. Elisa offers an alternative to microscopy because of its ease and speed. Radioimmuno assay techniques have been found to be much more specific and sensitive.

8. **Rapid antigen/antibody detection tests**. Species specific kits are available can detect one or a combination or all species in the same kit.

9. Species specific PCR/ nucleic acid amplification (very specific and sensitive) are available these days.

Treatment

1. **Primarily therapeutic:** (aiming at clinical cure). 4-aminoquinolines, e.g. chloroquine and amodiaquine (ideal), quinine (for drug resistant *P. falciparum*) and mepacrine (seldom used).

    These are potent schizonticidal drugs having effect on early erythrocytic phases of the parasite. For radical cure an 8-aminoquinoline, primaquine is used after the clinical cure. It acts on the exo-erythrocytic phases of parasites in the liver, therefore, it prevents relapses. It also acts on gametocytes but has minimal action on asexual blood parasites.

2. **Protective or prophylactic:** Proguanil (chlorguanide) pyrimethamine and trimethoprim combination (metakelfin). These are dihydrofolate reductase inhibitors and are mostly used to suppress clinical manifestations. These drugs can destroy pre-erythrocytic phase of the parasite in the liver and inactivate gametocytes, thereby preventing further development in mosquitoes. They also act on dividing schizonts.

    If the above mentioned drugs are not available or strains are resistant, one can use chloroquine or quinine. Cycloguanil, a metabolite of proguanil, may be used as a long-acting injectable prophylactic.

3. **Synergists (enhance the action of schizonticidal drugs):** Sulphonamides and sulfones (dapsone) are often used in conjunction with dihydrofolate reductase inhibitors.

    (Multiple drug regimens may be used in drug-resistant *P. falciparum* cases. G6PD deficiency should not be there in patients receiving primaquine)

ANTIMALARIALS

Class Summary

These agents inhibit growth by concentrating within acid vesicles of the parasite, increasing the internal pH of the organism. They also inhibit haemoglobin utilization and parasite metabolism.

Chloroquine Phosphate

Chloroquine phosphate is effective against *P. vivax*, *P. ovale*, *P. malariae*, and drug-sensitive *P. falciparum*. It can be used for prophylaxis or treatment. This is the prophylactic drug of choice for sensitive malaria.

Quinine

Quinine is used for malaria treatment only; it has no role in prophylaxis. It is used with a second agent in drug-resistant *P. falciparum*. For drug-resistant parasites, the second agent is doxycycline, tetracycline, pyrimethamine sulfadoxine, or clindamycin.

Quinidine Gluconate

Quinidine gluconate is indicated for severe or complicated malaria and is used in conjunction with doxycycline, tetracycline, or clindamycin. Quinidine gluconate can be administered IV and is the only parenterally available quinine derivative in the United States.

Doxycycline

Doxycycline is used for malaria prophylaxis or treatment. When it is administered for treatment of *P. falciparum* malaria, this drug must be used as part of combination therapy (e.g. typically with quinine or quinidine).

Tetracycline

Tetracycline may specifically impair the progeny of apicoplast genes, resulting in their abnormal cell division. Loss of apicoplast function in progeny of treated parasites leads to slow, but potent, antimalarial effect.

Clindamycin

Clindamycin is a part of combination therapy for drug-resistant malaria (e.g. typically with quinine or quinidine). It is a good second agent in pregnant patients.

Mefloquine

Mefloquine acts as a blood schizonticide. It may act by raising intravesicular pH within the parasite's acid vesicles. Mefloquine is structurally similar to quinine. It is used for the prophylaxis or treatment of drug-resistant malaria. It may cause adverse neuropsychiatric reactions and should not be prescribed for prophylaxis in patients with active or recent history of depression, generalized anxiety disorder, psychosis, or schizophrenia or other major psychiatric disorders.

Atovaquone and Proguanil

Atovaquone may inhibit metabolic enzymes, which in turn inhibits the growth of microorganisms.

Used for pediatric patients, this combination should be administered for uncomplicated *P. falciparum*; can also be used in combination with chloroquine.

This agent is approved in the United States for the prophylaxis and treatment of mild chloroquine-resistant malaria. It may be a good prophylactic option for patients who are visiting areas with chloroquine-resistant malaria and who cannot tolerate mefloquine. Each tab combines 250 mg of atovaquone and 100 mg of proguanil hydrochloride. The dosage for children is based on body weight; in children 40 kg (88 lb) or less, a lower-dose pediatric tablet (62.5 mg of atovaquone and 25 mg of proguanil hydrochloride) is available.

Primaquine

Primaquine is not used to treat the erythrocytic stage of malaria. Administer the drug for the hypnozoite stage of *P. vivax* and *P. ovale* to prevent relapse.

Artemether and lumefantrine

This drug combination is indicated for the treatment of acute, uncomplicated *P. falciparum* malaria. It contains a fixed ratio of 20 mg artemether and 120 mg lumefantrine (1:6 parts). Both components inhibit nucleic acid and protein synthesis. Artemether is rapidly metabolized into the active metabolite dihydroartemisinin (DHA), producing an endoperoxide moiety. Lumefantrine may form a complex with hemin, which inhibits the formation of beta hematin.

Artesunate

Artesunate, a form of artemisinin that can be used intravenously, is available from the CDC. It is not licensed for use in the United States but is available as part of an investigational new drug protocol.

Tafenoquine

Tafenoquine is an 8-aminoquinoline derivative. The 150 mg tablet (Krintafel) is indicated for the radical cure (prevention of relapse) of *P. vivax* malaria in patients aged 16 years or older who are receiving appropriate antimalarial therapy for acute *P. vivax* infection. Krintafel is administered as a single 300 mg dose coadministered on the first or second day of appropriate antimalarial therapy. The drug is active against all stages of the *P. vivax* life cycle, including hypnozoites.

Tafenoquine is also indicated for adults aged 18 years or older as prophylaxis when travelling to malarious areas. For this indication, the 100 mg tablet (Arakoda) is administered as a loading dose (before travelling to endemic area), a maintenance dose while in malarious area, and then a terminal prophylaxis dose in the week exiting the area.

Prophylaxis

Personal prophylaxis:
- (a) Protection against mosquito bites and
- (b) Systematic use of antimalaria] drugs as a chemoprophylactic measure (e.g. taking two tablets of chloroquine once every week). Other medications can also be used.

Community prophylaxis:
- (a) Prevention of carrier state by using drugs having gametocidal action (8-aminoquinoline).
- (b) Anti-mosquito measures. May be directed towards adult mosquitoes and their larvae

anti-adult:	insecticidal sprays
	DDT
	gammexane
anti-larval:	eliminating breeding places
	use of larvicides
	oil
	Paris-green
	DDT in oil

BLACKWATER FEVER

Acute haemolytic attacks in MT malaria; associated with taking of quinine; numerous theories as to mechanism

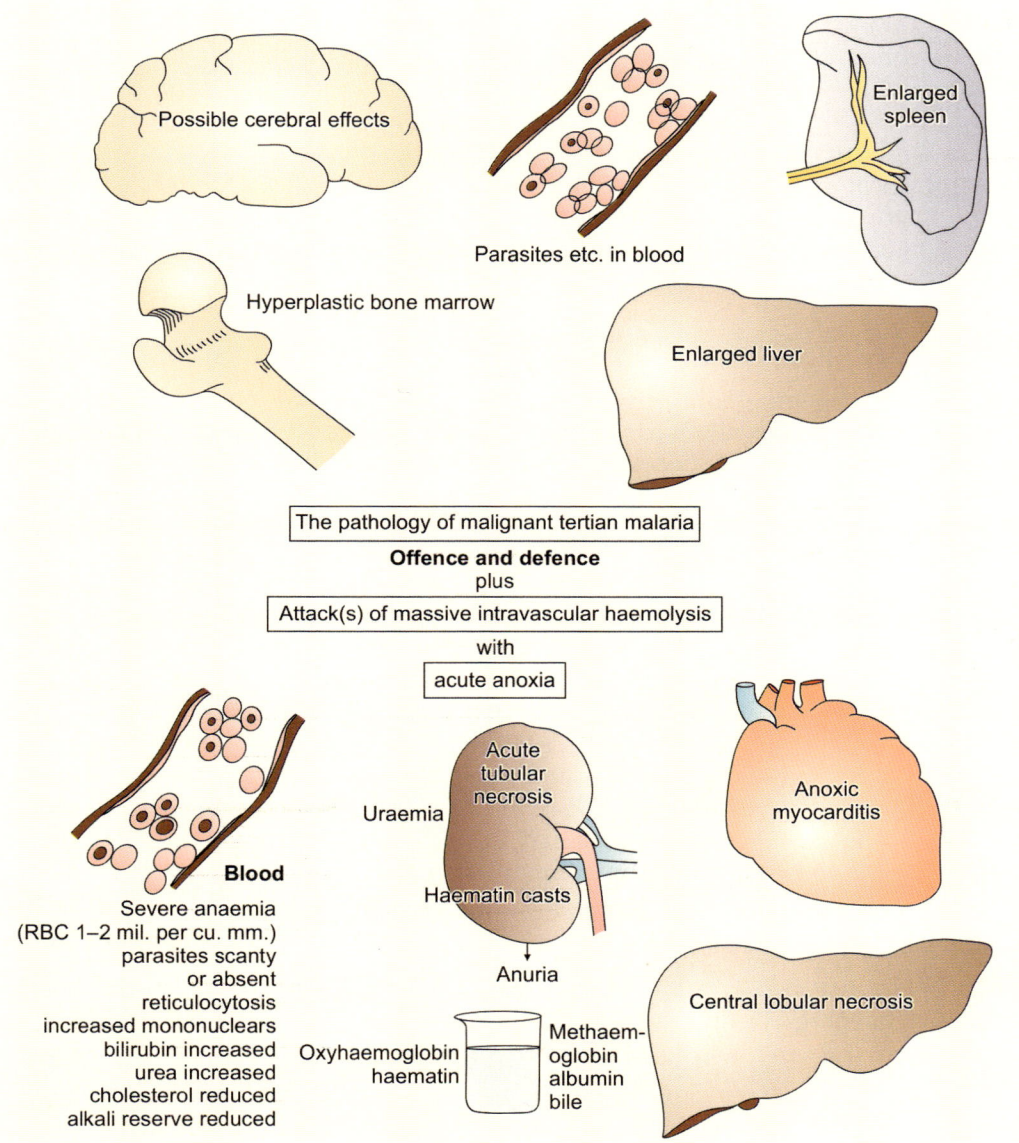

Possible cerebral effects

Parasites etc. in blood

Enlarged spleen

Hyperplastic bone marrow

Enlarged liver

The pathology of malignant tertian malaria

Offence and defence
plus

Attack(s) of massive intravascular haemolysis

with

acute anoxia

Acute tubular necrosis

Anoxic myocarditis

Uraemia

Blood

Haematin casts

Severe anaemia
(RBC 1–2 mil. per cu. mm.)
parasites scanty
or absent
reticulocytosis
increased mononuclears
bilirubin increased
urea increased
cholesterol reduced
alkali reserve reduced

Anuria

Central lobular necrosis

Oxyhaemoglobin
haematin

Methaem-
oglobin
albumin
bile

Blackwater fever is a manifestation of falciparum malaria in previously infected individuals and is characterised by sudden massive haemolysis followed by fever and haemoglobinuria.

Aetiology: Caused by *P. falciparum,* most commonly observed amongst the non-immune (not natives) persons who have stayed in malarious countries for 6 months to 1 year and have consumed inadequate doses of quinine for both suppressive prophylaxis and treatment of repeated clinical attacks. In such cases quinine consumption often precipitates the attack. Other factors that too can precipitate an attack of blackwater fever are—cold, heatstroke/exposure to sun, fatigue, trauma, pregnancy, parturition and X-ray treatment of spleen.

Pathogenesis: Intravascular haemolysis

Mechanism of haemolysis: Exact mechanism is not clearly understood. There is probably an involvement of a hemolytic agent that causes haemolysis of RBCs leading to liberation of vast quantities of oxyhaemoglobin into the blood stream. In falciparum malaria intravascular haemolysis occurs at the time of schizogony. Perhaps the RE system is stimulated to produce antibdies that act as haemolysins and lecitholysins. So with repeated attacks a hypersensitised state is evolved which when stimulated by any factor leads to an explosive outburst of haemolysin leading to the haemolytic crisis of blackwater fever. G6PD deficient individuals are particularly susceptible to haemolytic attacks.

EFFECTS OF INTRAVASCULAR HAEMOLYSIS

The excessive haemoglobin released in the circulation on account of intravascular haemolysis is either catabolised into methaemalbumin, or is converted by RE system into bilirubin and haemosiderin, or is excreted via the kidneys. The undermentioned effects are observed.

  (i) **Methaemalbuminemia:** Oxyhaemoglobin in blood is broken down into globin and haematin (ferrous form). Ferous form haematin is oxidised to ferric form haematin which combines with serum albumin to become methaemalbumin (it cannot go past the kidney and therefore does not appear in the urine but methaemalbuminemia occurs in blood).

 (ii) **Hyperbilirubinaemia:** Bilirubin formed by RE system is much too large for the liver to excrete and conjugate—leading to hyperbilirubinaemia.

(iii) **Haemoglobinuria:** The free circulating haemoglobin is bound to haptoglobin, whatever free haemoglobin remains is filtered through the kidney causing haemoglobinuria. Oxyhaemoglobin may be converted into methaemoglobin in the renal tubules or deposited in tubules as acid haematin. The various haemoglobin catabolism pigments that appear in blood and urine are

Blood: Oxyhaemoglobin, methaemalbumin and unconjugated/indirect bilirubin. Methaemalbumin does not pass the renal barrier and therefore does not appear in urine.

Urine: Oxyhaemoglobin makes urine red. Methaemoglobin gives it a dark brown/black colour (this pigment is not present in blood). Other pigments are haematin, urobilin.

Peripheral smear: P. falciparum parasites are not detected in the peripheral blood either during or after the attack as they are destroyed by the haemolytic crisis. However, the parasites appear within 1 to 2 weeks after the acute haemolytic crisis.

PATHOLOGY

Gross and microscopic features are identical with those seen in severe type of falciparum malaria (more so in liver and kidneys). Kidneys are enlarged and dark in colour (on account of congestion and pigmentation) and under the microscope one finds degenerative changes in distal convoluted tubules which are blocked with eosinophilic granular debris (haemoglobin casts). The liver is enlarged, soft and stained intensely yellow (due to haemosiderin), necrotic changes are most marked in the central zone of the liver lobule. Gall bladder is found to be filled with dark-green viscid bile. There is splenomegaly with blackish discolouration again on account of the malarial pigment.

Excessive haemosiderin pigment is seen in liver and kidneys also.

CLINICAL FEATURES

Beginning with fever and rigor, the attack is followed by aching pain in the loins, haemoglobinuria, icterus, bilious vomiting, circulatory and acute renal failure.

CLINICAL PATHOLOGY

Haematological changes: RBC count falls with a proportional decrease in haemoglobin. Shift to the left may be seen in peripheral smear (i.e. appearance of erythrocyte precursors). During recovery there is marked reticulocytosis (pointing to erythroid regeneration) with erythroid hyperplasia in the bone marrow. There is also neutrophilic leucocytosis.

Biochemical changes: Blood urea is increased while serum cholesterol is lowered.

Urinary changes: Colour changes from normal to red to dark brown (port-wine) and is acidic. Sediment shows heavy brown deposit. There is heavy albuminuria and urobilin test is markedly positive. Microscopically one finds haemoglobin casts and haematin crystals but no RBCs.

COMPLICATIONS

Include
- Uraemia (renal failure)
- Acute liver failure
- Circulatory collapse

Sequelae being—anaemia and pigment calculi.

Treatment

Treatment includes administration of chloroquin (or other drugs in resistant cases). The renal failure is of the reversible renal anoxia type, therefore, dialysis is essential and life-saving. Blood transfusion is necessitated because of marked anaemia that accompanies.

Prophylaxis: Chemoprophylaxis is important. If possible a patient of blackwater fever should not reside in the malarially endemic area and go elsewhere beyond the geographical zone supporting malaria.

MALARIA PROPHYLAXIS

Malaria prophylaxis is the preventive treatment of malaria. Several malaria vaccines are under development.

For pregnant women who are living in malaria endemic areas, routine malaria chemoprevention is recommended. It improves anaemia and parasite level in the blood for the pregnant women and the birthweight in their infants.

Strategies

Risk management

- Bite prevention—clothes that cover as much skin as possible, insect repellent, insecticide-impregnated bed nets and indoor residual spraying
- Chemoprophylaxis
- Rapid diagnosis and treatment

Recent improvements in malaria prevention strategies have further enhanced its effectiveness in combating areas highly infected with the malaria parasite. Additional bite prevention measures include mosquito and insect repellents that can be directly applied to skin. This form of mosquito repellent is slowly replacing indoor residual spraying, which is considered to have high levels of toxicity by WHO (World Health Organization). Further additions to preventive care are sanctions on blood transfusions. Once the malaria parasite enters the erythorocytic stage, it can adversely affect blood cells, making it possible to contract the parasite through infected blood.

Chloroquine may be used where the parasite is still sensitive, however, many malaria parasite strains are now resistant. Mefloquine (*Lariam*), or doxycycline (available generically), or the combination of atovaquone and proguanil hydrochloride (*Malarone*) are frequently recommended.

Medications

In choosing the agent, it is important to weigh the risk of infection against the risks and side effects associated with the medications.

Disruptive prophylaxis

An experimental approach involves preventing the parasite from binding with red blood cells by blocking calcium signalling between the parasite and the host cell. Erythrocyte-binding-like proteins (EBLs) and reticulocyte-binding protein homologues (RHs) are both used by specialized *P. falciparum* organelles known as rhoptries and micronemes to bind with the host cell. Disrupting the binding process can stop the parasite.

Monoclonal antibodies were used to interrupt calcium signalling between PfRH1 (an RH protein), EBL protein EBA175 and the host cell. This disruption completely stopped the binding process.

Suppressive prophylaxis

Chloroquine, proguanil, mefloquine, and doxycycline are suppressive prophylactics. This means that they are only effective at killing the malaria parasite once it has entered the erythrocytic stage (blood stage) of its life cycle, and therefore have no effect until the liver stage is complete. That is why these prophylactics must continue to be taken for four weeks after leaving the area of risk.

Mefloquine, doxycycline, and atovaquone-proguanil appear to be equally effective at reducing the risk of malaria for short-term travellers and are similar with regard to their risk of serious side effects. Mefloquine is sometimes preferred due to its once a week dose, however, mefloquine is not always as well tolerated when compared with atovaquone-proguanil. There is low-quality evidence suggesting that mefloquine and doxycycline are similar with regards to the number of people who discontinue treatments due to minor side effects. People who take mefloquine may be more likely to experience minor side effects such as sleep disturbances, depressed mood, and an increase in abnormal dreams. There is very low quality evidence indicating that doxycyline use may be associated with an increased risk of indigestion, photosensitivity, vomiting, and yeast infections, when compared with mefloquine and atovaquone-proguanil.

Causal prophylaxis

Causal prophylactics target not only the blood stages of malaria, but also the initial liver stage. This means that the user can stop taking the drug seven days after leaving the area of risk. Malarone and primaquine are the only causal prophylactics in current use.

Regimens

Specific regimens are recommended by the WHO, UK HPA and CDC for prevention of *P. falciparum* infection. HPA and WHO advice are broadly in line with each other (although there are some differences). CDC guidance frequently contradicts HPA and WHO guidance.

These regimens include:
- Doxycycline 100 mg once daily (started one day before travel, and continued for four weeks after returning);
- Mefloquine 250 mg once weekly (started two-and-a-half weeks before travel, and continued for four weeks after returning);
- Atovaquone/proguanil 1 tablet daily (started one day before travel, and continued for 1 week after returning). Can also be used for therapy in some cases.

In areas where chloroquine remains effective:
- Chloroquine 300 mg once weekly, and proguanil 200 mg once daily (started one week before travel, and continued for four weeks after returning);
- Hydroxychloroquine 400 mg once weekly (started one to two weeks before travel and continued for four weeks after returning)

What regimen is appropriate depends on the person who is to take the medication as well as the country or region travelled to. This information is available from the UK HPA, WHO or CDC (links are given below). Doses depend also on what is available (e.g. in the US, mefloquine tablets contain 228 mg base, but 250 mg base in the UK). The data is constantly changing and no general advice is possible.

Doses given are appropriate for adults and children aged 12 and over.

Other chemoprophylactic regimens that have been used on occasion:
- Dapsone 100 mg and pyrimethamine 12.5 mg once weekly (available as a combination tablet called Maloprim or Deltaprim): This combination is not routinely recommended because of the risk of agranulocytosis;
- Primaquine 30 mg once daily (started the day before travel, and continuing for seven days after returning): This regimen is not routinely recommended because of the need for G6PD testing prior to starting primaquine (*see the article on* primaquine for more information).

- Quinine sulfate 300 to 325 mg once daily: This regimen is effective but not routinely used because of the unpleasant side effects of quinine.

Prophylaxis against *Plasmodium vivax* requires a different approach given the long liver stage of this parasite. This is a highly specialist area.

VACCINES

In November 2012, findings from a Phase III trials of an experimental malaria vaccine known as RTS,S reported that it provided modest protection against both clinical and severe malaria in young infants. The efficacy was about 30% in infants 6 to 12 weeks of age and about 50% in infants 5 to 17 months of age in the first year of the trial.

The RTS,S vaccine was engineered using a fusion hepatitis B surface protein containing epitopes of the outer protein of *Plasmodium falciparum* malaria sporozite, which is produced in yeast cells.

RISK FACTORS

Most adults from endemic areas have a degree of long-term infection, which tends to recur, and also possess partial immunity (resistance); the resistance reduces with time, and such adults may become susceptible to severe malaria if they have spent a significant amount of time in non-endemic areas. They are strongly recommended to take full precautions if they return to an endemic area.

HISTORY

Malaria is one of the oldest known pathogens, and began having a major impact on human survival about 10,000 years ago with the birth of agriculture. The development of virulence in the parasite has been demonstrated using genomic mapping of samples from this period, confirming the emergence of genes conferring a reduced risk of developing the malaria infection. References to the disease can be found in manuscripts from ancient Egypt, India and China, illustrating its wide geographical distribution. The first treatment identified is thought to be Quinine, one of four alkaloids from the bark of the Cinchona tree. Originally it was used by the tribes of Ecuador and Peru for treating fevers. Its role in treating malaria was recognised and recorded first by an Augustine monk from Lima, Peru in 1633. Seven years later the drug had reached Europe and was being used widely with the name 'the Jesuit's bark'. From this point onwards the use of Quinine and the public interest in malaria increased, although the compound was not isolated and identified as the active ingredient until 1820. By the mid-1880s the Dutch had grown vast plantations of cinchona trees and monopolised the world market.

Quinine remained the only available treatment for malaria until the early 1920s. During the First World War German scientists developed the first synthetic antimalarial compound—Atabrin and this was followed by Resochin and Sontochin derived from 4-aminoquinoline compounds. American troops, on capturing Tunisia during the Second World War, acquired, then altered the drugs to produce Chloroquine.

The development of new antimalarial drugs spurred the World Health Organization in 1955 to attempt a global malaria eradication program. This was successful in much of Brazil, the US and Egypt but ultimately failed elsewhere. Efforts to control malaria are still continuing, with the development of drug-resistant parasites presenting increasingly difficult problems.

The CDC publishes recommendations for travels advising about the risk of contracting malaria in various countries.

Some of the factors in deciding whether to use chemotherapy as malaria pre-exposure prophylaxis include the specific itinerary, length of trip, cost of drug, previous adverse reactions to antimalarials, drug allergies, and current medical history.

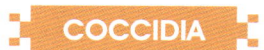

COCCIDIA

Classification

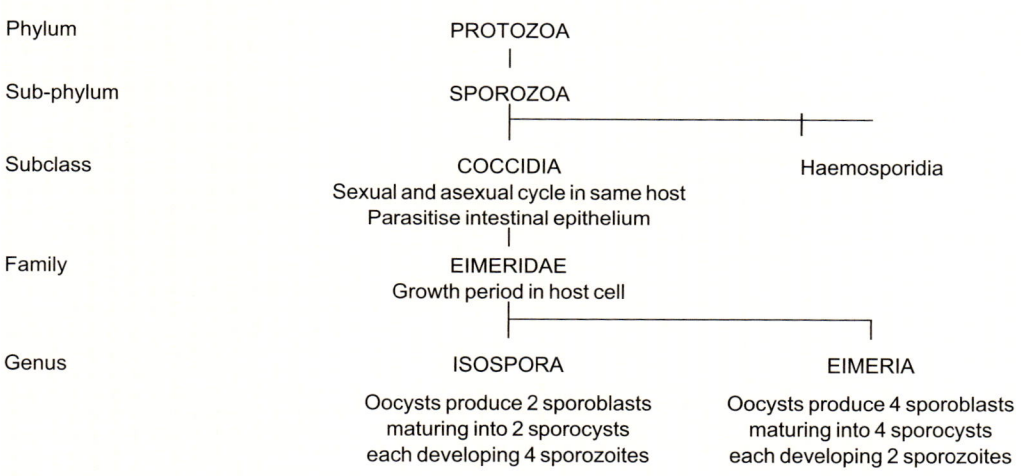

Phylum	PROTOZOA	
Sub-phylum	SPOROZOA	
Subclass	COCCIDIA Sexual and asexual cycle in same host Parasitise intestinal epithelium	Haemosporidia
Family	EIMERIDAE Growth period in host cell	
Genus	ISOSPORA	EIMERIA
	Oocysts produce 2 sporoblasts maturing into 2 sporocysts each developing 4 sporozoites	Oocysts produce 4 sporoblasts maturing into 4 sporocysts each developing 2 sporozoites

Oocyst Morphology

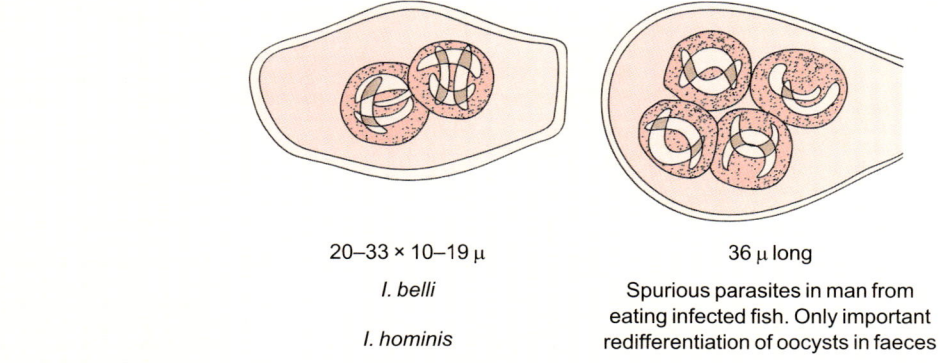

Species	20–33 × 10–19 μ	36 μ long
	I. belli	Spurious parasites in man from eating infected fish. Only important redifferentiation of oocysts in faeces
	I. hominis	

ISOSPORA (Causing Coccidiosis in man)

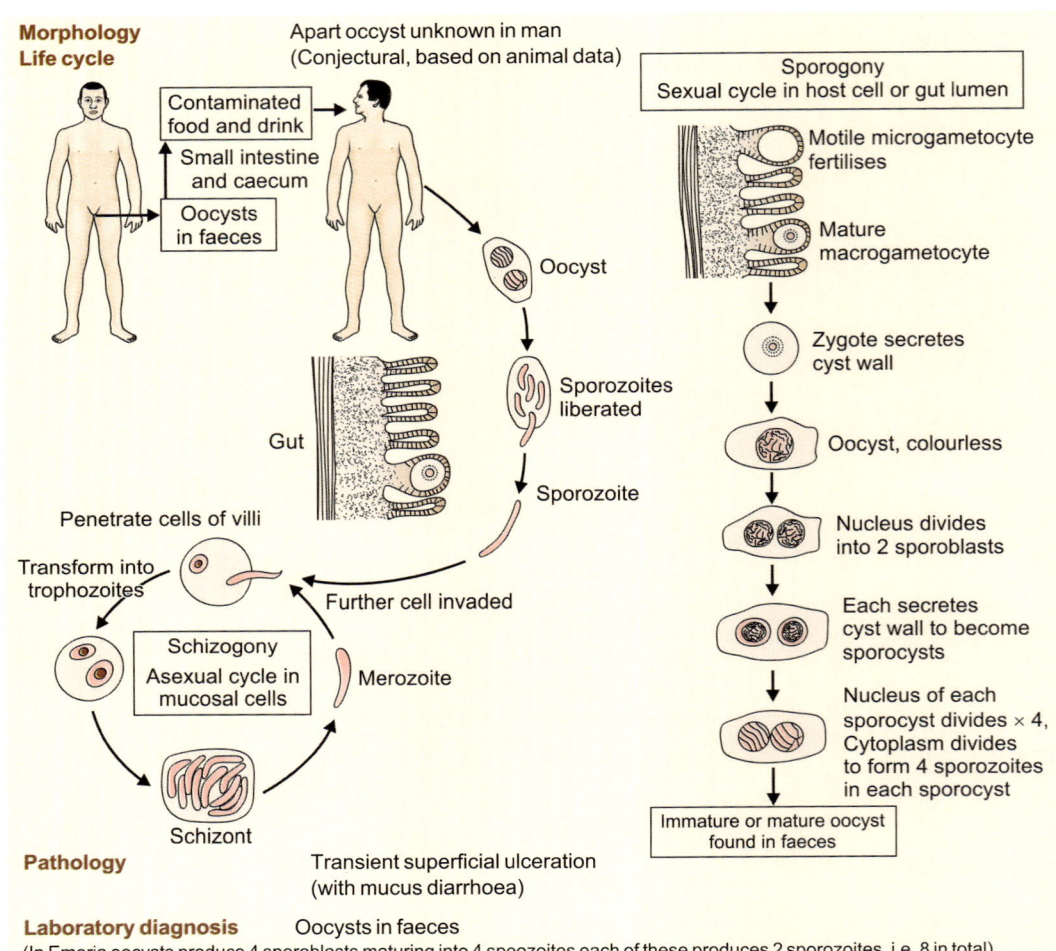

Morphology Life cycle

Apart occyst unknown in man (Conjectural, based on animal data)

Contaminated food and drink

Small intestine and caecum

Oocysts in faeces

Oocyst

Sporozoites liberated

Sporozoite

Gut

Penetrate cells of villi

Transform into trophozoites

Further cell invaded

Schizogony Asexual cycle in mucosal cells

Merozoite

Schizont

Sporogony Sexual cycle in host cell or gut lumen

Motile microgametocyte fertilises

Mature macrogametocyte

Zygote secretes cyst wall

Oocyst, colourless

Nucleus divides into 2 sporoblasts

Each secretes cyst wall to become sporocysts

Nucleus of each sporocyst divides × 4, Cytoplasm divides to form 4 sporozoites in each sporocyst

Immature or mature oocyst found in faeces

Pathology   Transient superficial ulceration (with mucus diarrhoea)

Laboratory diagnosis   Oocysts in faeces
(In Emeria oocysts produce 4 sporoblasts maturing into 4 spoozoites each of these produces 2 sporozoites, i.e. 8 in total)

Sarcocystis lindemanni

CLASSIFICATION

Phylum   Protozoa

Subphylum   Sporozoa

Class   Telosporidea   Sarcosporidea
Sexual spore (oocyst) simple   Sexual spore complex

Genus   Sarcocystis
Parasites in muscle, usually striated, in mammals, birds, reptiles

Species   *S. lindemanni*
A rare parasite of man

PROBABLE LIFE CYCLE

(Based on animal data)

Cyst in muscle or excreta of infected animal—ingested—spores freed—
enter intestinal epithelium—multiply—migrate to muscular tissue—grow into other cysts

Morphology

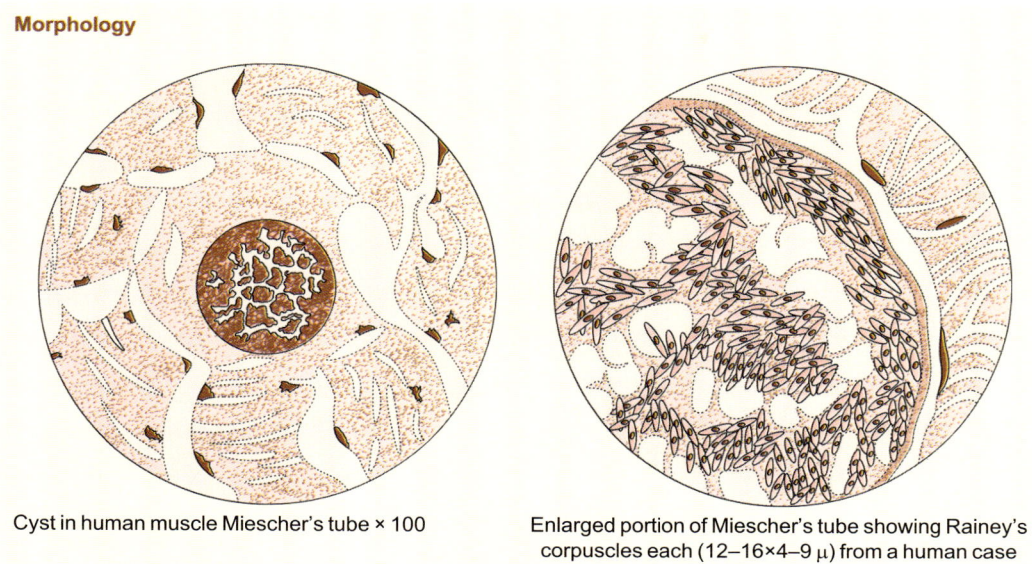

Cyst in human muscle Miescher's tube × 100

Enlarged portion of Miescher's tube showing Rainey's corpuscles each (12–16×4–9 μ) from a human case

Fig. 4.5: Cyst in muscle only known

Pathology

- Slight in man
- Allergy eosinophilia
- Muscular swellings

Laboratory Diagnosis

Histology of biopsy specimen

Protozoa of Uncertain Status

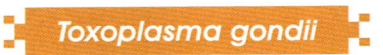

Toxoplasma gondii

Resembles *plasmodium* but:
1. Divides by binary fission rather than by schizogony.
2. Is non-specific with reference to host and tissue.
3. No evidence of an arthropod acting as biological vector
4. Lacks a sexual stage.

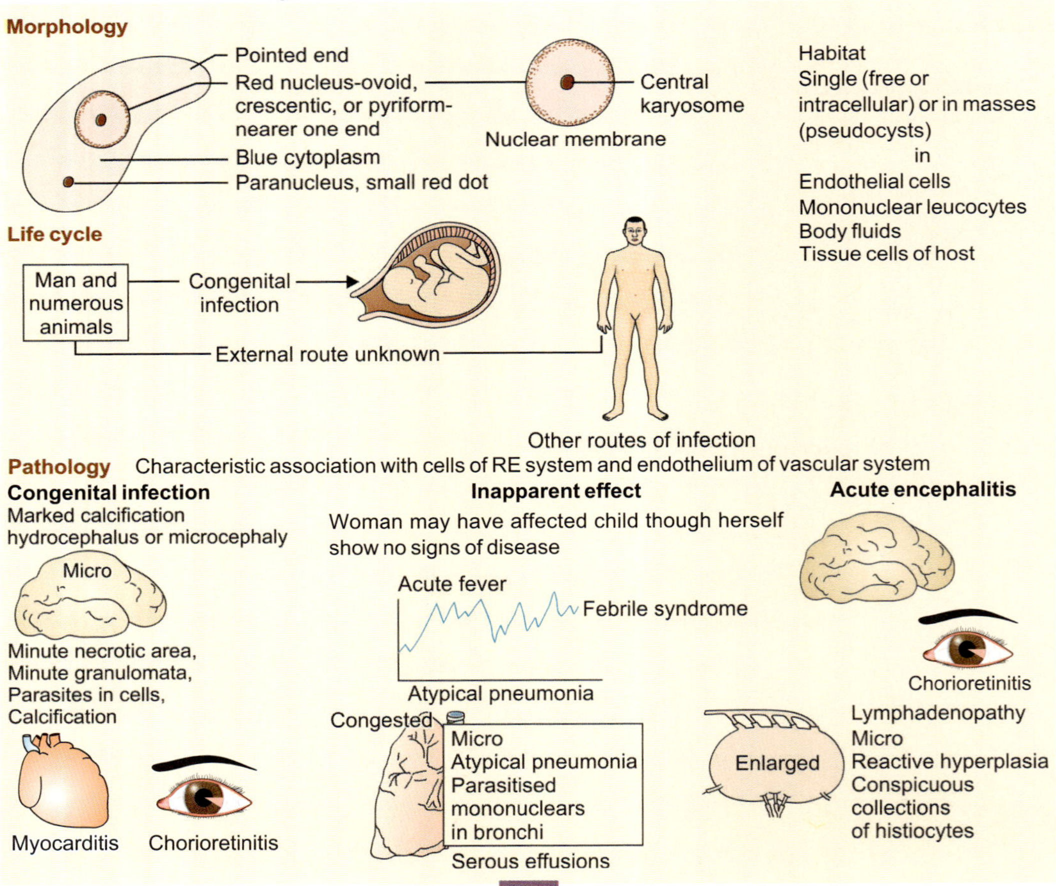

Morphology

Pointed end
Red nucleus-ovoid, ——— Central karyosome
crescentic, or pyriform-
nearer one end
Nuclear membrane
Blue cytoplasm
Paranucleus, small red dot

Habitat
Single (free or intracellular) or in masses (pseudocysts)
in
Endothelial cells
Mononuclear leucocytes
Body fluids
Tissue cells of host

Life cycle

Man and numerous animals	— Congenital infection →

External route unknown

Other routes of infection

Pathology Characteristic association with cells of RE system and endothelium of vascular system

Congenital infection
Marked calcification
hydrocephalus or microcephaly

Micro

Minute necrotic area,
Minute granulomata,
Parasites in cells,
Calcification

Myocarditis   Chorioretinitis

Inapparent effect
Woman may have affected child though herself show no signs of disease

Acute fever
Febrile syndrome

Atypical pneumonia
Congested
Micro
Atypical pneumonia
Parasitised
mononuclears
in bronchi
Serous effusions

Acute encephalitis

Chorioretinitis
Lymphadenopathy
Micro
Reactive hyperplasia
Conspicuous
collections
of histiocytes

Enlarged

Laboratory diagnosis

DEMONSTRATION OF PARASITE   SEROLOGICAL DEMONSTRATION OF SPECIFIC ANTIBODIES

From   Postmortem
        Ventricular aspirate   } by   Animal inoculation
        Biopsy liver and spleen

or

by   Complement fixation, ELISA
      Nutralisation
      Dye   } Tests
      Toxoplasmin (skin)
      test (unreliable)

Pneumocystis carinil causing interstitial plasma cell pneumonia

Morphology   **Pathology**

Foam-like masses in alveoli and bronchii

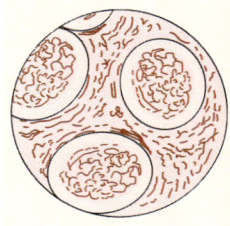

Cysts with up to 8 nuclei described
(special staining method)

Life cycle unknown

Laboratory diagnosis
Postmortem histology

Distended
thick pleura
cut surface grey
airless septae
thick

Micro
Alveolar epithelium
thick partly desquamated
Infiltration leucocytes
and plasma cells
Exudate, inflammatory
cells and *Pneumocystis
carinii* in lumen

Helminthology

Helminths are multicellular parasites, that are filaterally symmetrical animals having three germ layers (i.e. they are triploblastic metazoa).

Initial classification of worms of medical importance

SUBKINGDOM   **METAZOA**

1. Triploblastic
2. Possess a skin
3. Possess a mouth of sorts
4. Body systems mainly alimentary and reproductive
5. Possess primitive nervous and excretory systems
6. Sexes may be separate, hermaphroditism frequent

Phylum

Playtyhelminthes (Flat worms)
1. Flattened, segmented or unsegmented
2. Gut may or may not be present
3. No body cavity, viscera in gelatinous matrix

Nemathelminthes (Roundworms)
1. Unsegmented, cyclindrical, bilaterally symmetrical
2. Possess an alimentary system
3. Possess a body cavity

Class

Cestoda (tapeworms)
1. Segmented
2. Possess scolex, neck and proglottids

3. Hermaphroditic
4. Reproduction
   A. Oviparous
   B. Sometimes multiplication with larval forms

Trematoda (flukes)
1. Unsegmented
2. Leaf like or cylindrical

3. Generally hermaphroditic
4. Reproduction (digenetic)
   A. Oviparous
   B. Multiplication within larval forms
5. Infection mainly by larval stages entering intestinal tract, sometimes through skin

Nematoda (roundworms)
1. Unsegmented
2. Possess mouth, oeso-phagus and anus impor-tant in further diagnosis
3. In general sexes separate
4. Reproduction
   A. Oviparous
   B. Larviparous
5. Infection by
   A. Ingestion of eggs or
   B. Penetration of larvae through surfaces or
   C. Arthropod vector or
   D. Ingestion of encysted larvae

Plate IX

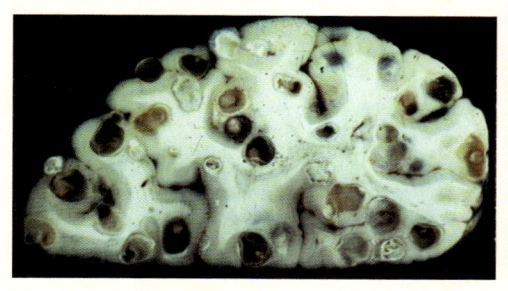

Cysticercosis of brain

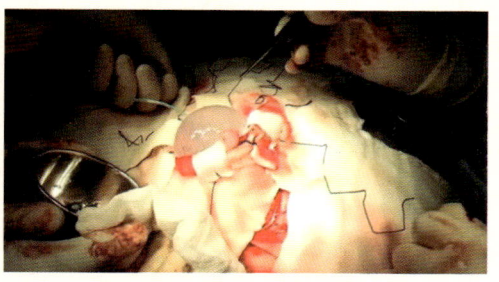

Hydatid cyst in brain

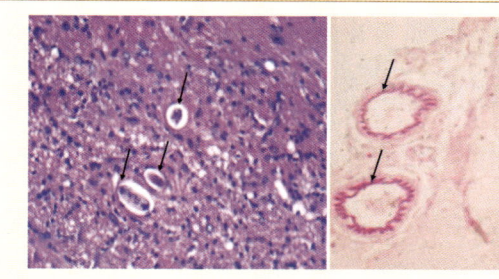

T. canis **larva in brain**

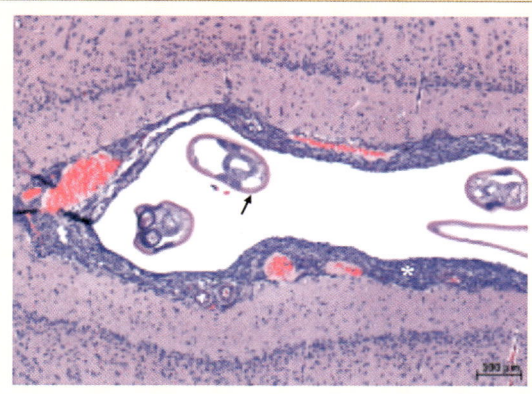

Angiostrongylus cantonesis young adulte worms (arrow) associated with meningitis, consisting of vascular congestion and intense macrophage infiltration (asterisk), with less number of lymphocytes (Rathus novergicus at 25 days post-infection)(HE, 100x)

A. Cantonensis **inmeninges of human brain**

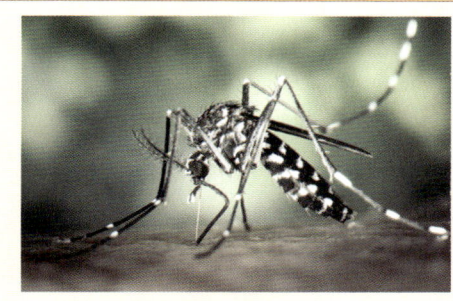

Aedes aegypti

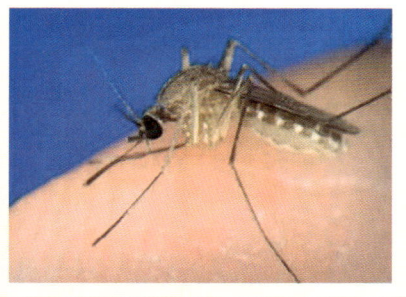

Culex mosquito

Plate X

Dog and Cat Hookworms: Cutaneous Larva Migrans

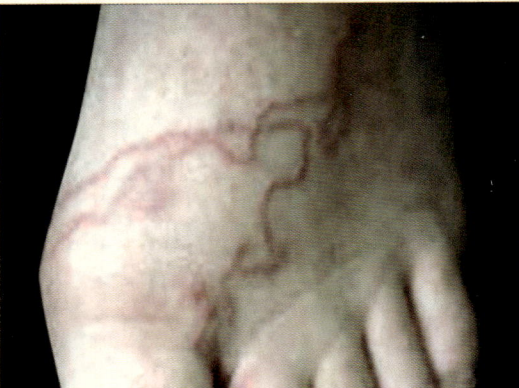

This is when a dog or cat hookworm gets into a human by accident. Since we are not the right kind of host, the worm dies under the skin and causes an allergic reaction.

Dog hookworm in human skin

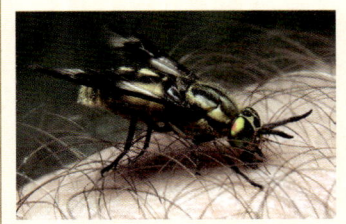

Chrysops

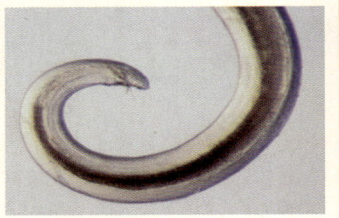

Loa loa tail

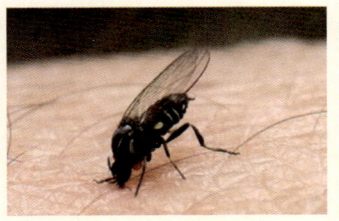

Simulium

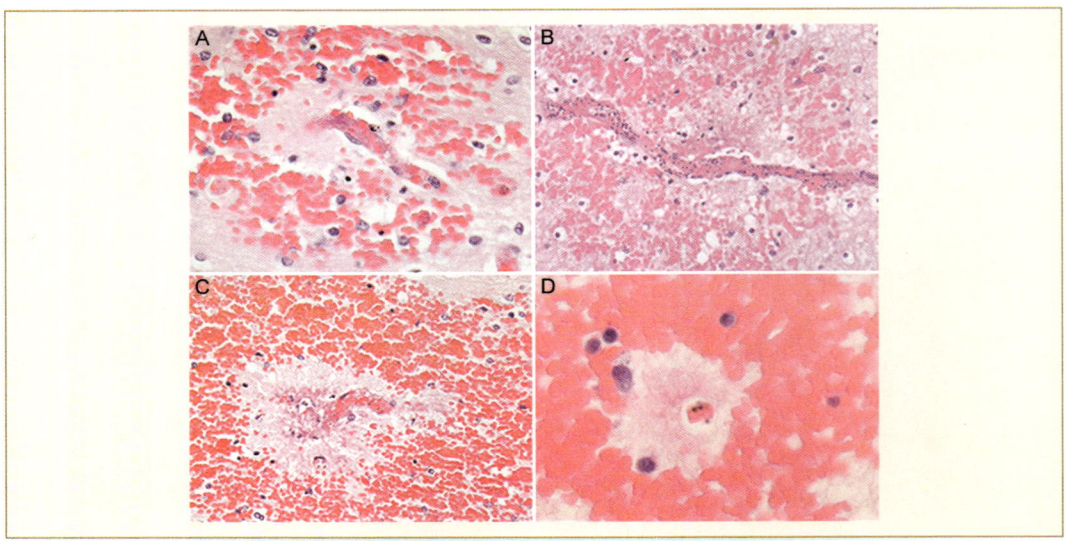

Cerebral malaria brain sections

Plate XI

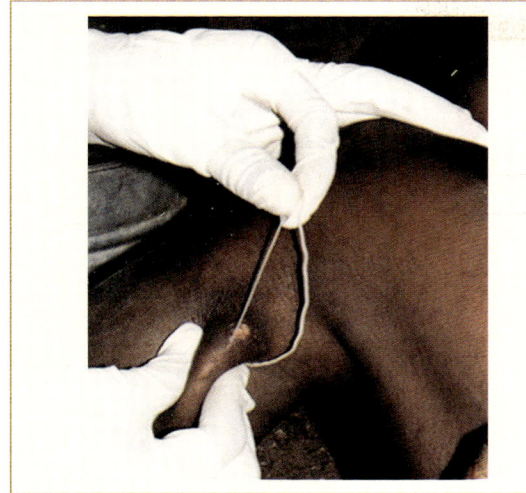

Guinea worm around knee

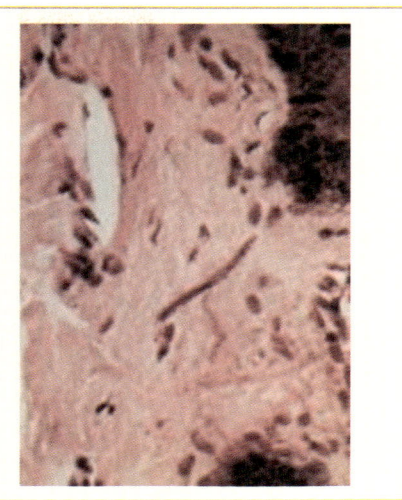

Microfilaria in skin biopsy

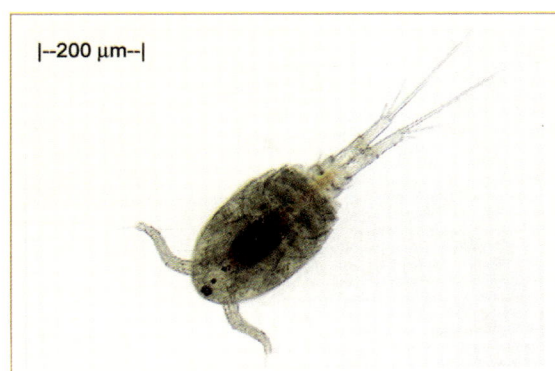

|--200 µm--|

Cyclops

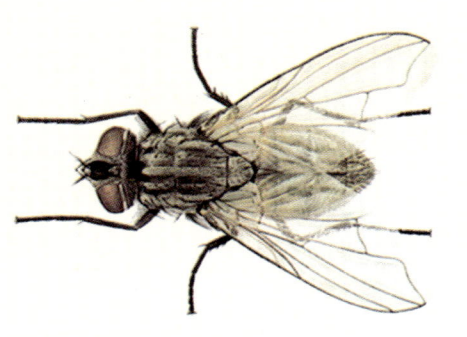

Housefly

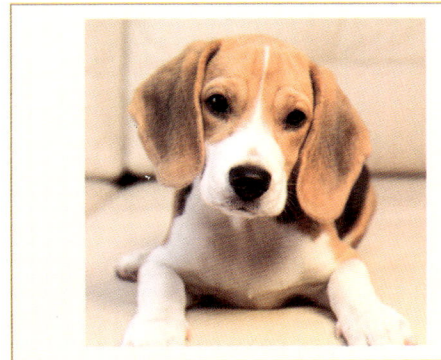

Dog

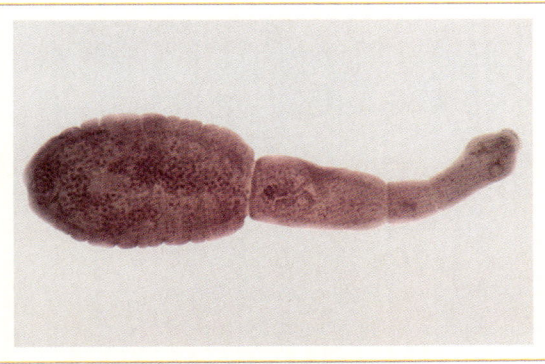

Adult echinococcus

Plate XII

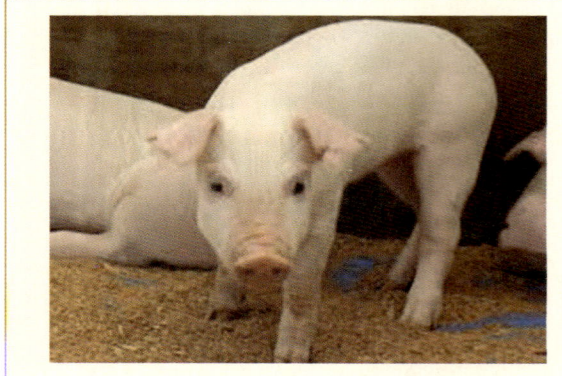

Pig

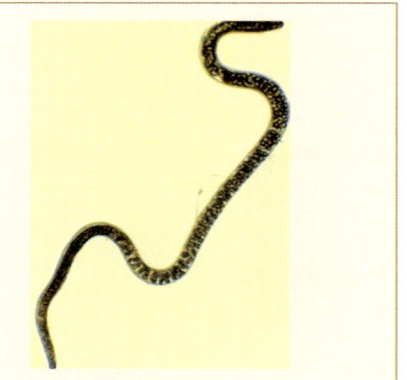

T. spiralis

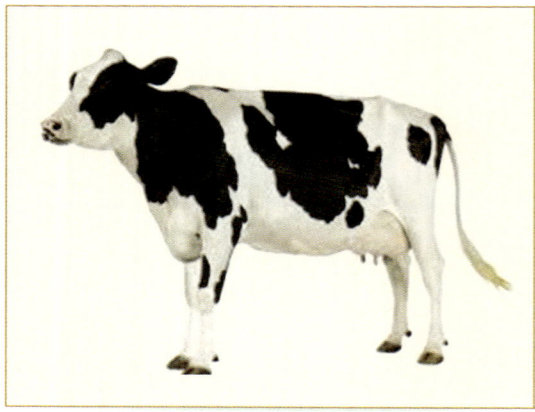

Cow

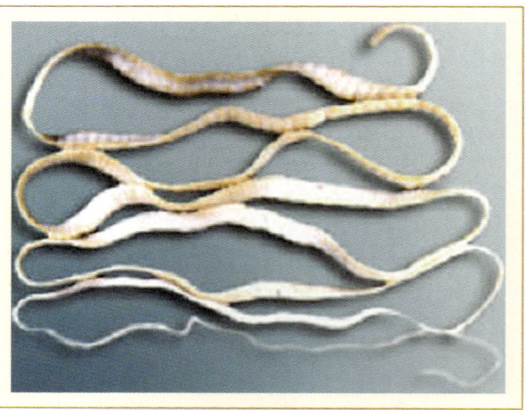

Adult *T. saginata*

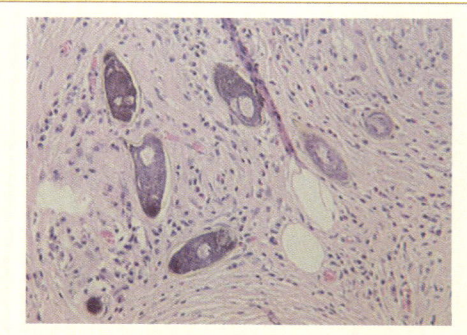

S. mansoni eggs in liver

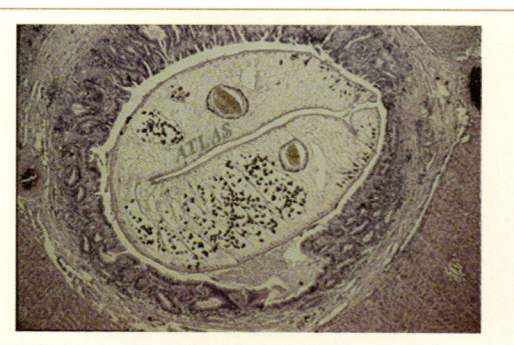

Sinensis in bile duct

Plate XIII

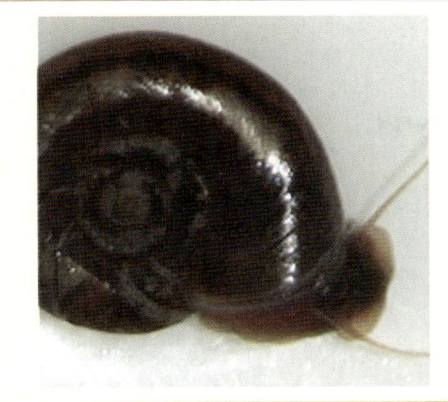

Biomphalaria snail

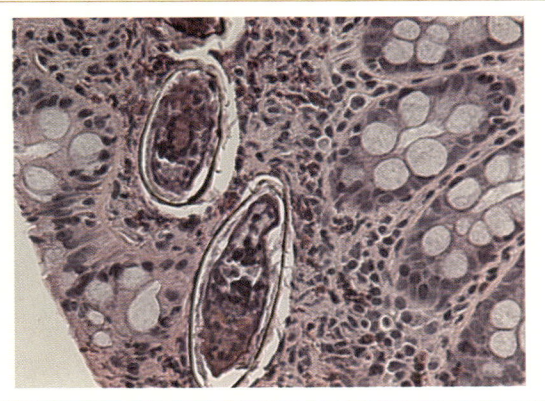

***S. mansoni* eggs in colonic biopsy**

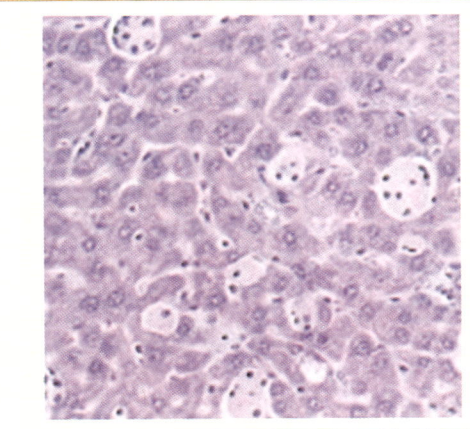

Kupffer cell hyperplasia in liver in malaria

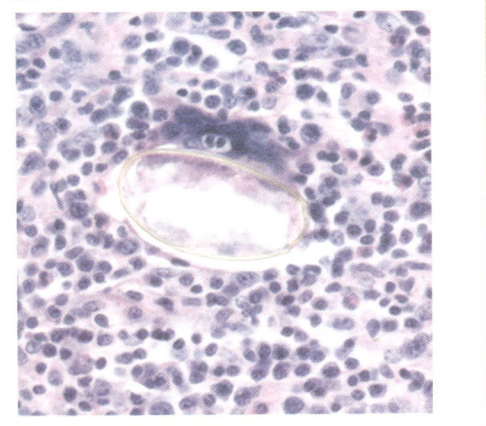

***P. westermani* in lymph node**

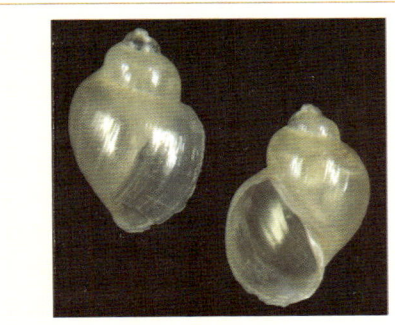

Bulinus snail

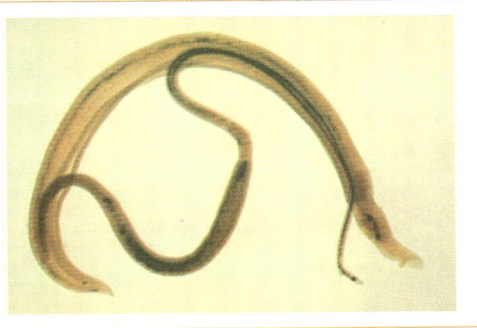

Adult *S. japonicum*

Plate XIV

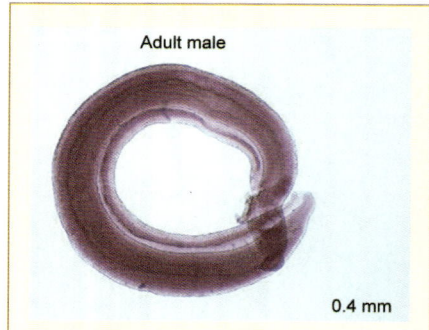

Adult male

0.4 mm

Adult *S. haematobium*

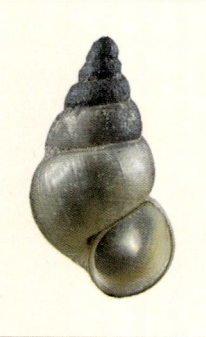

Oncomelania snail

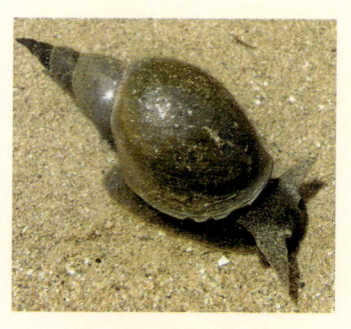

Lymnaea snail

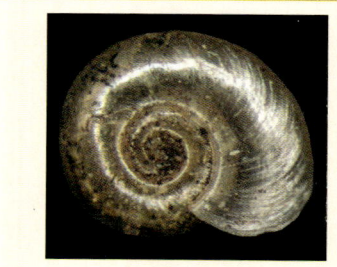

Segmentina snail

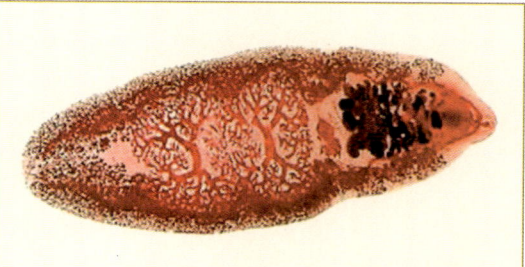

Adult *F. buski*

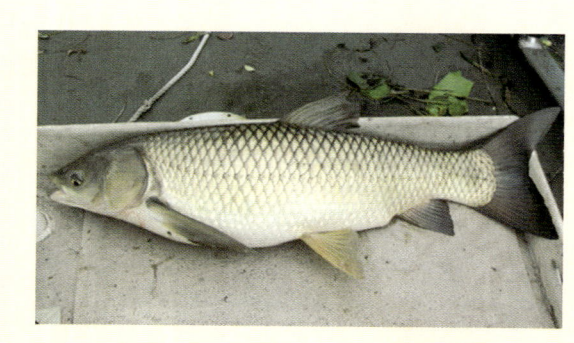

Ctenopharyngodon fish

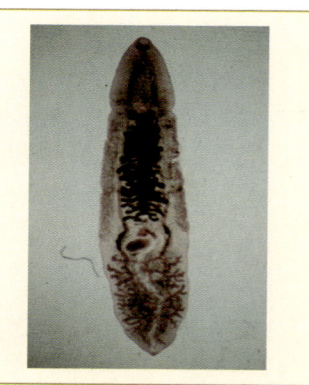

Adult *C. sinensis*

Plate XV

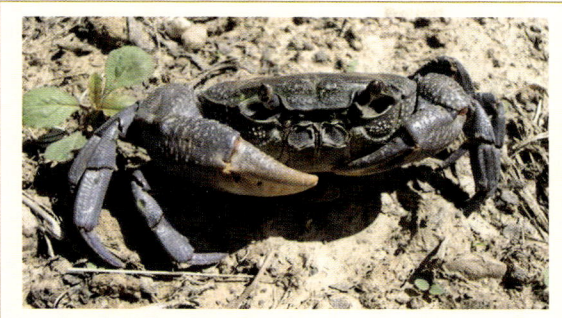

Potamon crab

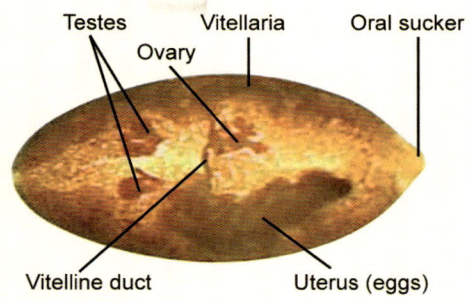

Testes · Ovary · Vitellaria · Oral sucker

Vitelline duct · Uterus (eggs)

Adult *P. westermani*

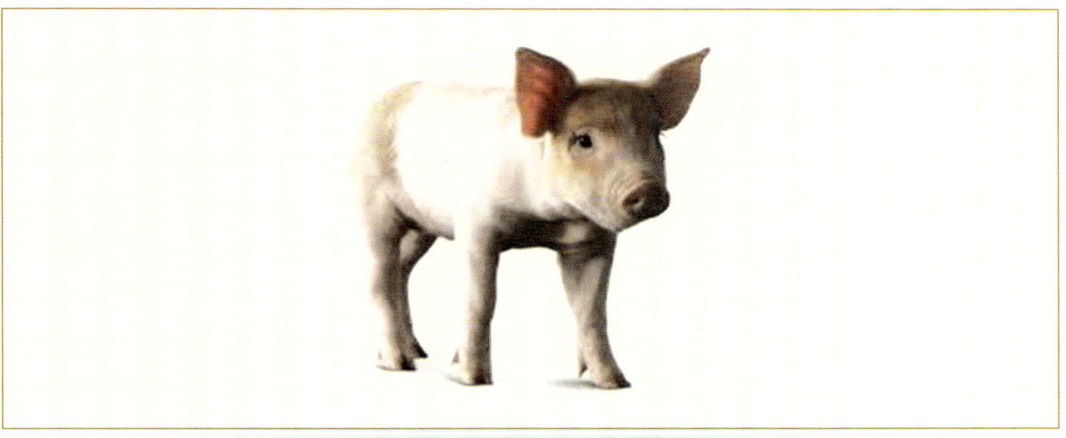

Pig

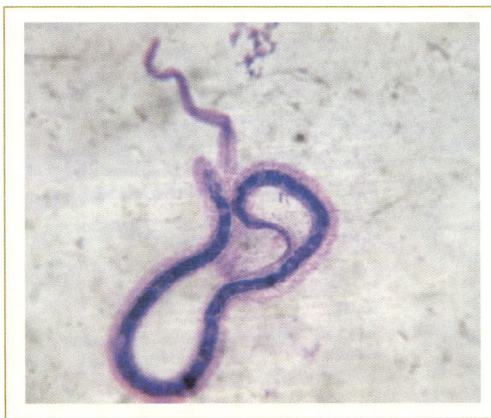
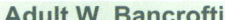

Adult W. Bancrofti

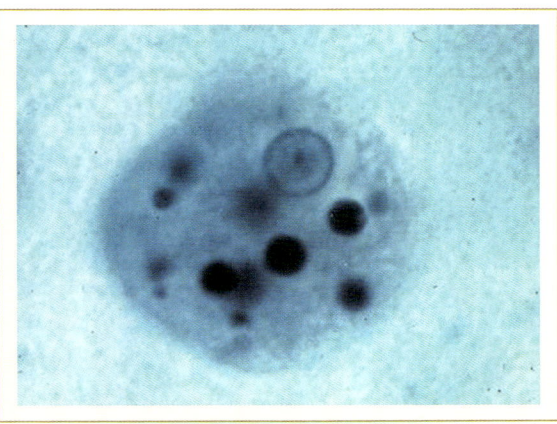

E. histolytica trophozoite

Plate XVI

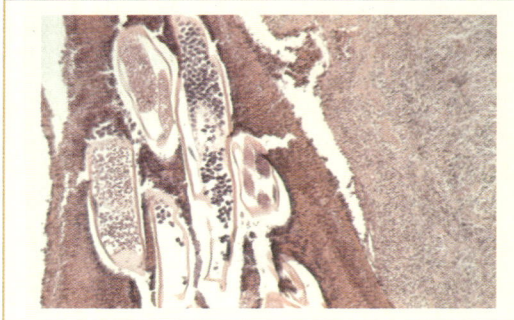

W. bancrofti in lymph node

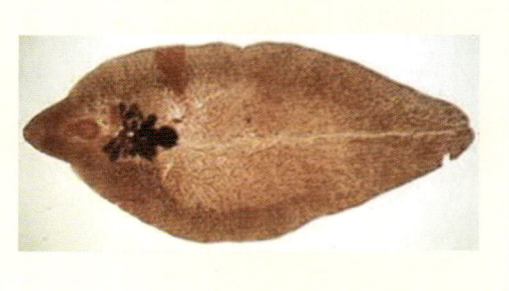

Adult F. hepatica

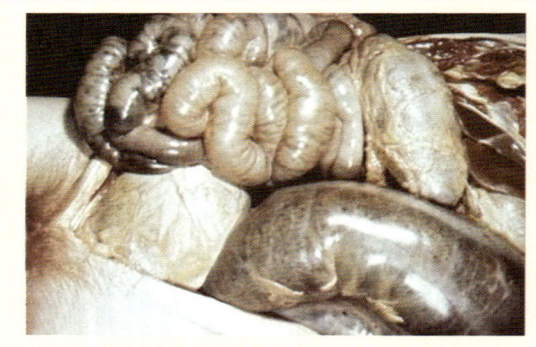

**Mega colon seen in
chronic Chagas' disease**

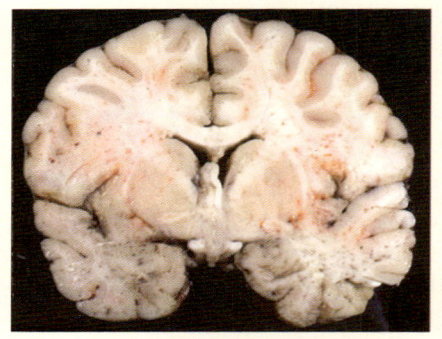

**Cross section of brain in
cerebral malaria**

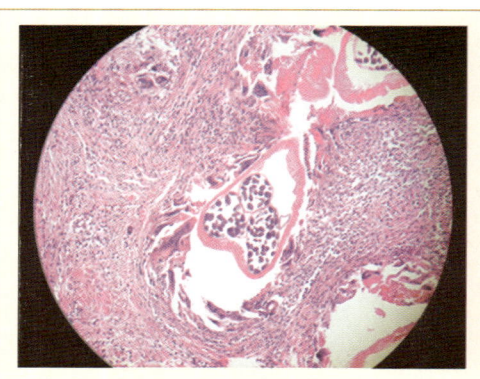

Cutaneous onchocerca

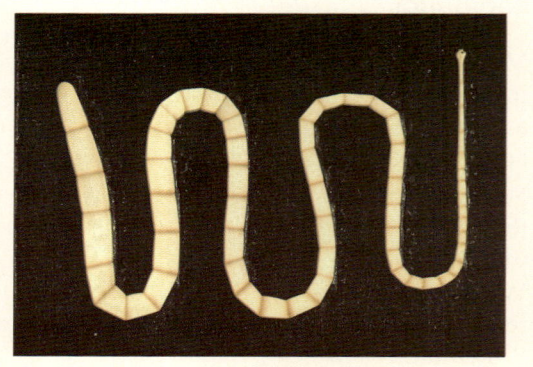

Adult T. solium

Phylum Nemathelminthes

CLASS NEMATODA

General Characteristics

Shape: Nematodes are elongated and cylindrical unsegmented worms without any appendage and tapering at both ends.

Size: Sizes are variable, e.g. *Trichinella spiralis* and *Stronglyloides stercoralis* measure less than 5 mm while the largest *Dracunculus medinensis* can measure up to 100 cm (1 metre) in length.

Body: Is covered by a tough protective covering or cuticle.

Body cavity: The body cavity of the worm houses the various organs—e.g. the digestive and reproductive systems. Their excretory and nervous systems are very basic and rudimentary. The systems float in the body cavity.

Alimentary canal: The alimentary canal is complete, consisting of an oral aperture, mouth cavity, oesophagus, intestine and a subterminal anus. When present, the mouth cavity may have teeth or cutting plates. When the mouth cavity is missing, the oral aperture is directly continuous with the oesophagus.

Sexes: Human nematodes are diecious helminths, i.e. the sexes are separate. Males being smaller than the females, and the reproductive organs are tubular and lie coiled within the body.

Reproductive System

Male genital system: It consists of a long convoluted tube that can be differentiated into testis, vas deferens, seminal vesicle and ejaculatory duct. The genital duct forms a common passage with the intestine and is designated as cloaca. In some males, accessory copulatory organs—spicule and gubernaculum may also be present.

Female genital system: This consists of a single or two convoluted tubes. Each half of the tube is differentiated into ovary, oviduct, terminal receptacle, uterus, vagina and vulva. The genital pore usually opens in the middle of the body or near the mouth. Where two tubes are present they may unite to form a common duct, vagina, before terminating in the genital pore.

Female nematodes may be further subdivided as (in contrast to trematodes and cestodes):

1. **Viviparous:** Giving birth to larvae (e.g. *Dracunculus medinensis, Wuchereria bancrofti, Brugia malayi* and *Trichinella spiralis*).
2. **Oviparous:** Egg laying *Ascaris lumbricoides, Trichuris trichiura, Ancylostoma duodenale, Necator americanus, Enterobius vermicularis.* In *T. trichiura*—eggs are unsegmented. *N. americanus* lays segmented eggs while *E. vermicular* lays eggs that contain larvae.
3. **Ova-viviparous:** Laying eggs containing larvae which are hatched out immediately as in *Strongyloides stercoralis*.

Life cycle: Most nematodes (except superfamilies filaroidea and dracunculoidea) pass their life cycles in one host—man is their optimum host. In Filaroidea the second host is an insect vector in which the larval development occurs. Where nematodes choose one host they localise in the GI tract and start developing. The eggs come out of the body and undergo certain morphological changes before they can enter a new host. In *T. spiralis,* however, pig is the optimum host, man being an alternative host only but the worm passes its adult and larval stages in the same host.

Modes of Infection

A. **By ingestion:**
   (i) Embryonated eggs contaminating food and drink, e.g.—*A. lumbricoides, T. trichiura* and *E. vermicularis*.
   (ii) Growing embryos present in an intermediate host (infected cyclops) as in *D. medinensis*.
   (iii) Encysted embryos in infected pig's flesh, as in *T. spiralis*.
B. **By cutaneous penetration:** The filariform larvae bore through the skin, as in *N. americanus, A. lumbricoides* and *S. stercoralis*.
C. **By blood sucking insects**—as in superfamily Filorioidea.
D. **By inhalation of infected dust** containing embryonated eggs—*A. lumbricoides* and *E. vermicularis*.

Larval stages of nematodes of lower animals capable of infecting man				
Definitive host	Adult worm	Normal habitat	Mode of infection	Disease caused
1. Hookworm of dogs and cats	*A. braziliense A. caninum*	Small intestine	Filariform larva enters skin	Cutaneous larva migrans
2. Ascarids of dogs and cats	*Toxocara canis and T. cati*	Small intestine	Ingestion of eggs	Visceral larva migrans and granalomatous ophthalmitis
3. Ascarids of sea mammals	*Anisakis marina*	Small intestine	Larva eaten with marine fish	Eosinophilic granuloma of bowel
4. Rat lungworm	*Angiostrongylus cantonensis*	Pulmonary artery	Ingestion of larvae in molluscs or carrier hosts	Eosinophilic meningoencephalitis
5. Spiruroid worm of dogs and cats	*Gnasthostoma spinigerum*	Gastric wall tumor	Larva ingestion in fish	Cutaneous larva migrans
6. Filarial worms of dogs and cats	*Brugia pahangi*	Lymphatics	Bite of an infected vector	Tropical pulmonary eosinophilia

Nematoda (Contd.)

| | | Class: APHASMIDIA | | | PHASMIDIA | |
| | | No caudal chemoreceptor organs | | | With caudal chemoreceptor organs | |

ABRIDGED CLASSIFICATION

Super family	Size and shape	Mouth and oesophagus	Tail in ♂	Reproduction	Genus	Species
APHASMID NEMATODES						
Trichinelloidea	Small, delicate, may be attenuated anteriorly	No buccal capsule, oesophagus degenerate	No bursa oviparous	Larviparous or Trichuris	Trichenella, Trichura, Capillaria	spiralis, trichiura, hepatica
Mermithoidea	Long, pointed anteriorly	Non-muscular oesophagus	Oviparous		Spurious infections in man	
Dioctophyma-toidea	Large, attenuated ends	No buccal capsule	Bursa present	Oviparous	Dioctophyma	renale
PHASMID NEMATODES						
Rhabditoidea	Parastic ♀ thin, ♂ stout	No buccal capsule. Oesophagus filariform in ♀, muscular buibous in ♂	No bursa	Larviparous	Strongyloides	stecoralis
Strongyloidea	Small, delicate	Well-developed buccal capsule	Bursa with rays present	Oviparous	Ancylostoma, Ancylostoma, Ancylostoma, Necator, Ternidens, Oesopha-gostomum, Sayngamus	duodenale, braziliense, caninum, americanus, deminutis, apiostomum, laryngeus
Note: Does NOT include the genus Strongyloides, see above						
Trichostrongloidea	Small, slender	Capsular rudimentary or absent	Conspicuous bursa	Oviparous	Trichostrongylus, Haemonchus	spp., contortus

Nematoda (Phasmid Nematodes) (Contd.)						
Super family	Size and shape	Mouth and oesophagus	Tail in ♂	Reproduction	Genus	Species
Metastrongyloidea	Small filiform	Capsule rudimentary or absent Pair of lateral trilobed lips	Bursa present, rays striated	Oviparous	Metastrongylus	elongatus
Oxyuroidea	Small, ♀ pin shaped	No true capsule 3 lips Distinct posterior bulb in oesophagus	Bursa poorly developed or absent	Oviparous	Entrobius	vermicularis
Ascaroidea	Large, stout	No buccal capsule 3 lips	No bursa	Oviparous	Ascaris Toxocara Tooxocara	lumbricoides canis cati
Spiruroidea	Filiform to robust	No capsule various lips	No bursa various papille	Oviparous	Gongylonema Gnasthostoma Physaloptera Thelazia	pulchrum spinigerum caucasica callipseda
Filarioidea	Filiform	Rudimentary capsule No lips	Various papillae	Larviparous	Wuchereria Brugia Brugia Brugia Onchocerca Loa Acanthochie-lonema Dipetalonema Mansonella Dirofilaria	bancrofti malayi pahangi patei volvulus loa perstans streptocerca ozzardi spp.
Dracunculoidea	Long, cord-like	Mouth simple Oesophagus and intestine rudimentary		Larviparous	Dracunculus	medinesis

Classification of Nematodes

According to habitat: Are intestinal and somatic.
- A. **Intestinal:**
  Small intestine only
  - *Ascaris lumbricoides* (roundworm)
  - *Ancylostoma duodenale* (hookworm)
  - *Necator americanus* (American hookworm)
  - *Strongyloides stercoralis*
  - *Trichinella spiralis* (Trichina worm)
  - *Capillaria philippinensis*

  Caecum and appendix
  - *Trichuris trichiura* (Whipworm)
  - *Enterobius vermicularis* (Threadworm or pinworm)
- B. **Somatic:** (Within the tissues and organs)
  Subcutaneous tissues
  - *Loa loa* (African eye worm)
  - *Onchocerca volvulus*
  - *Dracunculus medinensis* (Guinea worm)

  Lymphatic system
  - *Wuchereria bancrofti*
  - *Brugia malayi*

  Lungs
  - *Strongyloides stercoralis*

  Mesentery
  - *Dipetalonema perstans*
  - *Mansonella ozzardi*

  Conjunctiva
  - *Loa loa*

Systematic classification of nematodes				
Subclass	*Order*	*Superfamily*	*Genus*	*Species*
Phasmidia	Rhabditida	Rhabditoidea	Strongyloldes	*S. stercoralis*
		Strongyloldea	Ancylostoma	*A. duodennal*
			Necator	*N. americanus*
		Metastrongyloidea	Angiostrongylus	*A.cantonensis*
		Oxyuroidea	Enterobius	*E.vermicularis*
		Ascaridoidea	Ascaris	*A.lumbricoides*
	Spirurida	Filarioidea	Wuchereria	*W.bancrofti*
			Brugia	*B.malayi*
			Onchocerca	*O. volvulus*
			Dipetatonema	*D.perstans*
		Filarioidea	Mansonella	*M.ozzardi*
			Dirofilaria	*D. conjunctivas*
				D.immitis

Contd.

Systematic classification of nematodes (*Contd.*)				
Subclass	*Order*	*Superfamily*	*Genus*	*Species*
			Loa	*L. loa*
		Dracunculoidea	Dracunculus	*D.medinensis*
		Spiruroidea	Gnasthostoma	*G.spinigerum*
Aphasmidia	Enoplida	Trichinelloidea	Tnchinella	*T.spiralis*
(Caudal			Trichuris	*T.trichiura*
chemoreceptors			Capillaria	*C.phillipinensis*
missing/absent)				

Important Terms Employed in the Description of Nematodes

Buccal capsule: Where the oral aperture leads to mouth cavity, it may contain teeth or cutting organs.

Cuticle: Outer hyaline, non-cellular layer forming nematodal integument.

Cervical alae: Wing-like cuticular expansion near the mouth.

Cloaca: A conjoint passage in male nematodes where the genital duct and rectum open.

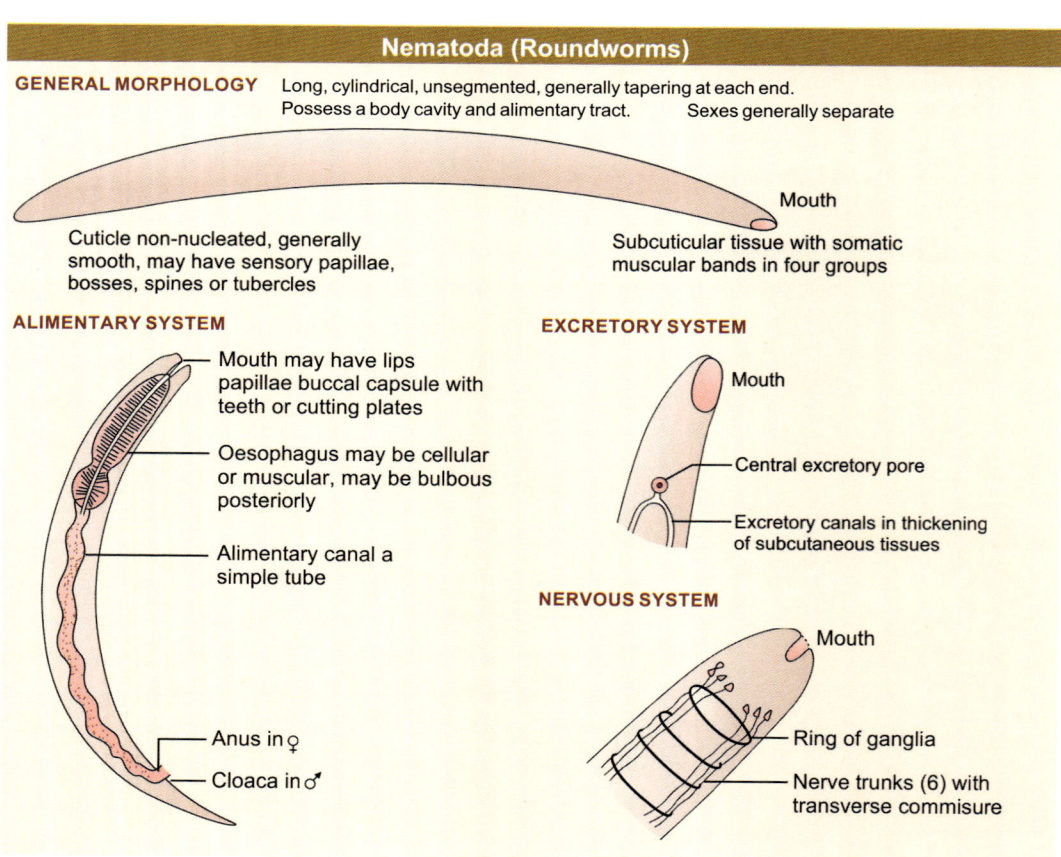

Nematoda (Roundworms)

GENERAL MORPHOLOGY   Long, cylindrical, unsegmented, generally tapering at each end.
Possess a body cavity and alimentary tract.   Sexes generally separate

Mouth

Cuticle non-nucleated, generally smooth, may have sensory papillae, bosses, spines or tubercles

Subcuticular tissue with somatic muscular bands in four groups

ALIMENTARY SYSTEM

Mouth may have lips papillae buccal capsule with teeth or cutting plates

Oesophagus may be cellular or muscular, may be bulbous posteriorly

Alimentary canal a simple tube

Anus in ♀

Cloaca in ♂

EXCRETORY SYSTEM

Mouth

Central excretory pore

Excretory canals in thickening of subcutaneous tissues

NERVOUS SYSTEM

Mouth

Ring of ganglia

Nerve trunks (6) with transverse commisure

REPRODUCTIVE SYSTEM

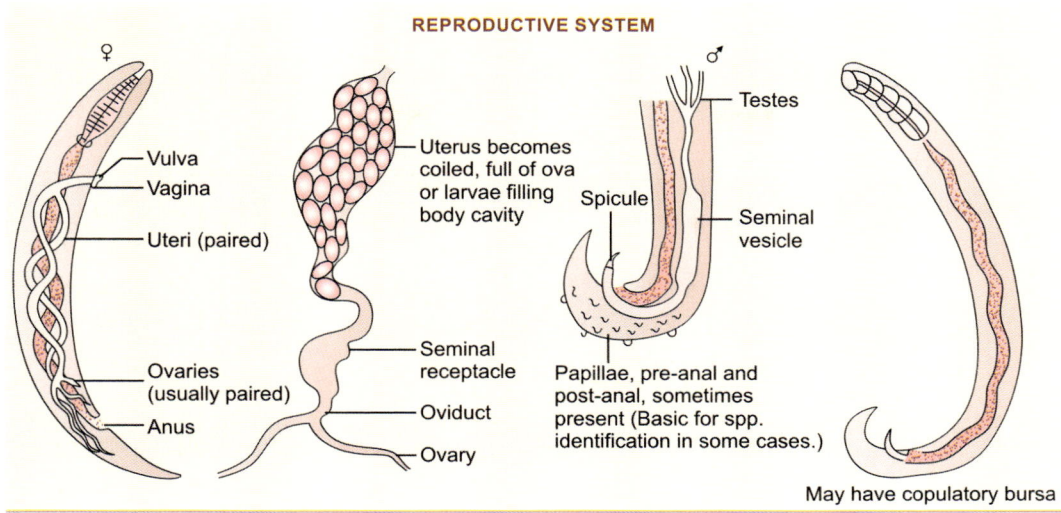

Female labels: Vulva, Vagina, Uteri (paired), Ovaries (usually paired), Anus

Uterus becomes coiled, full of ova or larvae filling body cavity

Seminal receptacle, Oviduct, Ovary

Male labels: Testes, Spicule, Seminal vesicle

Papillae, pre-anal and post-anal, sometimes present (Basic for spp. identification in some cases.)

May have copulatory bursa

Nematoda (Life cycle in general)			
A. NO INTERMEDIATE HOST REQUIRED			
Outside man	*Infection by*	*Inside man*	*Species*
Embryonated ova to environment	Ingestion	Develop to adult in intestine	*Enterobius vermicularis*
Non-embryonated ova to environment		Develop to adult in intestine	*Trichuris trichiura*
	Ingestion	Respiratory tree — Lung, Blood, Ova hatch, LARVAL CYCLE, Oesophagus, Develop to adult in intestine	*Ascaris lumbricoides* Toxocara spp. in animals Larval stage only in man
Mature in damp soil / Mature in hatch / Encyst on vegetation	Ingestion — Encysted	Develop to adult in intestine	*Trichostronglus* spp *Haemonchus contortus*
Mature and hatch in damp soil	Piercing skin	LARVAL CYCLE — Blood, Skin, Develop to adult in intestine	Hookworms, i.e. *Ancylostoma duodenate* *A. brazillense* (human strains) *Necator americanus*

Contd.

Nematoda (Life cycle in general) (*Contd.*)

Ova laid in tissues In liver	Ingestion of infected tissue	 Intestine to liver		*Capillaria hepatica*
Wall larvae to gut lumen In intestinal larvae re-enter host Infect new host Larvae to environment Become free living Larvae from free cycle	Piercing mucosa or anal skin Piercing skin Piercing skin	 LARVAL CYCLE Develop to adult in intestine		*Strongyloides stercoralis*

B. INTERMEDIATE HOST(S) REQUIRED

Outside man	Intermediate host	Infection of man by	Inside man	
Embryonated ova to environment	Ingested by beetles Larvae hatch and encyst	Ingestion of infected beetles	Intestine to buccal cavity	*Gongylonema pulchrum*
Hatch in soil	Ingested by earthworms	Ingestion of earthworms	Intestine to lungs	*Metastrongylus elongatus*
Non-embryonated ova to environment	Ingested by leech Larvae developed Ingested by	Ingestion of fish	Intestine to Renal pelvis	*Dioctophyma renale*
Mature and hatch in damp soil	Ingested by Cyclops Larvae develop Cyclops ingested by Frogs Fish Snakes	Ingestion of infected flesh	Mature in stomach wall	*Gnathostoma spinigerum* Larval stage only in man
Larviparous In blood or tissue juices	Ingested by insects Cyclical development	Bite of insect	Mature in lymph vessels subcutaneous tissue	Filarial worms *Wuchereria bancrofti* *Brugia malayi* *Loa loa* *Onchocerca volvulus*
Through skin to water	Ingested by Cyclops	Ingestion of cyclops	Retroperitoneal then subcutaneous issue	*Dracunculus medinensis*

Contd.

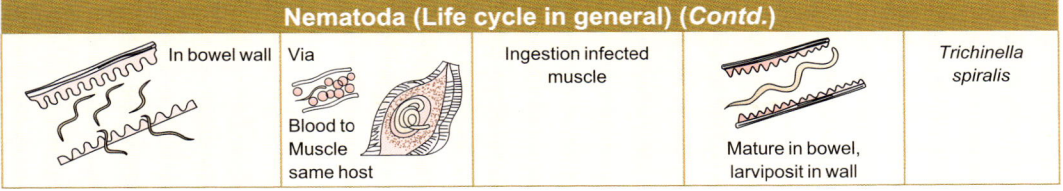

Nematoda (Life cycle in general) (*Contd.*)				
In bowel wall	Via Blood to Muscle same host	Ingestion infected muscle	Mature in bowel, larviposit in wall	*Trichinella spiralis*

C. LIFE CYCLE OBSCURE				
Outside man	*Conjectural cycle*		*Inside man and other hosts*	
Embryonated ova to environment	Beetles 2nd intermediate host	Fly	Matures in intestine / Matures in conjunctiva	*Physaloptera caucasia* / *Thelazia callipaeda*
Non-embryonated ova to environment	Matures and hatches in soil / larvae swallowed		Matures in intestine / Matures in wall of caecum then in lumen	*Ternidens deminutus* / *Oesopha-gostomun apostomum*
	Earthworm		Matures in respiratory passage	*Syngamus laryngeus*

Filariform larva: Has a rather long esophagus not proportional to the length of the larva and its posterior end does not show a bulbous dilatation.

Rhabditiform larva: Esophageal length short as compared to the larval length, posterior end shows a bulbous dilatation.

Gulbernaculum: Elevation on dorsal wall of cloaca which guides the spicule during copulation.

Spicule: Is the accessory copulatory organ, it is rod-like and protrusible.

Copulatory bursa: Is an umbrella-like cuticular expansion surrounding the cloaca of the male nematode of certain species.

TRICHINELLOIDEA

Worm body divided into a hair-like (filariform) anterior end and a stout posterior end.

Oesophagus is rudimentary and consists of a narrow channel running through a column of large cells; intestine is cellular. Females are uniovarian.

TRICHINELLA SPIRALIS

(The Trichina Worm)

Geographical distribution: Cosmopolitan, frequent in temperate climates. Common in Europe and United States. Also seen in some regions of Africa, China and Western Middle East.

Habitat: Commences as an intestinal parasite and stays buried in duodenal or jejunal mucosa (where its adult life is passed but period of stay is short). Fertilised female discharges embryos into circulation which ultimately encyst in the striated muscles of animal harboring the adult worm (pig/rat/man).

Morphology: It is amongst the smallest nematodes infecting man. Morphological features and relative sizes of male, female worms and larva are given for comparison. In male spicule and copulatory sheath are missing but there are two prominent cervical papillae on either side.

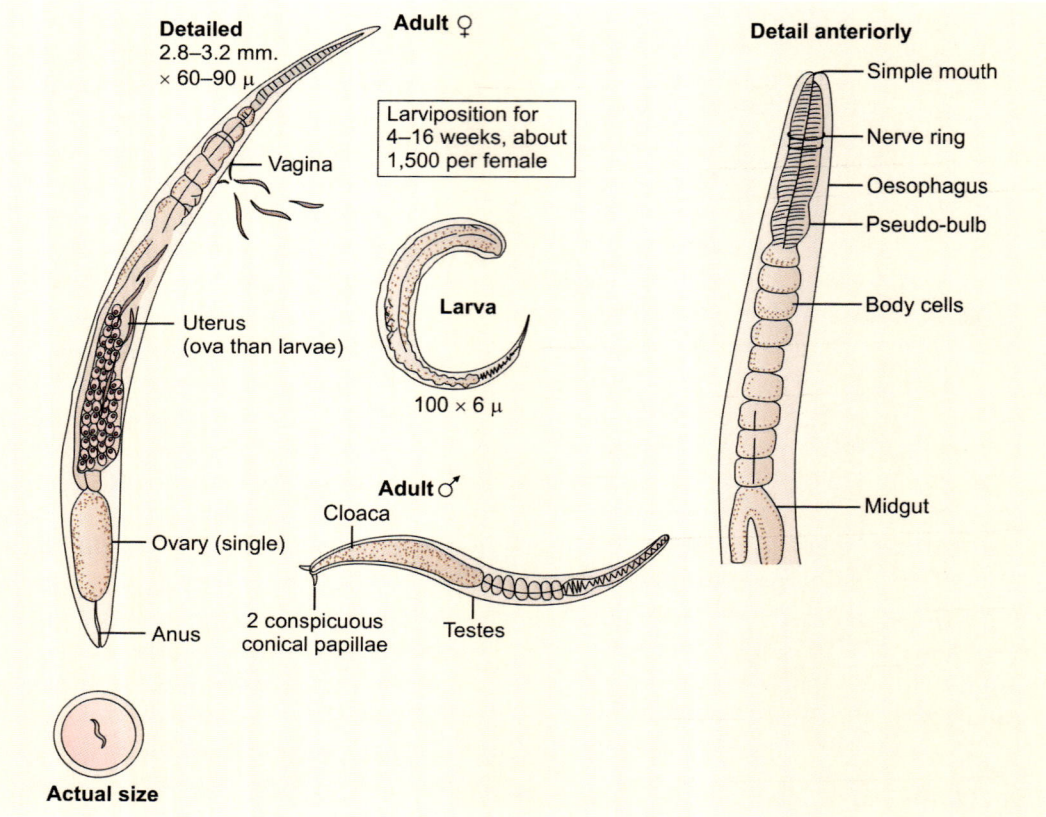

The *females* discharge embryos and not eggs (they are viviparous). *Larvae* remain encysted in the striated muscles (do not go to cardiac or involuntary muscles). Within the cyst the larva matures to sexual differentiation and increases from 100 μ to 1000 μ by 35th day. Usually a cyst shows a single larva. The long axis of the cyst capsule is parallel to that of the muscle fibre. It gets calcified by 6–18 months. Muscles most commonly involved are intercostals, diaphragm, deltoid, pectoralis major, biceps and gastrocnemius. Most encysted larvae die within 6 months, however, some may live up to 30 years.

Morphology

Trichinella spiralis

Although a single individual animal serves both as definitive and intermediate host, two hosts are needed to complete the life cycle. The parasite cannot complete its life cycle in man. Primary host of *T.spiralis* in pig which serves as the reservoir host for man. Infection normally passes from pig to pig and rat, and from rat to rat. Infection of a new host is brought about by ingestion of raw flesh of the trichinosed animal containing the viable encysted larvae.

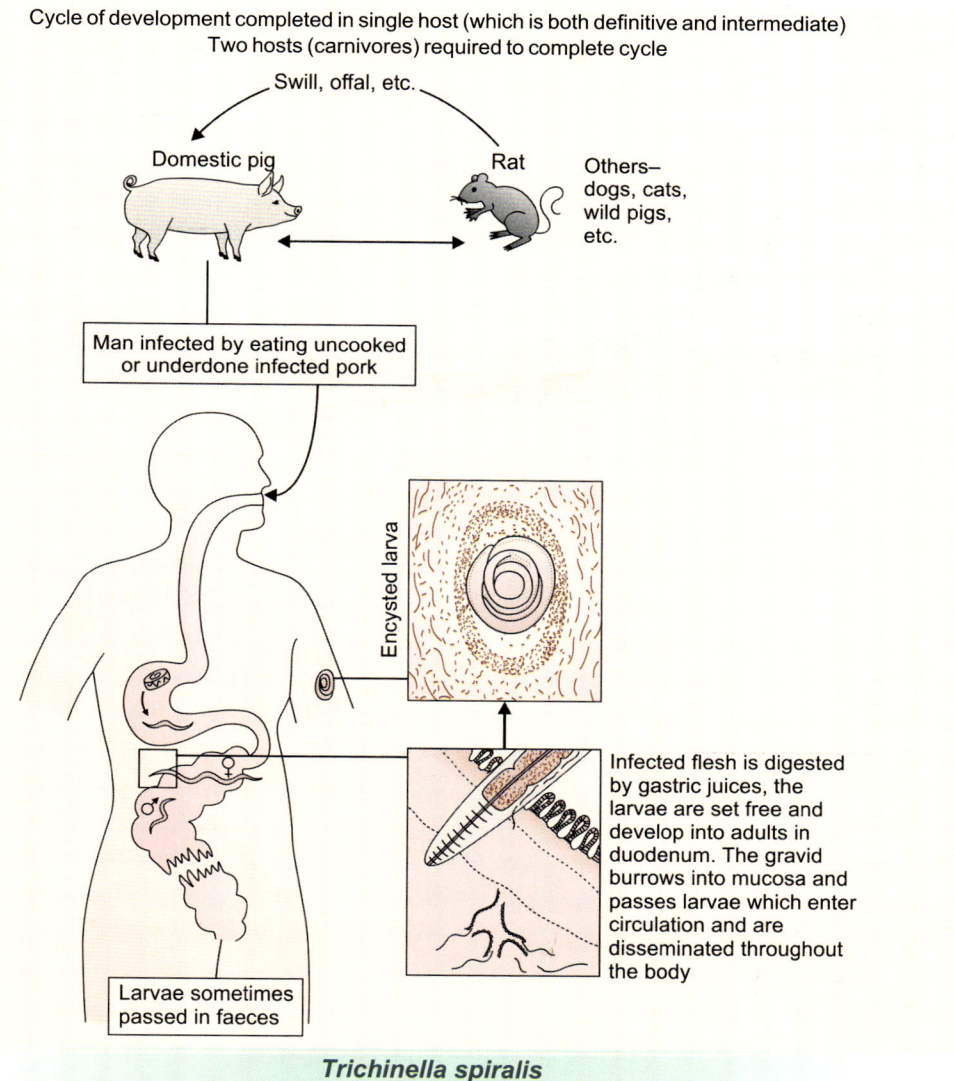

Cycle of development completed in single host (which is both definitive and intermediate)
Two hosts (carnivores) required to complete cycle

Swill, offal, etc.

Domestic pig

Rat

Others—
dogs, cats,
wild pigs,
etc.

Man infected by eating uncooked
or underdone infected pork

Encysted larva

Infected flesh is digested
by gastric juices, the
larvae are set free and
develop into adults in
duodenum. The gravid
burrows into mucosa and
passes larvae which enter
circulation and are
disseminated throughout
the body

Larvae sometimes
passed in faeces

Trichinella spiralis

The subsequent course is:
Trichinella larvae remaining encysted in rat's muscle are consumed by a healthy rat.
↓

Post-ingestion, male and female larvae within 48 hours develop into adults. After fertilisation the larvae are liberated 24 hours later.
↓

Larvae reach blood circulation and finally get deposited in muscles. Further maturation into adult worms occurs only if they are taken up by another rat or pig.

$\downarrow$

A similar process is repeated when they are consumed by a pig.

$\downarrow$

Infected pig's muscle are eaten by man. Larvae are released in the duodenum/jejunum, become adults and mature sexually in about a weeks time. The male dies after fertilising the female. Fertilised female burrows deep into intestinal mucosa and a thousand or more larvae are discharged into lymphatic or vascular channels, this continues for 1 to 4 months. Subsequently the female also dies after discharging the larvae. The larvae finally settle down in striated muscles at which point the cycle ends in man.

Immunity: Both CMI and humoral immunities come into play. Immunised mice when exposed to an infection eliminate the adult worms by CMI. Humoral antibodies, however, are not protective but are useful for serological diagnostic techniques. Serum IgE is markedly increased.

Pathology

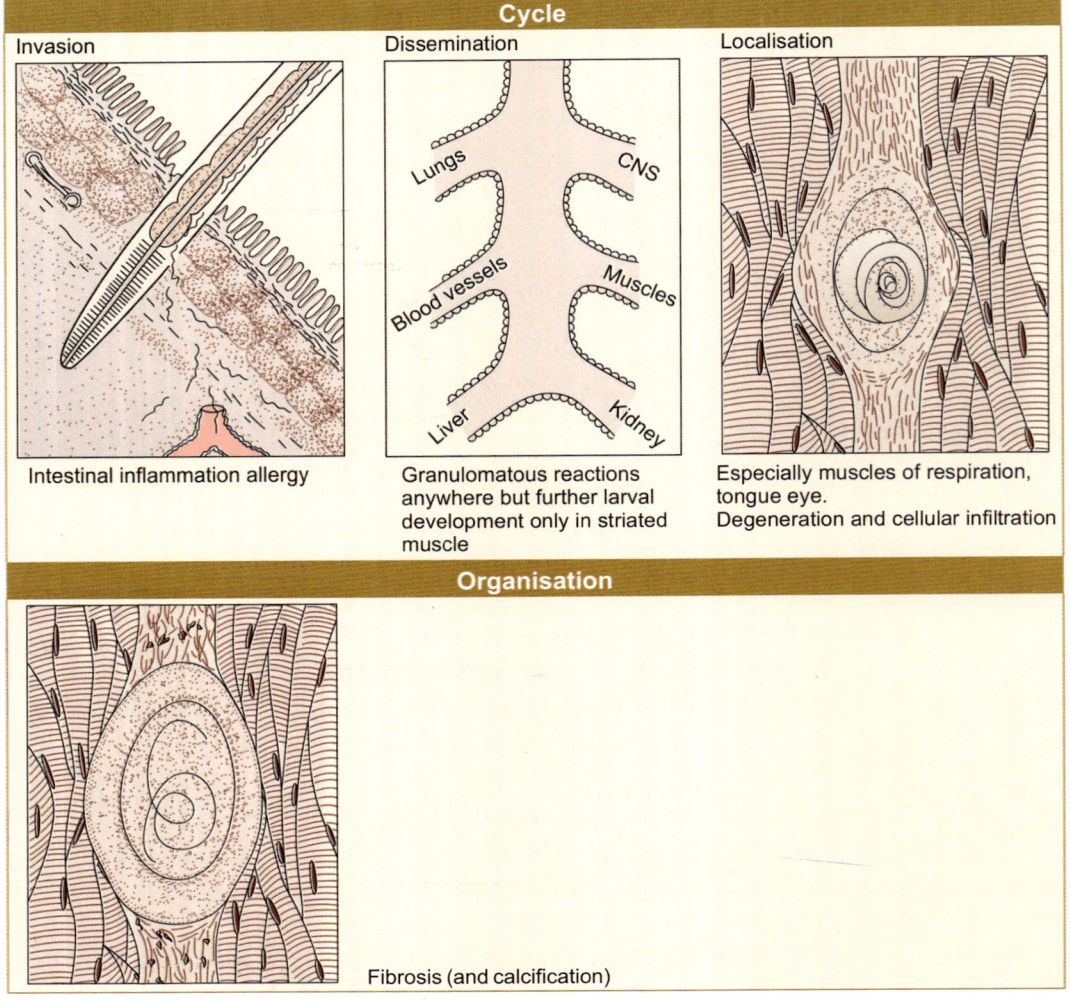

Cycle

Invasion

Intestinal inflammation allergy

Dissemination

Lungs   CNS
Blood vessels   Muscles
Liver   Kidney

Granulomatous reactions anywhere but further larval development only in striated muscle

Localisation

Especially muscles of respiration, tongue eye.
Degeneration and cellular infiltration

Organisation

Fibrosis (and calcification)

Diagnosis: Most certain diagnosis is demonstration of larvae in muscles obtained either from biopsy or autopsy.

1. **During diarrhoeal stages**—adult worms/larvae in stool are rarely found.
2. **Eosinophilia in blood**—moderate to severe.
3. **Serological tests**—CFT, precipitin and bentonite flocculation test. Latex agglutination test and ELISA techniques can also be used. After about 7 weeks of infection—fluorescent antibody technique test can also be used.
4. **Muscle biopsy**—by third or fourth week of infection. Ideal sites for biopsy are tendinous insertions of deltoid or gastrocnemius muscle.
5. **Skin test**—intradermal injection of 0.1 ml of 1 : 10,000 dilution of Bachman's antigen (prepared from trichinella larvae obtained from infected rabbit's muscle) bring about an immediate (15–20 minutes) erythematous patch. The test remains positive for one to two decades.
6. **X-rays** can reveal calcified cysts.

Treatment: Thiabendazole has been found to be useful. Clinical symptoms can be reduced by administering corticosteroids.

Prophylaxis: Careful selection of pigs at slaughter houses and avoiding eating raw or ill-cooked pork.

Trichuris trichiura (Whipworm)

(Also known as *Trichocephalus trichiura*)

Historical: Commonly known as whipworm, was first identified by Linnaeus in 1771 and later by Stiles in 1901.

Geographical distribution: Worldwide, commoner in moist regions.

Habitat: Adult worm lives in colon, especially the caecum and also in the appendix.

Morphology: Adult worm looks like a whip with anterior 3/5 hairy and thin and posterior 2/5 thick and stout. Almost the complete anterior part lies embedded in the colonic mucosa. The anterior part is just a long esophagus lined by a single layer of large secretory cells. The thicker posterior portion contains the rest of the GI tract and sexual organs.

Morphology

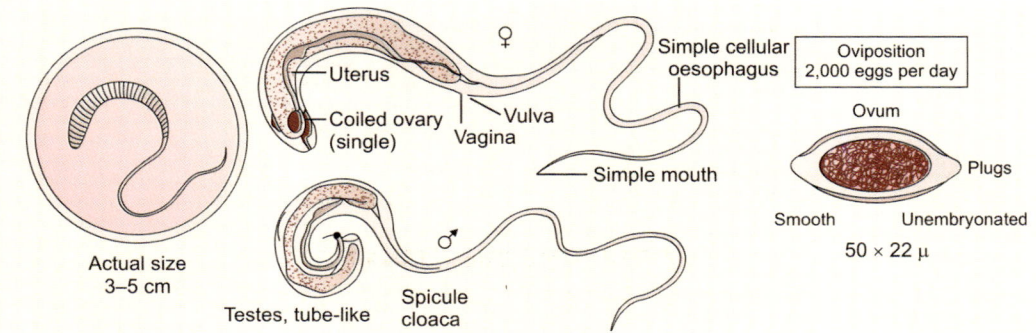

Male: Male is 3–4 cm with a ventrally coiled caudal end.

Female: Female is 4–5 cm long and the caudal extremity is comma shaped. They are oviparous. Eggs measure 50 × 25 μ, are bile stained (brownish) with a double shell, shaped like a barrel with a mucous plug at each pole. On leaving the human body it contains an unsegmented ovum and it floats in a saturated solution of common salt (sodium chloride).

Worm passes its complete life cycle in a single host—man. No intermediate host needed. However, a change of host is necessary for propagation of species. With defaecation eggs come out and develop gradually in moist earth or in water. In tropical climates a rhabditiform larva develops within a months time (whereas in temperate climates it may take 6–12 months). These embryonated eggs are infective to man when ingested. Shell gets digested and a larva comes out through either pole and gets localised in caecum. They get embedded in colonic mucosa and become sexually mature in about a month and the gravid female starts laying eggs—the cycle is then repeated.

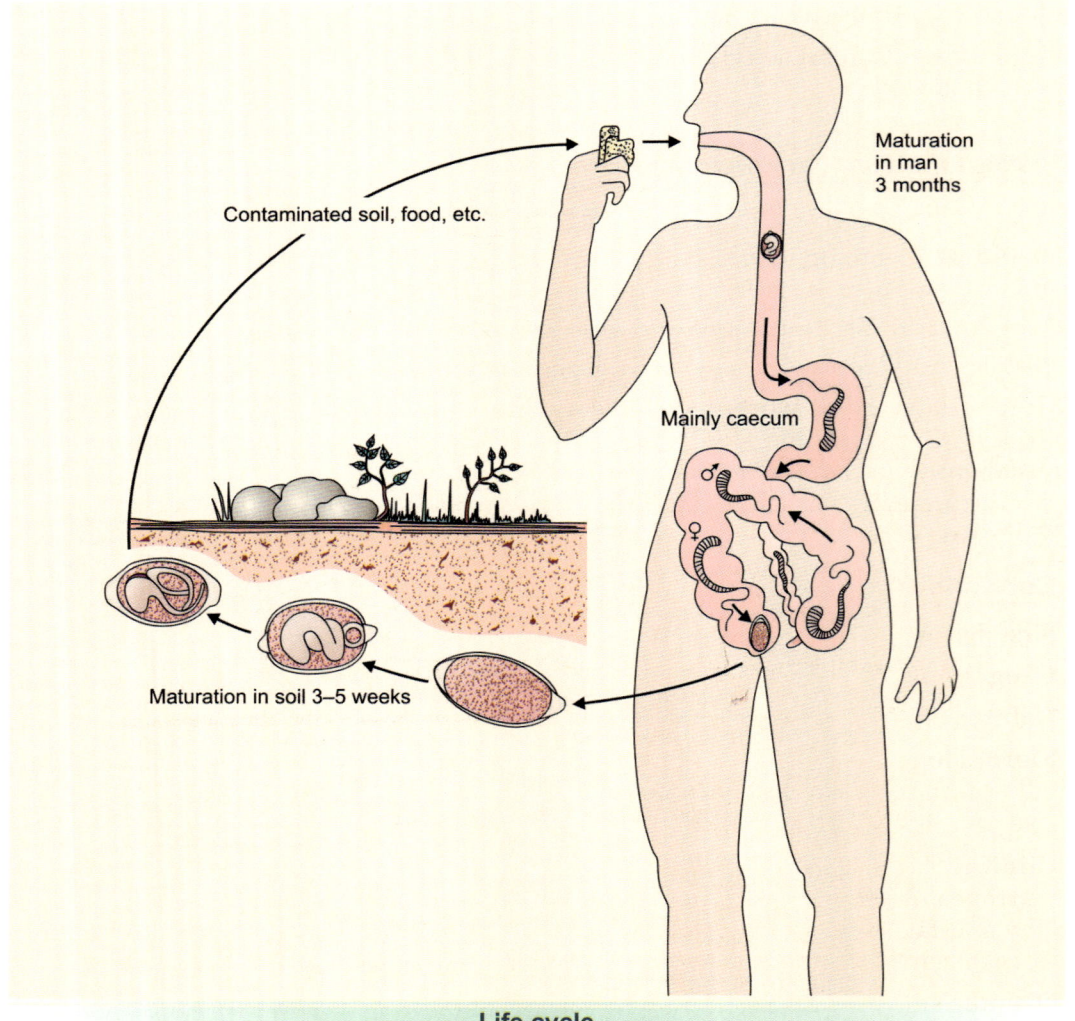

Contaminated soil, food, etc.

Maturation
in man
3 months

Mainly caecum

Maturation in soil 3–5 weeks

Life cycle

Pathology: Generally there are no effects, however, in the appendix they may simulate symptoms of acute appendicitis. Very heavy infection leads to local inflammation causing abdominal discomfort and diarrhoea.

Diagnosis: Blood may show eosinophilia up to 25%. Ova are seen in the stools. Sometimes adult worms may be seen in the stool.

Treatment: Drugs available are stilbazium iodide, difetarsone, thiabendazole, meben-dazole, pyrantel and albendazole.

Prophylaxis: Includes proper disposal of night-soil and prevention of consumption of raw and uncooked vegetables and fruits.

Capillaria hepatica

(The capillary liver worm)

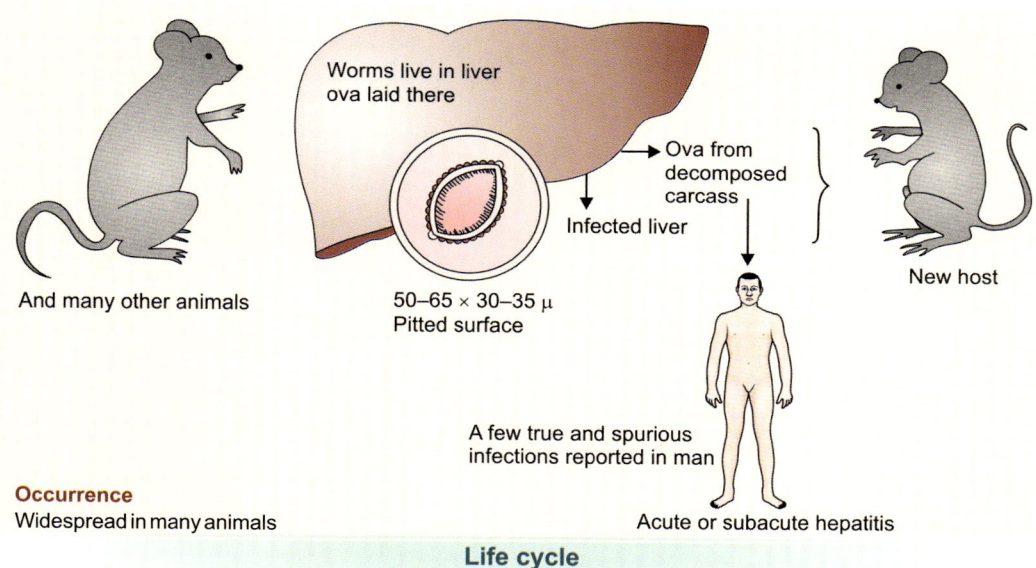

Worms live in liver ova laid there

Ova from decomposed carcass

Infected liver

50–65 × 30–35 µ
Pitted surface

New host

And many other animals

A few true and spurious infections reported in man

Acute or subacute hepatitis

Occurrence
Widespread in many animals

Life cycle

Capillaria philippinensis

First discovered in Philippines by Chitwood in 1968.

Geographical distribution: Reported chiefly from Northern Philippines.

Habitat: Small intestine, especially jejunum.

Morphology: Dimensions—2–4 mm × 0.03–0.04 mm. Eggs resemble *T.trichiura* eggs but are smaller, more oval with flattened and less prominent bipolar mucous plugs. Life cycle is not clearly understood.

Clinical: Patient gets colicky abdominal pain, borborgymi and chronic watery diarrhoea, muscle wasting and oedema. These result from protein-losing enterop-athy and fat and sugar malabsorption. There is increased fat excretion. There is also hypokalaemia and hypocalcemia.

Diagnosis: Is established by demonstration of eggs in the stool. Adults and larvae may also be detected in stool. Jejunal biopsy might show embedded worms in mucosa.

Treatment: Usual drugs thiabendazole, albendazole, etc. can be given for prolonged periods.

Capillaria hepatica involves liver and diagnosis can be established by finding Trichuris-like eggs encapsulated in the liver.

Other Aphasmid Nematodes of Lesser Importance

Mermithid worms (including cabbage snakes)

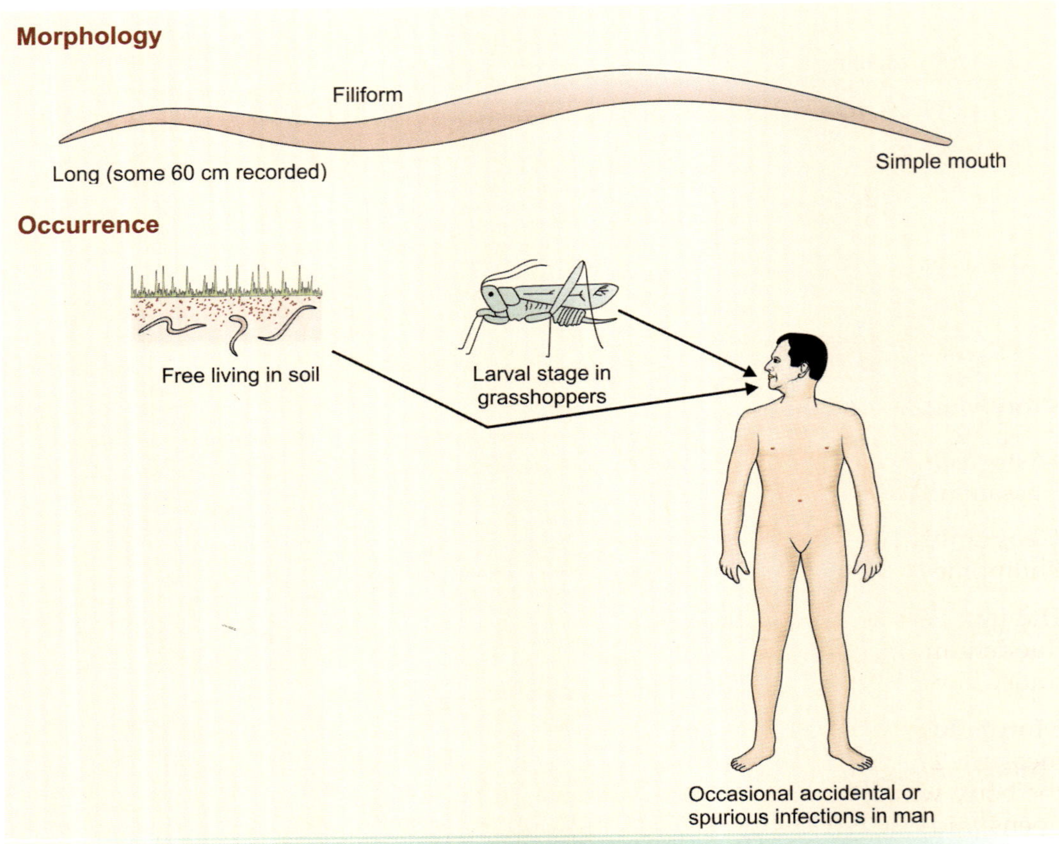

Morphology

Filiform

Long (some 60 cm recorded)

Simple mouth

Occurrence

Free living in soil

Larval stage in grasshoppers

Occasional accidental or spurious infections in man

Mermithid worms

Dioctophyma renale (The giant kidney worm)

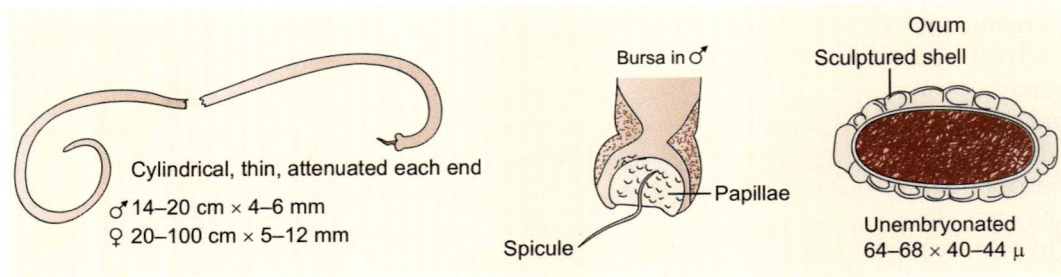

Cylindrical, thin, attenuated each end

♂ 14–20 cm × 4–6 mm
♀ 20–100 cm × 5–12 mm

Bursa in ♂

Papillae

Spicule

Ovum
Sculptured shell

Unembryonated
64–68 × 40–44 μ

Life Cycle

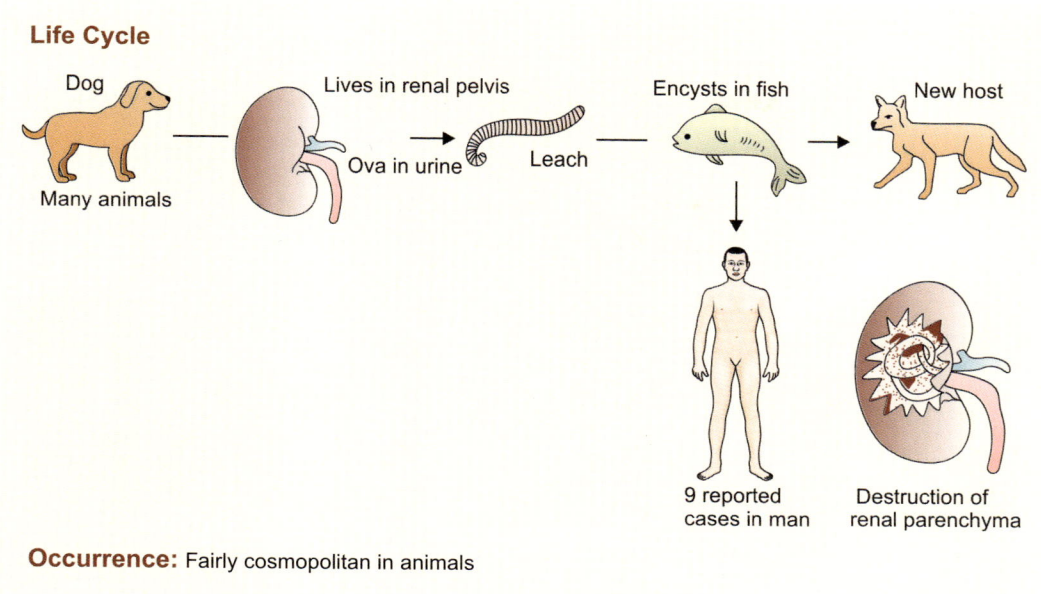

Dog — Many animals — Lives in renal pelvis — Ova in urine — Leach — Encysts in fish — New host — 9 reported cases in man — Destruction of renal parenchyma

Occurrence: Fairly cosmopolitan in animals

Dioctophyma renale

Strongyloides stercoralis

Historical: First detected by Bavay in 1876 and later demonstrated by Stiles and Hassall in 1902.

Geographical distribution: Cosmopolitan. Common in Far East (Cambodia and Philippines), Africa and Brazil.

Habitat: Female parasites live in the mucosa of small intestine, particularly in the duodenum and jejunum. At post-mortem by scraping mucosa, one can show parasites under low-power magnification of the microscope.

Morphology: Males are less easily distinguished in parasitism. The *parasitic females* measure 2.5 mm x 40–50 μ. The cylindrical oesophagus occupies anterior third of the body while the intestine extends through the posterior two-thirds and the anus opens mid-ventrally, a little before the caudal end. The posterior tip is pointed and the vulval opening is found at the junction of middle and posterior thirds of the body. Paired genitalia are attached at right angles to the vulva and disposed anteriorly and posteriorly (one set each). Females are ovo-viviparans. The *parasitic males* are shorter and broader as compared to the females. They lack penetrating capacity and stay parasitic in the bowel-lumen. *Eggs* lie anteroposteriorly in a single row (5–10 eggs in each uterus) and measure 55 × 30 μ are thin shelled, transparent and oval. They contain ready to hatch larvae and as soon as they are laid, the rhabditiform larvae emerge and wriggle their way out of the mucosa to be ultimately passed out with the faeces. The *rhabditiform larvae* seen in the bowel lumen, have a short mouth and double-bulb oesophagus. While in the lumen they are metamorphosed into filariform larvae which may penetrate the peri-anal or perineal skin, thus providing a source of auto-infection (hyperinfection).

Morphology

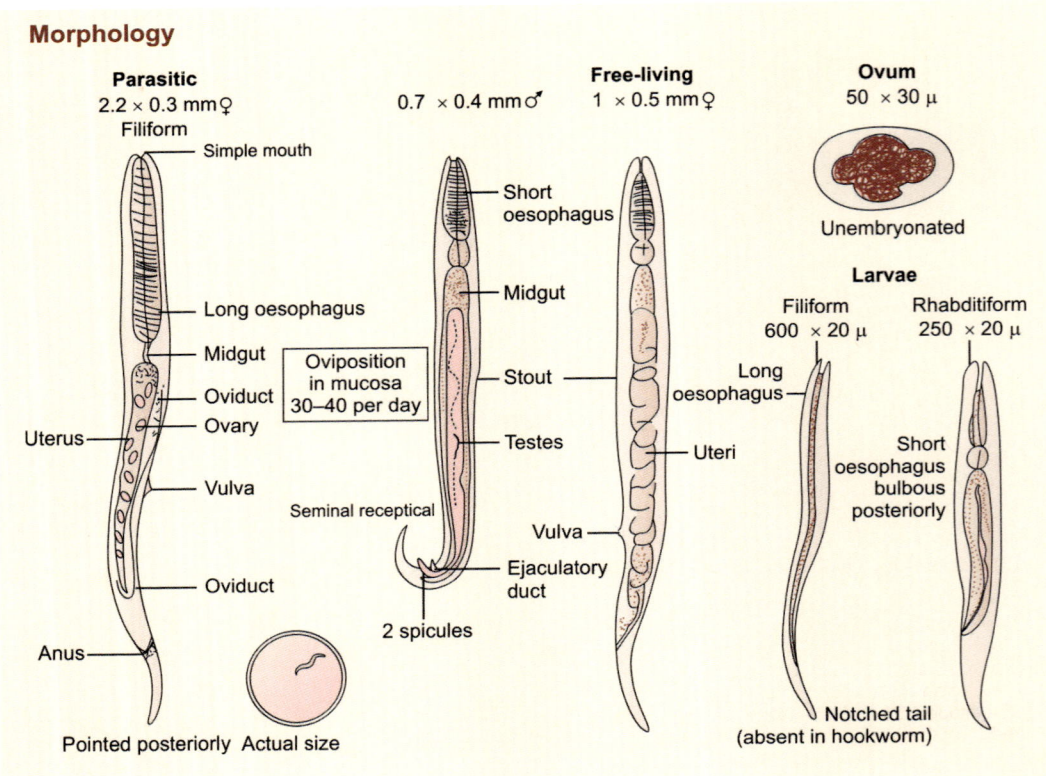

Parasitic
2.2 × 0.3 mm♀
Filiform
— Simple mouth
— Long oesophagus
— Midgut
— Oviduct
— Ovary
Uterus—
— Vulva
       Oviposition
       in mucosa
       30–40 per day
— Oviduct
Anus—
Pointed posteriorly Actual size

Free-living
0.7 × 0.4 mm♂   1 × 0.5 mm♀
— Short oesophagus
— Midgut
— Stout
— Testes
Seminal receptical
— Ejaculatory duct
2 spicules
Long oesophagus —
— Uteri
Vulva —

Ovum
50 × 30 μ
Unembryonated

Larvae
Filiform   Rhabditiform
600 × 20 μ   250 × 20 μ
Long oesophagus —
Short oesophagus bulbous posteriorly
Notched tail
(absent in hookworm)

This explains the heavy worm-load in some individuals and their persistence even 2–3 decades after the person has left the endemic region. The rhabditiform larvae may be expelled with the faeces and may undergo development in the soil: Direct (host-soil-host) or Indirect cycle. In the *indirect (heterogenetic) development*— the rhabditiform larvae mature in 24–30 hours into free-living sexual generations (males = 0.7 mm and females = 1 mm). Copulation between these produces a second generation of rhabditiform larvae. In 3–4 days' time they are transformed into filariform larvae. Each original pair of rhabditiform larvae produces 30 second generation 30 filariform larvae. *Direct development* involves maturation of rhabditiform larvae into filariform ones in 3–4 days' time (the sexual phase here is omitted). So here one rhabditiform larva produces a single filariform larva only. *Filariform larvae* are thinner and larger than rhabditiform ones. They possess short mouths and cylindrical oesophagus. They constitute the infective stage and enter the body through the skin as do the ancylostomes.

Strongyloides infected patients if put on steroids develop severe strongyloidiasis (hyperinfection syndrome) which may turn fatal. Secondary bacterial infection may lead to Gram-negative bacteriaemia.

The females may sometimes enter the bronchial columnar epithelium, where they deposit ova but most of the females, however, pass up the respiratory tract to enter the GI tract. Fertilisation (rarely occurs in respiratory tract) may take place in bronchi or trachea.

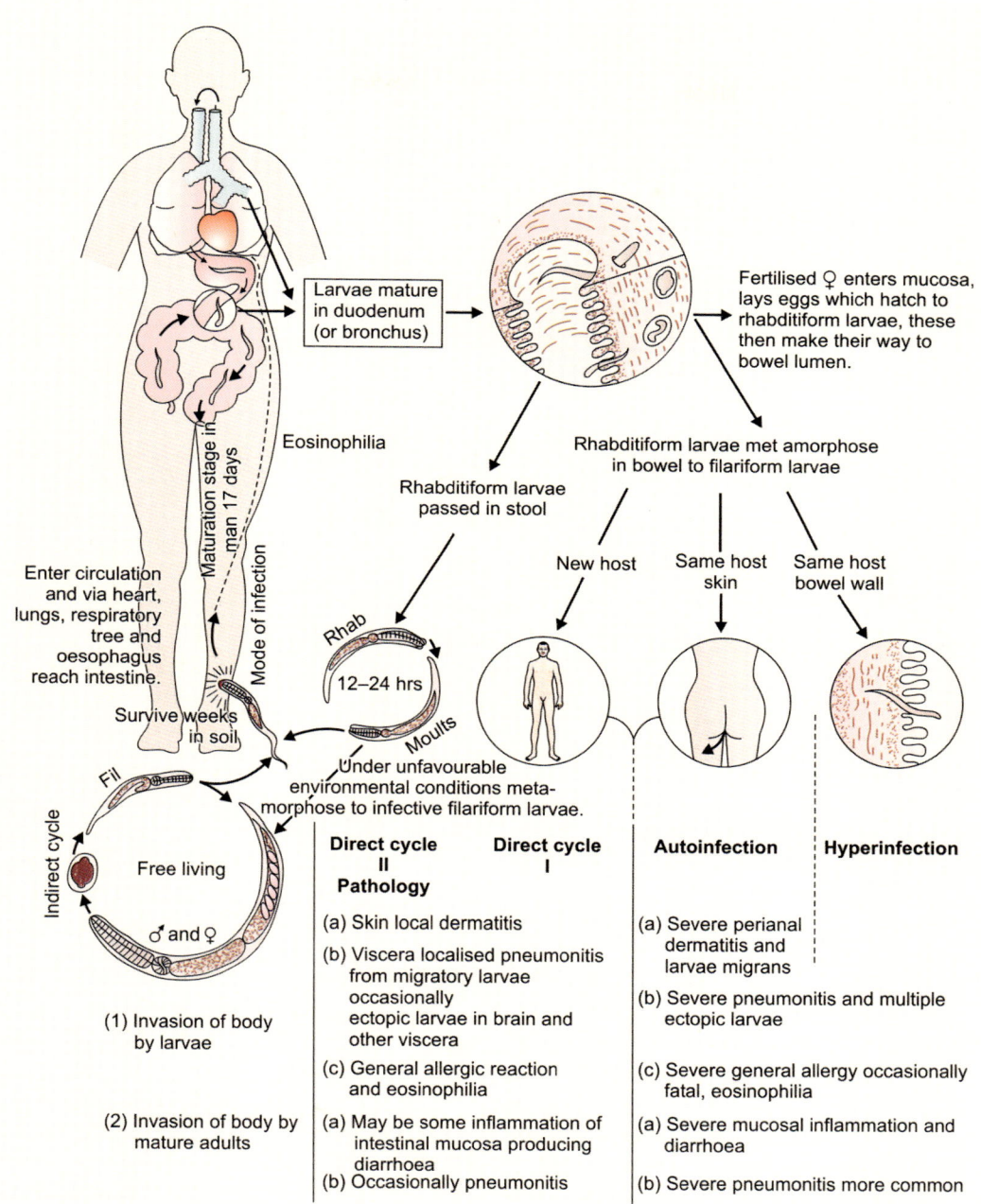

Larvae mature in duodenum (or bronchus)

Fertilised ♀ enters mucosa, lays eggs which hatch to rhabditiform larvae, these then make their way to bowel lumen.

Eosinophilia

Rhabditiform larvae met amorphose in bowel to filariform larvae

Rhabditiform larvae passed in stool

New host   Same host skin   Same host bowel wall

Enter circulation and via heart, lungs, respiratory tree and oesophagus reach intestine.

Maturation stage in man 17 days

Mode of infection

Survive weeks in soil

Rhab

12–24 hrs

Moults

Under unfavourable environmental conditions meta-morphose to infective filariform larvae.

Fil

Indirect cycle

Free living

♂ and ♀

(1) Invasion of body by larvae

(2) Invasion of body by mature adults

Direct cycle II
Pathology

(a) Skin local dermatitis
(b) Viscera localised pneumonitis from migratory larvae occasionally ectopic larvae in brain and other viscera
(c) General allergic reaction and eosinophilia

(a) May be some inflammation of intestinal mucosa producing diarrhoea
(b) Occasionally pneumonitis

Direct cycle I

Autoinfection

(a) Severe perianal dermatitis and larvae migrans
(b) Severe pneumonitis and multiple ectopic larvae
(c) Severe general allergy occasionally fatal, eosinophilia

(a) Severe mucosal inflammation and diarrhoea
(b) Severe pneumonitis more common

Hyperinfection

Life cycle and pathology

Diagnosis: Is established by demonstrating typical rhabditiform larvae in freshly evacuated stool. There is eosinophilia in peripheral blood. In pulmonary infections rhabditiform larvae may be seen in sputum. Duodenal/jejunal washings or biopsies may reveal larvae of *S. stercoralis*. Over 3/4th cases show a positive filarial complement fixation test (CFT).

Treatment: Specific anthelmintic for strongyloidiasis is thiabendazole.

Prophylaxis

(i) **Attack on adult parasite:** Anthelmintic treatment of carriers and diseased individuals.

(ii) **Attack on larvae:** Proper sewage disposal. Dis-infection of faeces or soil.

(iii) **Personal protection:** Wearing boots and gloves.

STRONGYLOIDEA

(Superfamily)

Superfamily	Family	Subfamily	Features	Genus species
Strongyloidea	Ancylostomatidae (Have teeth or cutting plates in the mouth cavity)	Ancylosto-matinae (Tooth-like processes)	Two pairs of teeth	Ancylostoma duodenale
			One pair of teeth	Ancylostoma brazilense
			Three pairs of teeth	Ancylostoma caninum
		Uncinariinae (Cutting plates)	Cutting plates	Necator americanus
	Strongyloidea			Oesopha-gostomum apiostomum
	No teeth or cutting plates			Ternidens deminutus

These organisms possess a well-developed buccal capsule or mouth cavity that may contain teeth or cutting organs. Males possess bursa copulatrix that surrounds the cloaca. The eggs have a transparent shell and are hatched in a segmented condition. The larva develops in moist soil.

Ancylostoma Duodenale

(Old World Hookworm)

Historical: First detected by Agelo Dubini in 1838. Portal of entry and pathogenesis were first described by Looss in 1898.

Geographical distribution: Widely distributed in tropical and subtropical countries, i.e. occurs in regions where humidity and temperature are appropriate for the development of larvae in the soil. It is found in India (especially Punjab and Uttar Pradesh), Sri Lanka, Central and North China, North Africa (especially Egypt), Southern Europe, Pacific Islands and Southern States of America.

Habitat: Small intestine, particularly in jejunum and less often in duodenum and rarely in ileum.

Morphology

Adult worm: When freshly passed are reddish brown due to ingested blood. Otherwise they are greyish white, small and cylindrical. Anterior end is bent and hence the name hookworm. The bend is in line with the body curvature. Oral aperture is not terminal but directed towards the dorsal surface. The buccal capsule is lined with a hard substance and six teeth, of which four are hook-like on the ventral surface and two are knob-like on the dorsal surface. There are 5 glands connected with the digestive system; one of them labelled as oesophageal gland secretes an anti-clotting substance. The sexes are easily differentiated.

	Male	*Female*
Size	Length = 8 mm	Length = 12.5 mm
Posterior end	Shows copulatory bursa. Expanded umbrella-like	No bursa, tapering end
Genital opening	Opens with cloaca posteriorly	Opens at the junction of posterior and middle third of the body

The life span of an adult worm is 3–4 years.

Eggs: Oval or elliptical, 60 × 40 μ, colourless, surrounded by a transparent hyaline shell-membrane, contain a segmented ovum with 4 blastomeres; has a clear space between the egg-shell and ovum. It floats in saturated solution of common salt. Eggs are initially unsegmented but develop segmentation as they pass through the bowel. These eggs are not infective to man.

Immunology: Complete immunity may develop as a result of successive small infections. In endemic regions most individuals suffer from minimal intestinal infection without any significant symptoms. A heavy infection with anaemia symptoms may result from lack of immunity.

Life cycle: Man is the only definitive host for *A. duodenale* and no intermediate host is necessary. Various life cycle stages are:

The segmented ova are passed out with faeces

Each egg produces a rhabditiform larva (250 μ) which hatches out in 48 hours. It then moults on 3rd and 5th days to develop into a filariform larva (600–700 μ) which is infective to man. It takes 8–10 days time to reach this stage after laying down of eggs.

The filariform larvae shed off their sheaths and penetrate the skin of a new host.

Having entered the skin they reach the subcutaneous lymphatics or small venules to reach the venous circulation and via the right heart reach the pulmonary capillaries where they break through the capillary wall to enter the alveolar spaces and migrate via bronchi, trachea, larynx and epiglottis to the back of the pharynx to be ultimately swallowed. During this migratory phase or on entering the oesophagus, a third moulting occurs and a terminal buccal capsule is formed. This migratory phase lasts for about 10 days.

The growing larvae settle in small intestine and undergo a final fourth moulting to mature into adolescent worms, the definite buccal capsule is formed (replacing the provisional toothless buccal capsule). In about a months' time they mature sexually and the fertilised females start laying eggs that are evacuated with the faeces. The cycle is repeated. Time lapse between skin penetration and egg appearance in faeces is about 6 weeks.

Pathology and Clinical Features

Chief feature of ancylostomiasis is iron deficiency anaemia.

Mode of infection: Portal of entry is skin especially:
  (a) the thin skin between the toes,
  (b) dorsum of the feet, and
  (c) the inner side of soles.

Any thin part of skin can be penetrated. Skin over hands may serve as entry portal in gardeners and miners. Very rarely drinking water contaminated with filariform larvae may cause hookworm infection.

Pathogenic Effects

Caused by Ancylostoma larvae

  A. **Ground itch or dermatitis:** Occurs at entry site. Common with Necator than with Ancylostoma and disappears in less than 15 days' time. Subsequent general symptoms appear 2–4 months later.
  B. **Creeping eruption:** As the larvae wander about (may do so for weeks, months or up to 2 years), they produce reddish itchy papule along the path (called larva migrans). Noted more so with *A. braziliense* and *A. caninum*. The filaform larvae of non-human hookworms hardly ever penetrate below the stratum germinativum of human skin. The larvae migrate between the corium and stratum granulosum in tunnels at the rate of 1–2 cm/day. Migration persists for months till the larva dies. Larvae of *S. stercoralis* move faster 3–4 cm/day.
  C. **Pulmonary lesions:** Bronchitis and broncho-pneumonia may occur associated with marked eosinophilia.

Effects caused by adult worms

By using the strong buccal capsule they attach usually to the jejunal mucosa. As time passes microcytic hypochromic anaemia gradually develops which may be very severe. This occurs on account of blood sucking by the worm and certain other factors:
  (i) **Chronic blood loss:** Occurs due to blood ingestion by parasites and haemorrhages from the puncture sites. *A. duodenale* sucks up more blood (0.2 ml/day) than *N. americanus* (0.03 ml/day).
  (ii) **Nutritional defects:** Deficiency of iron or other haematopoietic vitamins is usually associated with hookworm infections. So one can get microcytic hypochromic or macrocytic or a dimorphic anaemia.

Clinical Features of Hookworm Associated Anaemia

  A. **Gastrointestinal manifestations:** Dyspepsia, epigastric tenderness may simulate duodenal ulcer. Pica or geophagy may also be associated. Acid secretion is diminished (hypoacidity and not achlorhydria is usually seen). There is associated constipation, sometimes there may be steatorrhoea (fatty diarrhoea the cause of which cannot be explained).
  B. **Symptoms related to anaemia:** Skin takes up a sallow colour; mucous membranes of eyes, lips and tongue show extreme pallor. Face appears puffy with oedema

in the lower eyelids, feet and ankle. Koilonychia is frequent. Patient appears pale plumpy with a protruding abdomen and dry lustreless hair. Cardiovascular effects include hyperkinetic circulatory state that ultimately leads to circulatory failure. In children growth may be hampered and stunted.

Laboratory Diagnosis

Direct methods

A. **Stool examination**—may find adult worms. Microscopic examination will reveal eggs. Concentration method may be necessitated. Intensity of hookworm infection can be assessed by egg-counting methods.
B. **Duodenal content examination**—aspiration of duodenal contents may reveal eggs or adult worms.

Indirect methods

A. **Blood**—shows anaemia and eosinophilia.
B. **Stool**—occult blood test is usually positive. Charcot-Leyden crystals are often found in the stool.

Differentiation between Ancylostoma or Necator cannot be made by looking at the eggs. Distinction can be made by studying the morphology of adult worms and the mature infective filariform larvae.

Treatment: Includes removal of worms and treatment of anaemia. Specific anthelmintic treatment should not be commenced if haemoglobin level is 30% less than the normal. Various anthelmintics that can be used are tetrachloroethylene (more specific against *N.americanus),* bephenium hydroxynaphthoate (more specific against *A. duodenale),* thiabendazole, tetramisole, pyrantel pamoate, mebendazole and alben-dazole or combinations thereof. For mixed infections combination drugs or broad-spectrum anthelmintics should be used. If associated with anaemia, appropriate haematinics should also be added after assessing the type of anaemia.

Prophylaxis: Is identical to that for *S. stercoralis.*

Necater americanus

(American hookworm on new world hookworm)

Geographical distribution: First discovered in America (most likely of African origin though), it has spread to India, Far East, Australia and is found in America too. It is the commonest species found in India (except in Punjab and Uttar Pradesh) and Sri Lanka. Barring the morphological features (specific details), the pathogenicity, diagnosis and treatment are identical to those for *Ancylostoma duodenale.*

The differentiating features are given diagrammatically in the Figure as follows.

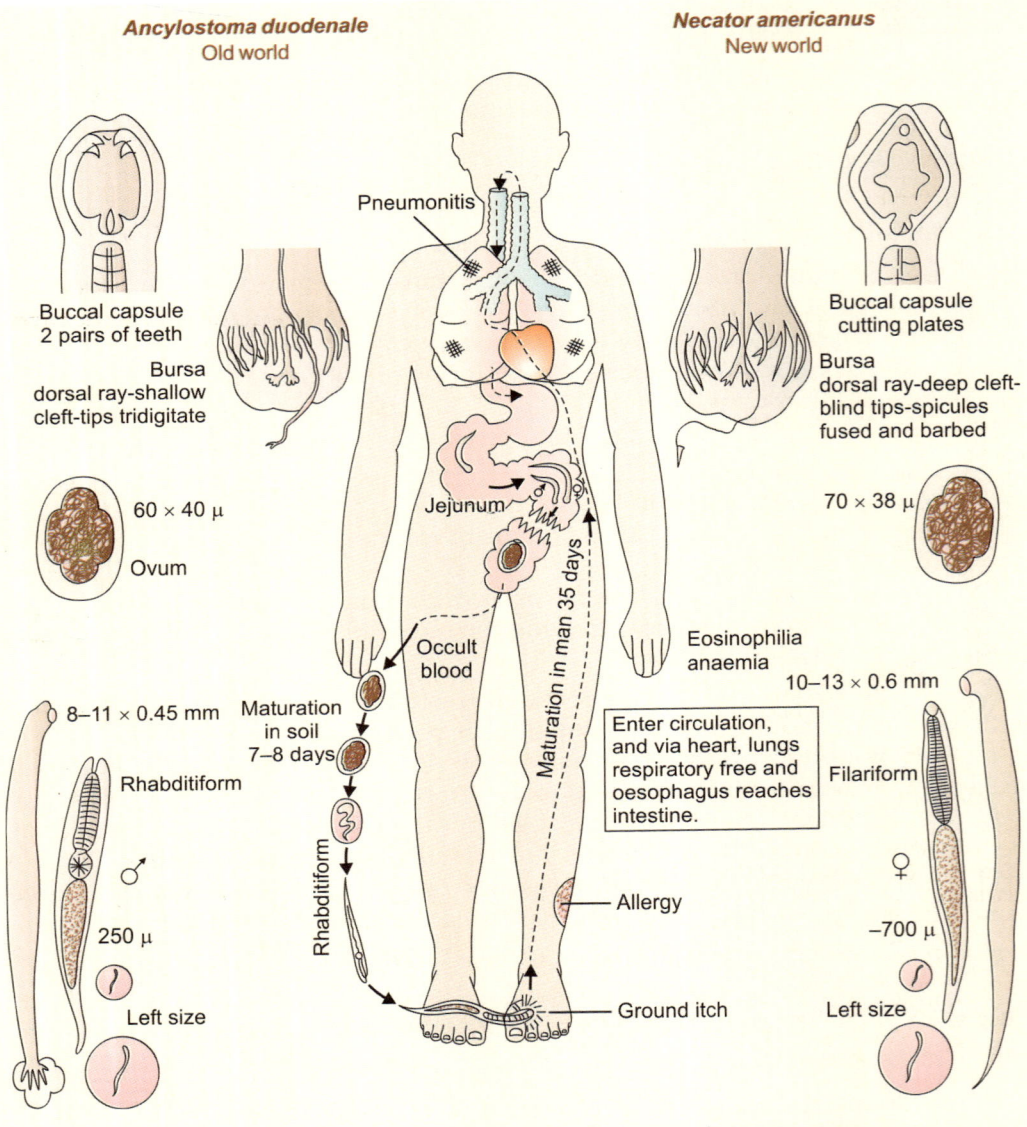

Ancylostoma duodenale
Old world

Buccal capsule
2 pairs of teeth

Bursa
dorsal ray-shallow
cleft-tips tridigitate

60 × 40 μ

Ovum

8–11 × 0.45 mm

Maturation
in soil
7–8 days

Rhabditiform

♂

250 μ

Left size

Necator americanus
New world

Buccal capsule
cutting plates

Bursa
dorsal ray-deep cleft-
blind tips-spicules
fused and barbed

70 × 38 μ

Eosinophilia
anaemia

10–13 × 0.6 mm

Filariform

♀

−700 μ

Left size

Pneumonitis

Jejunum

Occult
blood

Maturation in man 35 days

Rhabditiform

Enter circulation,
and via heart, lungs
respiratory free and
oesophagus reaches
intestine.

Allergy

Ground itch

Geographical distribution
Europe - N. Africa - India - S.E. Asia

Geographical distribution
USA - Central America-Central & SW Africa-Oceania-SE
Asia

CYCLE AND PATHOLOGY IN MAN

1. **Infection:** General allergic reactions—ground itch—cutaneous larva migrans in non-human ancylostomes.

2. **Migration:** Long involvement—localised pneumonitis—eosinophilia-allergy

3. Localisation in jejunum—ingestion of blood by parasites—occult bleeding from intestinal mucosa—anaemia
(and sequelae)

LABORATORY DIAGNOSIS Ova in stools

HOOKWORMS

GENERAL MORPHOLOGY

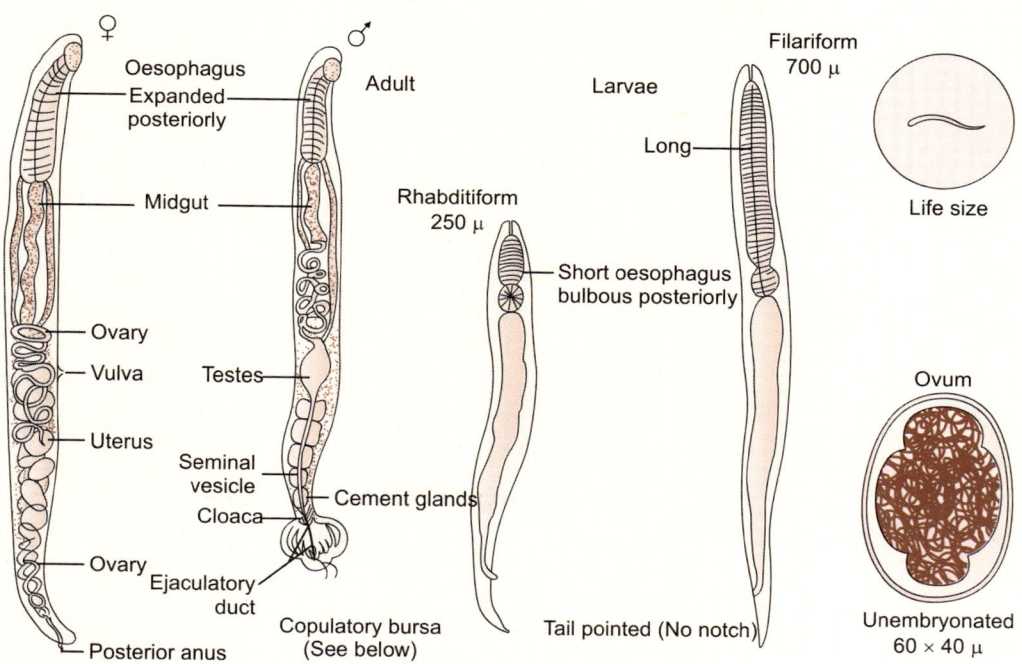

♀
Oesophagus
Expanded posteriorly

♂ Adult

Larvae

Filariform
700 µ

Midgut

Rhabditiform
250 µ

Long

Life size

Short oesophagus bulbous posteriorly

Ovary
Vulva   Testes
Uterus
Seminal vesicle
Cloaca   Cement glands
Ovary
Ejaculatory duct
Posterior anus
Copulatory bursa
(See below)

Tail pointed (No notch)

Ovum

Unembryonated
60 × 40 µ

PARTICULAR MORPHOLOGY

	Ancylostoma duodenale	*A. braziliense*	*A. caninum*	*Necator americanus*
Size in mm	♂ 8–11 × 0.45 ♀ 10–13 × 0.6	7.5–8.5 × 0.35 9–10.5 × 0.375	10 × 0.4 14 × 0.6	7–9 × 0.3 9–11 × 0.4

Buccal capsule

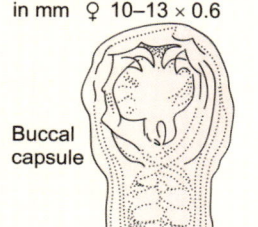 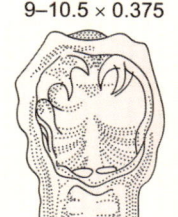 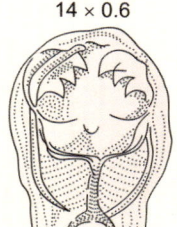 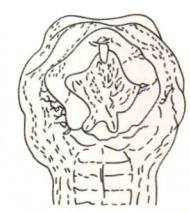

Two fused teeth, outer the larger 2 inconspicuous teeth	Pair of small median teeth Pair of large outer teeth	Three pairs of teeth	Cutting plates Dorsal teeth

Copulatory bursa

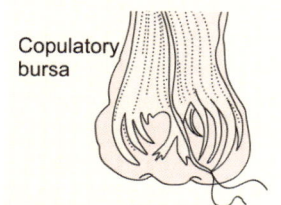 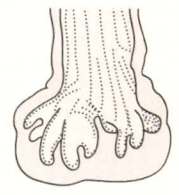 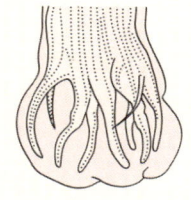 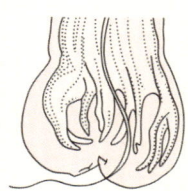

Spicules Dorsal ray. Shallow cleft Tips tridigitate	As broad as long Ray stunted	Large, flame-shaped Rays long and slender	Spicules fused and barbed Dorsal ray. Deep cleft. Tips bifid

Hookworms

Ancylostoma braziliense

This is a parasite of domestic animals (dogs and cats) in India, Malaysia and Brazil. Adult worm is smaller than *A. duodenale*. The buccal capsule has a small orifice and the ventral dental plate contains a pair of large teeth. Man is only an accidental host unsuitable for its growth and development and it causes creeping eruption mainly. *A. ceylanicum* is supposed to be identical to *A. braziliense* and is found in Sri Lanka, it does not cause cutaneous larva migrans in man.

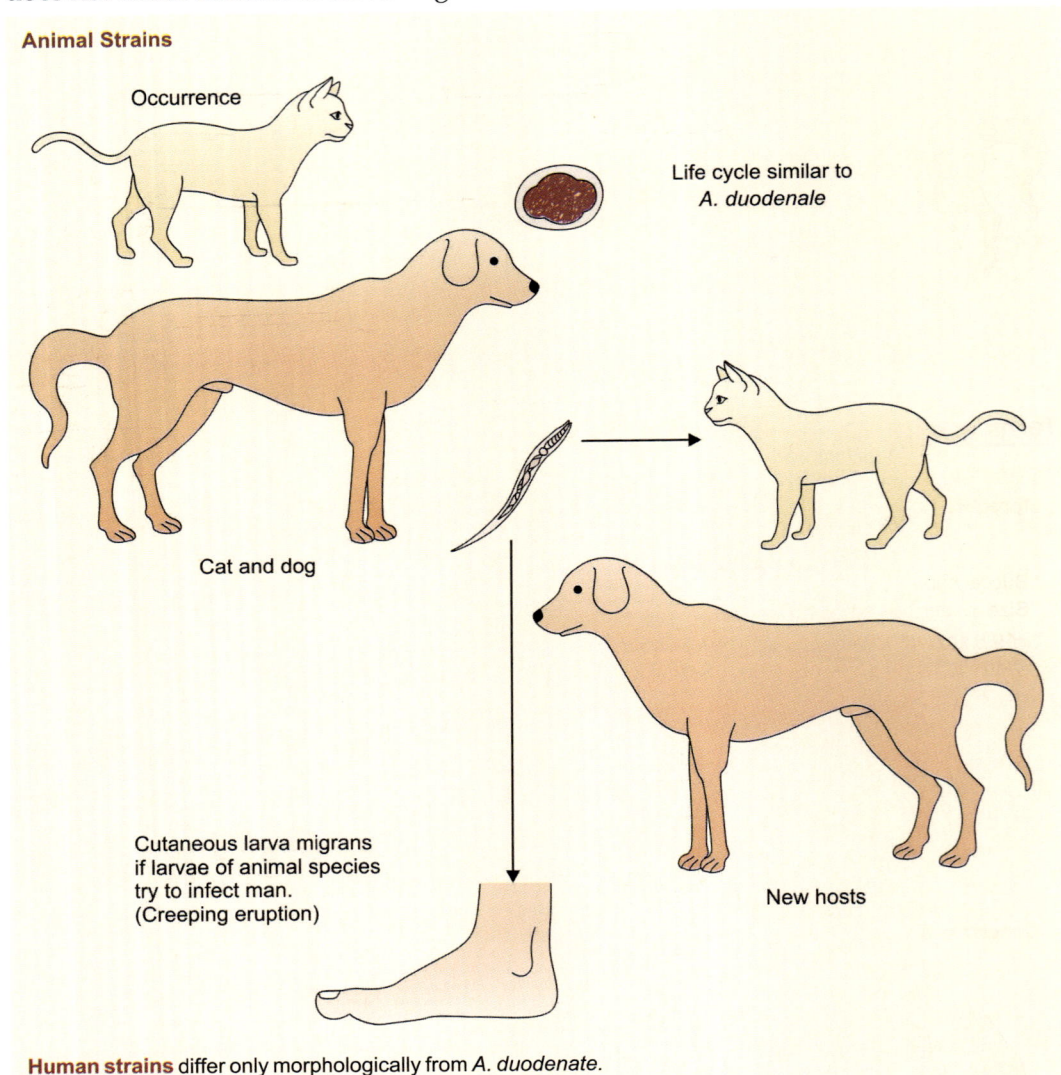

Animal Strains

Occurrence

Life cycle similar to *A. duodenale*

Cat and dog

Cutaneous larva migrans if larvae of animal species try to infect man. (Creeping eruption)

New hosts

Human strains differ only morphologically from *A. duodenate*.

Ancylostoma caninum

A common dog parasite with a worldwide distribution. Buccal capsule has the largest orifice and each of the paired ventral plates contains 3 teeth, increasing in size from within outwards. Life cycle is same as for other Ancylostomes. The infective filariform larvae can cause creeping eruption in man.

Occurrence

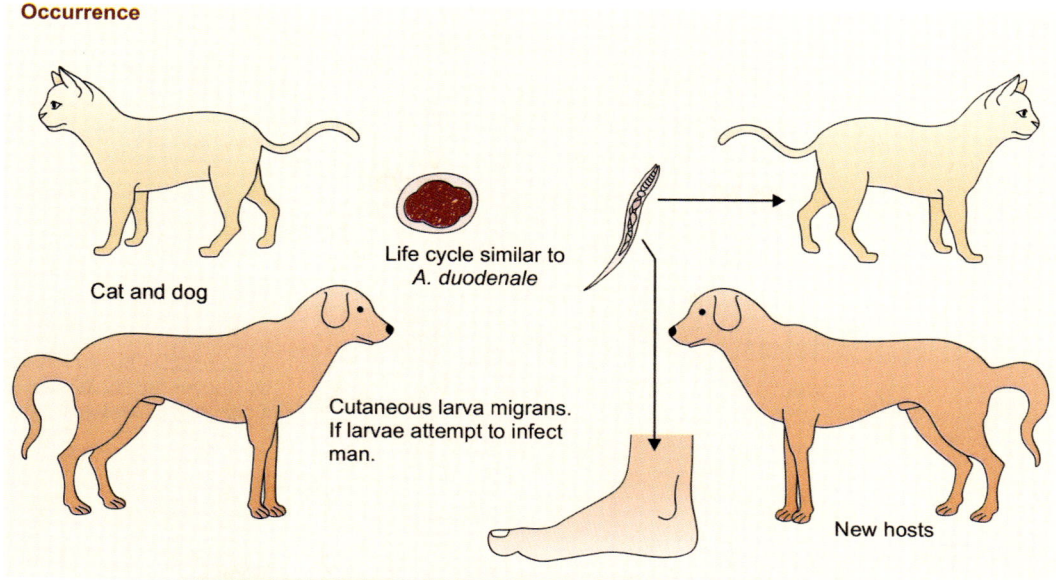

Cat and dog

Life cycle similar to *A. duodenale*

Cutaneous larva migrans. If larvae attempt to infect man.

New hosts

Members of family stronglyloidea of lesser importance

Ternidens deminutus

Morphology: Resemble hookworms

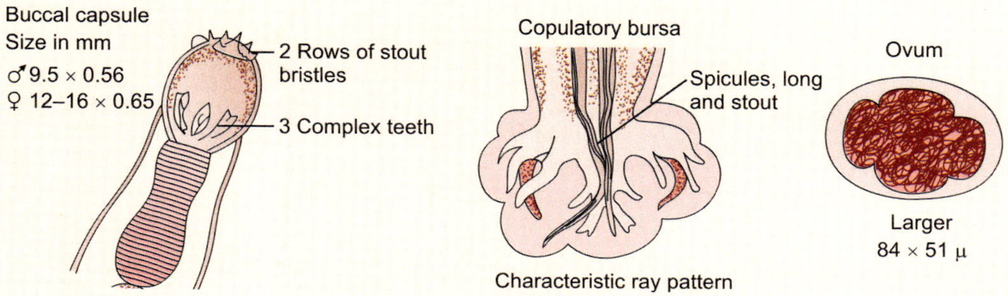

Buccal capsule
Size in mm
♂ 9.5 × 0.56
♀ 12–16 × 0.65

2 Rows of stout bristles

3 Complex teeth

Copulatory bursa

Spicules, long and stout

Characteristic ray pattern

Ovum

Larger
84 × 51 μ

Occurrence

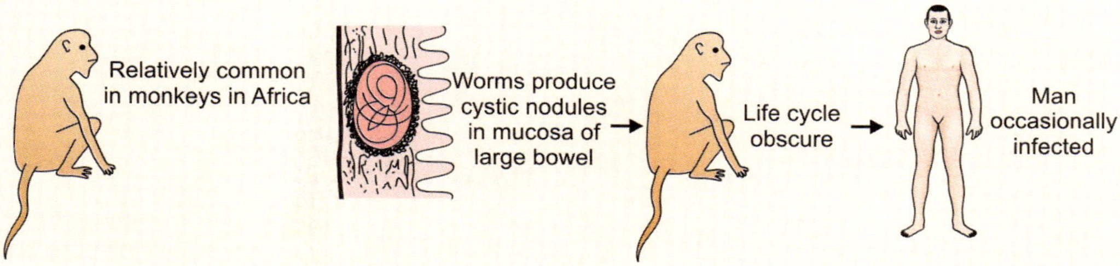

Relatively common in monkeys in Africa

Worms produce cystic nodules in mucosa of large bowel

Life cycle obscure

Man occasionally infected

Oesophagostomum apiostomum

Morphology: Like hookworms

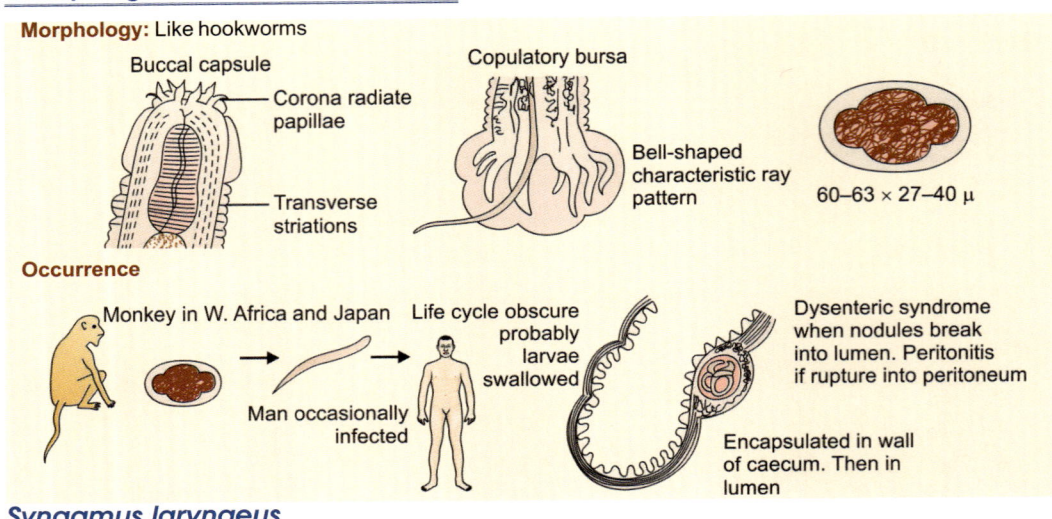

Buccal capsule
— Corona radiate papillae
— Transverse striations

Copulatory bursa
Bell-shaped characteristic ray pattern

60–63 × 27–40 μ

Occurrence

Monkey in W. Africa and Japan   Life cycle obscure probably larvae swallowed

Man occasionally infected

Dysenteric syndrome when nodules break into lumen. Peritonitis if rupture into peritoneum

Encapsulated in wall of caecum. Then in lumen

Syngamus laryngeus

Morphology Like hookworm

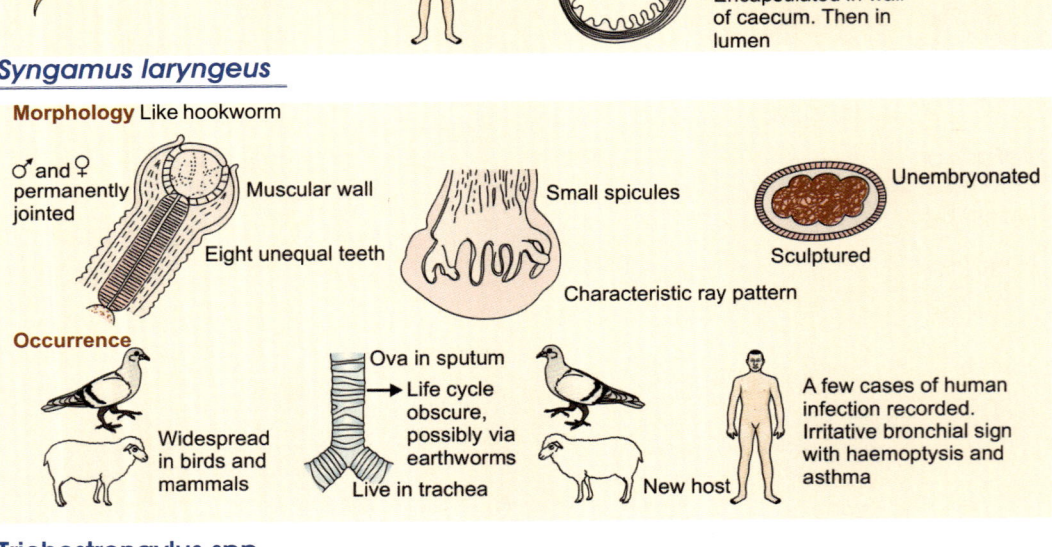

♂ and ♀ permanently jointed   Muscular wall
Eight unequal teeth

Small spicules
Characteristic ray pattern

Unembryonated
Sculptured

Occurrence

Ova in sputum
Life cycle obscure, possibly via earthworms
Live in trachea

Widespread in birds and mammals

New host

A few cases of human infection recorded. Irritative bronchial sign with haemoptysis and asthma

Trichostrongylus spp.

Morphology

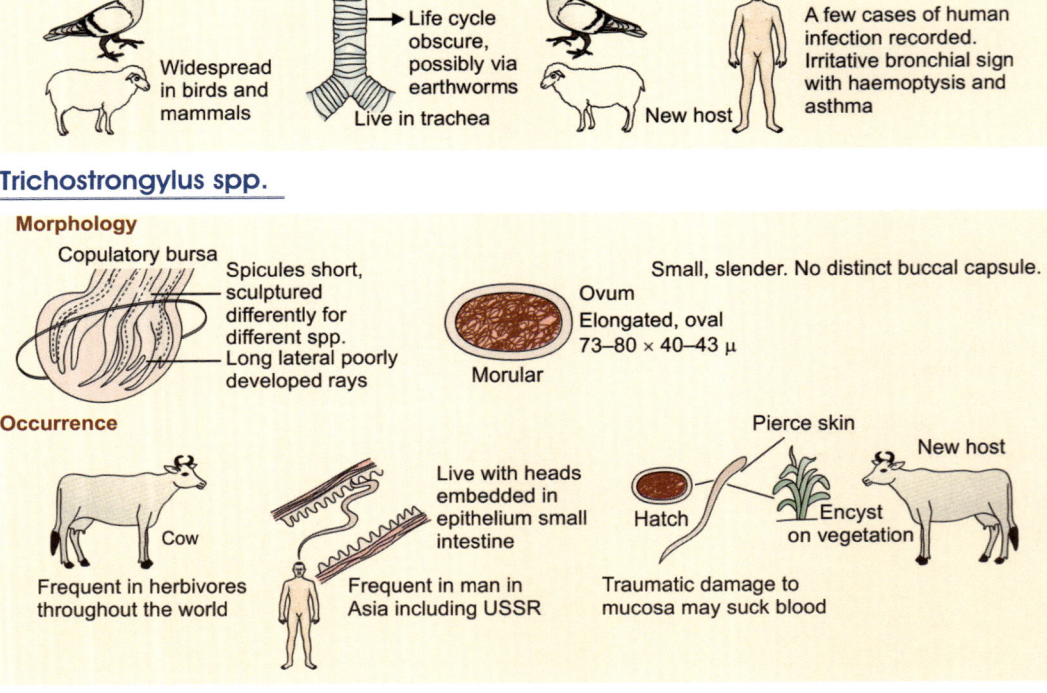

Copulatory bursa
Spicules short, sculptured differently for different spp.
Long lateral poorly developed rays

Ovum
Elongated, oval
73–80 × 40–43 μ
Morular

Small, slender. No distinct buccal capsule.

Occurrence

Cow

Frequent in herbivores throughout the world

Live with heads embedded in epithelium small intestine

Frequent in man in Asia including USSR

Hatch

Pierce skin
New host
Encyst on vegetation

Traumatic damage to mucosa may suck blood

Haemonchus contortus (The sheep wire worm)

Morphology

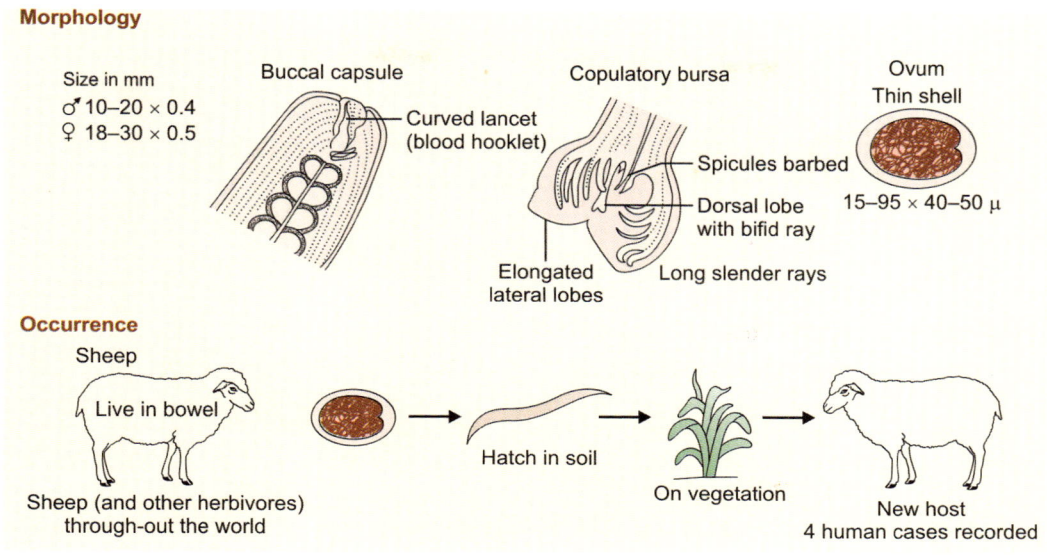

Size in mm
♂ 10–20 × 0.4
♀ 18–30 × 0.5

Buccal capsule

Curved lancet
(blood hooklet)

Copulatory bursa

Spicules barbed

Dorsal lobe
with bifid ray

Elongated
lateral lobes

Long slender rays

Ovum
Thin shell

15–95 × 40–50 µ

Occurrence

Sheep

Live in bowel

Sheep (and other herbivores)
through-out the world

Hatch in soil

On vegetation

New host
4 human cases recorded

Metastrongylos elongastos (The porcine lung worm)

Morphology

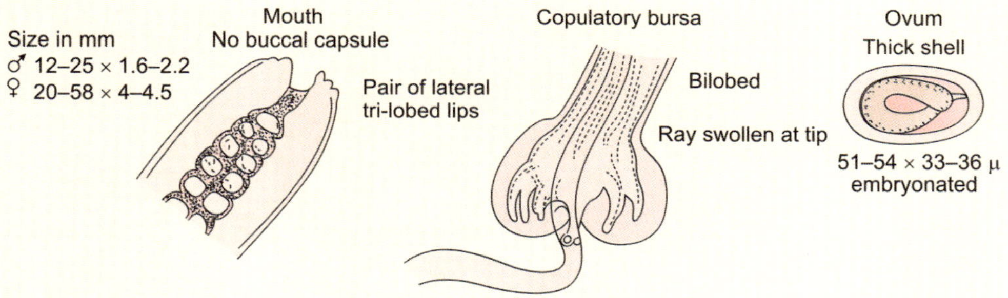

Size in mm
♂ 12–25 × 1.6–2.2
♀ 20–58 × 4–4.5

Mouth
No buccal capsule

Pair of lateral
tri-lobed lips

Copulatory bursa

Bilobed

Ray swollen at tip

Ovum
Thick shell

51–54 × 33–36 µ
embryonated

Occurrence

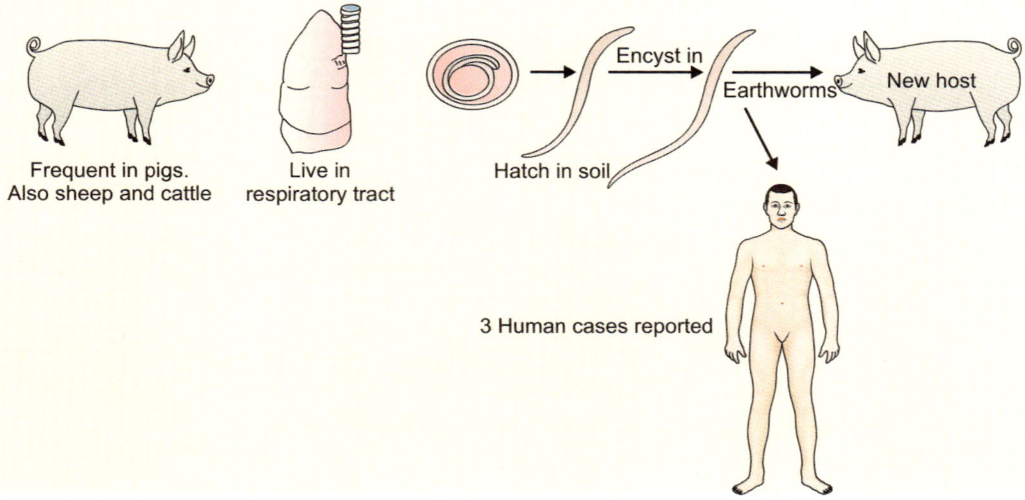

Frequent in pigs.
Also sheep and cattle

Live in
respiratory tract

Hatch in soil

Encyst in
Earthworms

New host

3 Human cases reported

OXYUROIDEA

(Superfamily)

Tiny pin-shaped nematodes. Cuticle near the mouth forms a wing-like expansion. They show a globular enlargement in the posterior end of the oesophagus. Males possess caudal pipillae while the posterior extremity of females is long, tapering and finely pointed tail that constitutes a third of the worm's length *Enterobius vermicularis* was first identified by Linnaeus in 1758 and later by Leach in 1853.

Enterobius vermicularis

(Threadworm, pinworm or seatworm)

Geographical distribution: Cosmopolitan distribution.

Habitat: Adult worms (gravid females) live in the caecum and vermiform appendix of man and remain there until eggs are produced. Usually they remain on mucosal surface but may occasionally encyst in the submucosa.

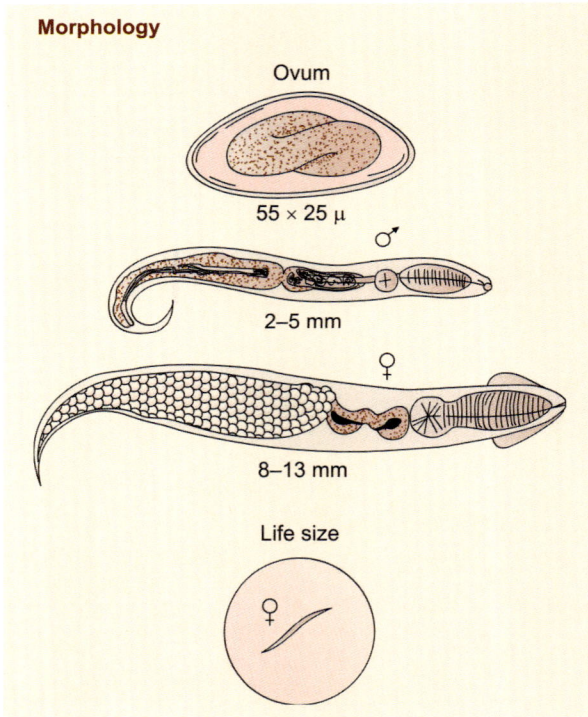

Morphology

Ovum

55 × 25 µ

♂

2–5 mm

♀

8–13 mm

Life size

♀

Adult worm is small, white and spindle-shaped resembling a tiny piece of thread. Both the sexes show cervical alae at the anterior extremity but do not have any buccal cavity. The posterior oesophageal end is globular in shape. *Males* measure 2–5 mm in length with curvature of the posterior third of the body length. Males usually die after fertilising the females. *Females* measure 8–13 mm in length and show a long drawn out, tapering and finely pointed tail. The gravid female, after oviposition, dies within 2–3 weeks. *Eggs* 55 × 25 µ, are colourless, asymmetrical (plano-convex), surrounded by a transparent shell, contain a coiled tadpole-like larva and float on the saturated solution of common salt.

Morphology
(detailed)

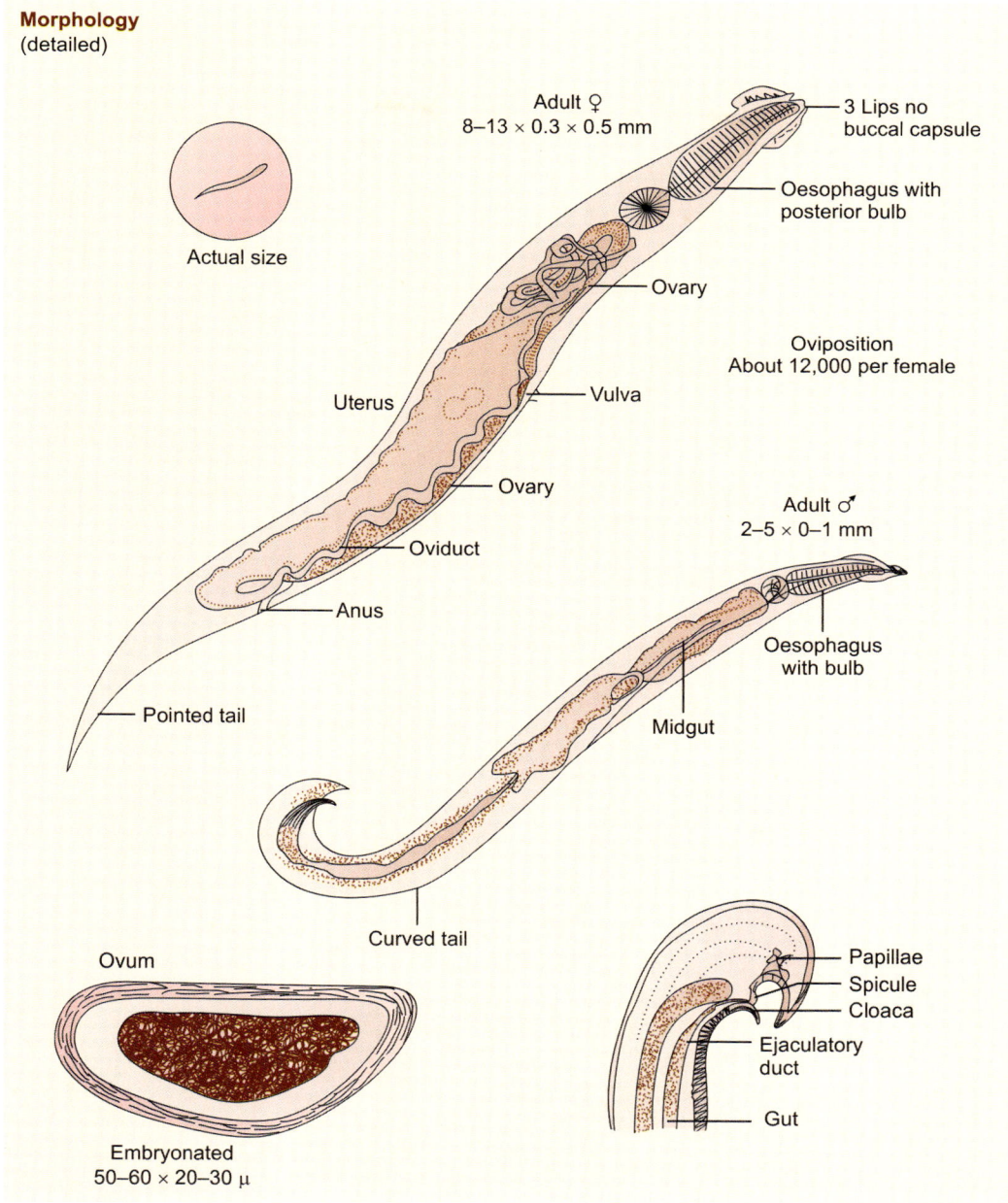

Actual size

Adult ♀
8–13 × 0.3 × 0.5 mm

3 Lips no
buccal capsule

Oesophagus with
posterior bulb

Ovary

Oviposition
About 12,000 per female

Uterus

Vulva

Ovary

Adult ♂
2–5 × 0–1 mm

Oviduct

Anus

Oesophagus
with bulb

Midgut

Pointed tail

Curved tail

Ovum

Papillae
Spicule
Cloaca

Ejaculatory
duct

Gut

Embryonated
50–60 × 20–30 µ

Life cycle: No intermediate host is needed. The eggs, newly-laid on the perianal skin and containing a tadpole-like larva complete their development in 24–36 hours in the presence of oxygen. Infection occurs by ingestion of these eggs. The shells are dissolved by digestive juices and the larvae escape in the small intestine to mature into adolescent worms. Males fertilise the females and die. Gravid female then migrates through the small intestine to the caecum, colon and appendix. They stay there till the eggs develop. At night the fertilised female reaches the peri-anal skin and deposits the eggs there. The whole cycle takes 2–4 weeks' time.

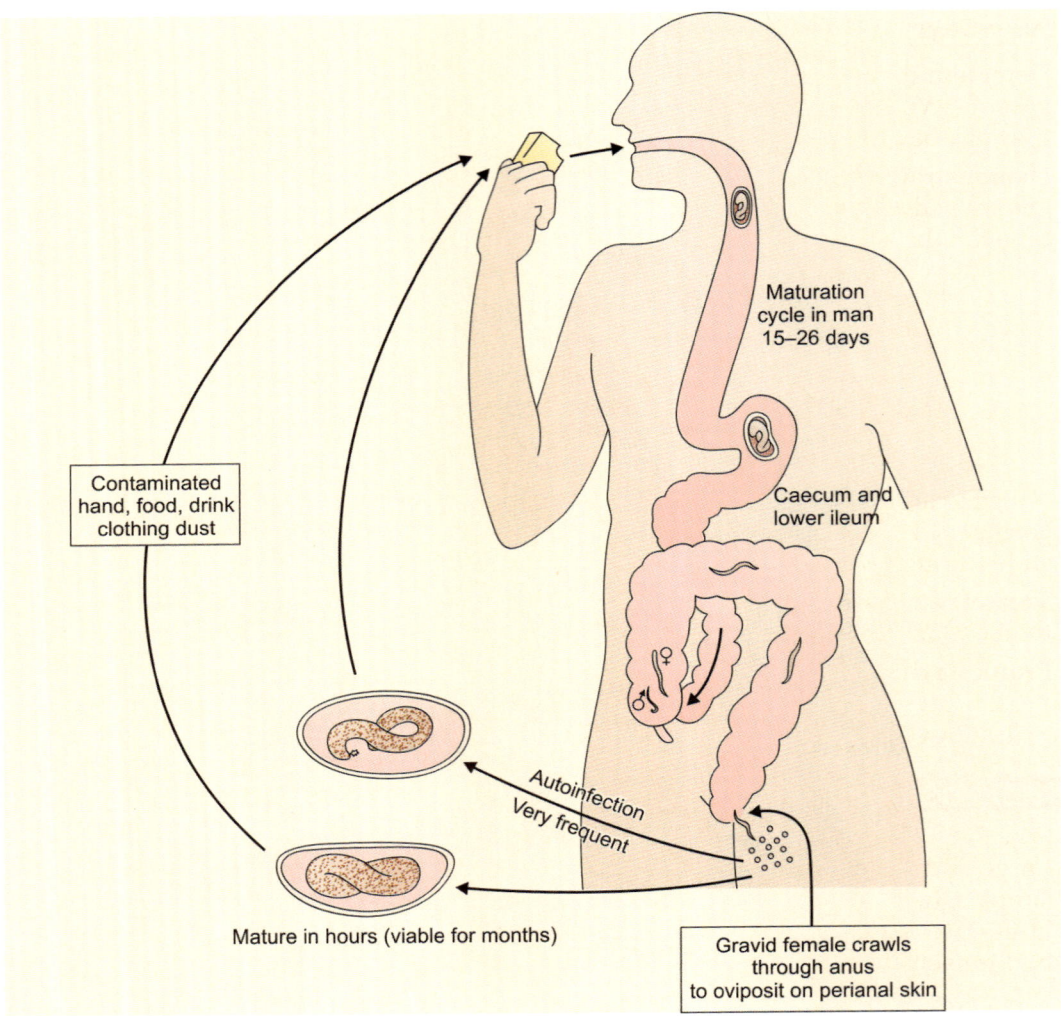

Maturation cycle in man 15–26 days

Contaminated hand, food, drink clothing dust

Caecum and lower ileum

Autoinfection Very frequent

Mature in hours (viable for months)

Gravid female crawls through anus to oviposit on perianal skin

Pathology

E. vermicularis infection is known as oxyuriasis or enterobiasis.

Mode of infection: Common among children, transmission is effected by ingestion of eggs. Persons handling the night clothes or bed linens of infected patients are more susceptible. Rarely, however, the infection can also be airborne. *Autoinfection:* The movement of egg-laying females causes intense itching, the patient scratches and transfers the eggs from anus to mouth and ingests them. *Retrofection:* The hatched eggs in the perianal skin migrate upwards through the anus and later mature in the colon.

Pathogenesis: Besides causing itching the gravid females often enter the female genital tract and urethra causing inflammation and in the fallopian tube can even enter the peritoneal cavity.

Clinical

Pruritis periani et perinei and eczematous lesions around the anus and perineum, salpingitis, nocturnal enuresis and sometimes inflammation of appendix (appendicitis).

Laboratory Diagnosis

Detection of adult worms: Can be seen around the anus by patient himself or by the parents. Worms may also be observed in the stool. If necessary, an enema or a purgative may be given. Lastly the anal region can be inspected to reveal the gravid females.

Demonstration of eggs: Very rarely the eggs may be found in the stool. Eggs are generally demonstrated in the scrapings from the perianal skin by an NIH swab, ideal time to take the scrapings is when the patient gets up in the morning.

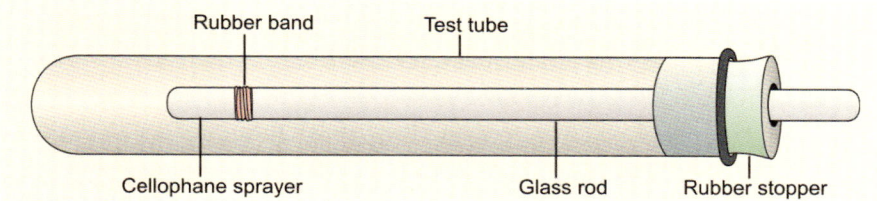

Eggs can also be recovered from under the finger-nails and the washings from garments. Examination of scotch tape first stuck around the anus and then seen on a slide through the microscope.

Treatment: Piperazine salts, pyrvinium pamoate, pyrantel pamoate, stilbazium iodide, thiabendazole, mebendazole and albendazole.

Prophylaxis:
  (i) Prevention of re-infection of the individual already infected, and
  (ii) Prevention of the infection by contact for which mass treatment may be needed.

ASCARIDOIDEA
(Superfamily)

Large and stout worms. No buccal capsule but the mouth has three lips. Possess a simple digestive tube. Male has one or two copulatory spicules. Females are a little larger than males. *Ascaris lumbricoides* (the common roundworm) was first discovered by Linnaeus in 1758.

Ascaris lumbricoides

Geographical distribution: Cosmopolitan distribution. More prevalent in India, South-East Asia and China. Unhygienic habits are partly responsible for its spread.

Habitat: Adult worm survives in the small intestine (mainly in jejunum) of man and maintain its position on account of its muscle tone.

Morphology: These are the largest intestinal nematodes of man and resemble the ordinary earthworm. Freshly evacuated they are light brown or pink in colour but gradually turn white. It is rounded with tapering ends (anterior end being thinner). Mouth opens at the anterior end and possesses three finely toothed lips, one dorsal and two ventral. The digestive and reproductive organs float inside the body cavity containing an irritating fluid (irritant being *ascaron or ascarase).* The allergic reactions seen in infected individuals and laboratory workers are due to this ascaron. Total life span of an adult worm is about 12 months within the human host.

Male: 15–20 cm × 2–4 mm. Tail end is curved ventrally in the form of a hook. Genital pore opens into the cloaca from which two curved copulatory spicules protrude. Both, the anus and the ejaculatory duct open into the cloaca.

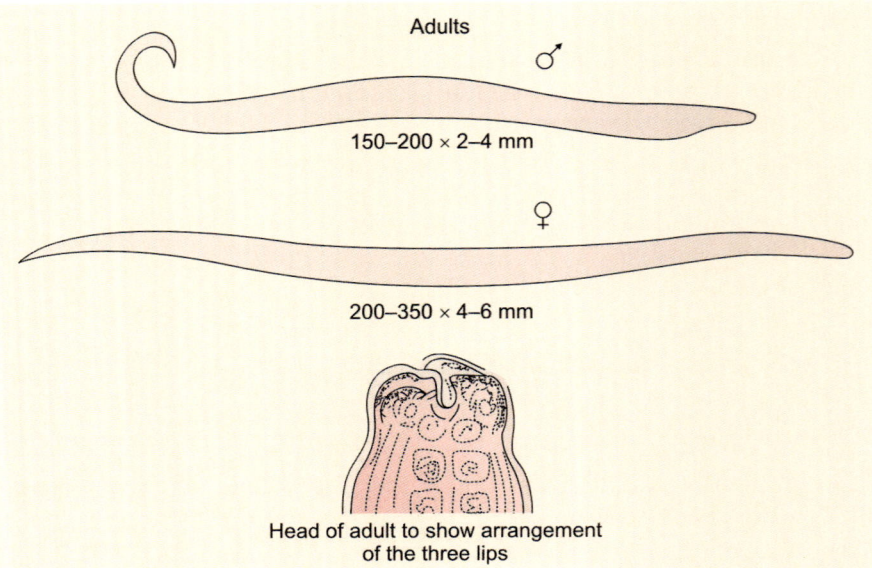

Adults

150–200 × 2–4 mm

200–350 × 4–6 mm

Head of adult to show arrangement
of the three lips

Female: Longer and stouter than male, measures 200–350 × 4–6 mm. The posterior extremity is neither curved nor pointed. Anus opens via a transverse slit on the ventral aspect a little before the posterior end.

Vulva opens at the junction of anterior and middle thirds on the mid-ventral aspect. A mature female can discharge up to 2 lakh eggs a day.

Eggs

The *fertilised egg* measures 60 × 45 μ, and is always bile stained. It is surrounded by a thick smooth translucent shell with an outer albuminous coat that is thrown into rugosities, when this outer coat is lost, it is labelled as a decorticated egg. It contains a large prominent unsegmented ovum (nucleus is masked by tremendous amount of coarse yolk granules); there is a clear crescentic area at each pole. This egg floats on a saturated solution of common table salt. An *unfertilised* female too can discharge eggs which are narrower, larger (80 × 55 μ) and more elliptical. These too are bile stained and exhibit a thinner shell with an irregular albuminous coating. It contains a small atrophied ovum with a mass of disorganised, highly refractile granules of differing sizes. It does not float on saturated common salt solution (it is the heaviest of all helminthic eggs).

Life cycle: Only a single host is required obviating the necessity of an intermediate host. Species is maintained by transference from one host to another. When freshly passed, they are not infective to man.

Mode of infection: Infection occurs by swallowing mature ascaris eggs (embryonated eggs) with raw vegetables cultivated on soil manured by infected human excreta. Contaminated water supply can also infect. Dirty fingers with attached eggs can also transmit infection. Dessicated eggs inhaled can also reach pharynx and be swallowed, they can also reach moist mucous surface of upper respiratory tract and the hatched larvae may directly penetrate into the blood stream. The important features are infecting agent = embryonated egg, portal of entry = alimentary canal, migration of larvae = through lungs and site of localisation = small intestine.

Morphology

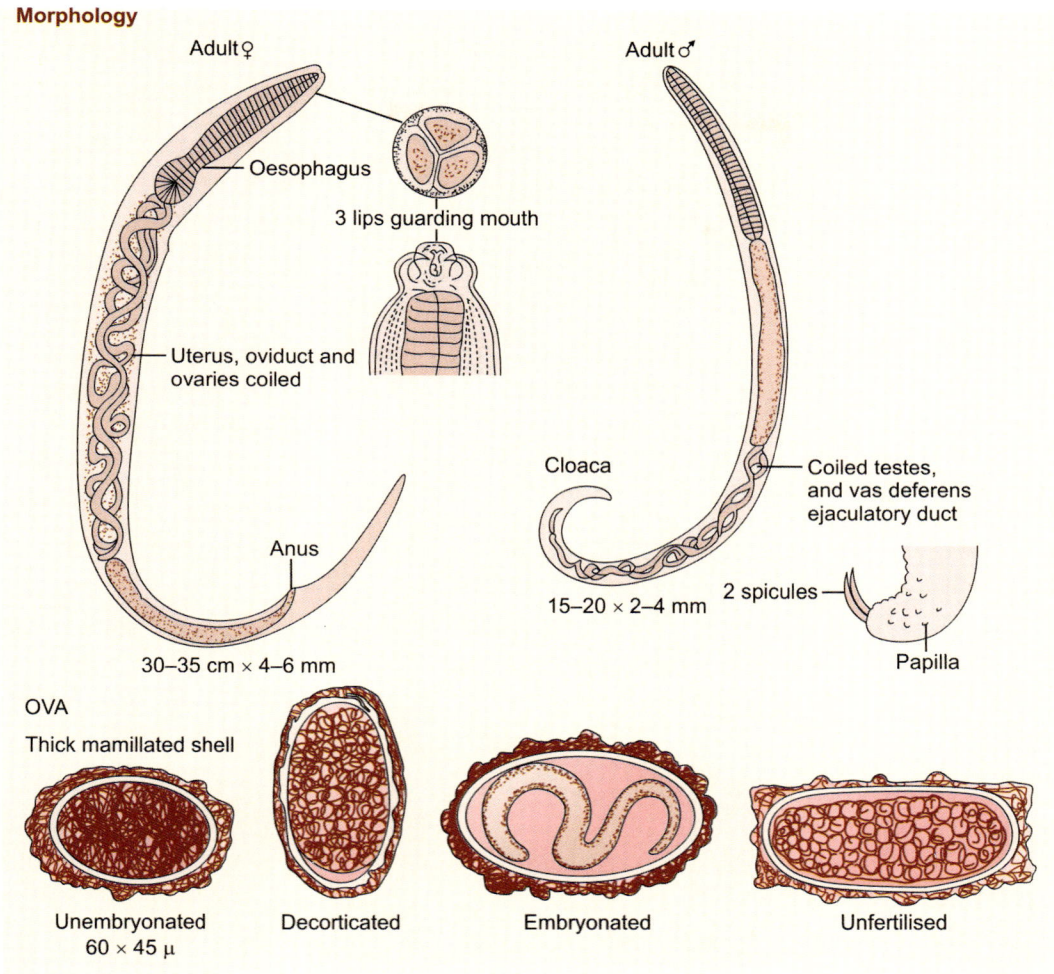

Adult ♀

Adult ♂

Oesophagus

3 lips guarding mouth

Uterus, oviduct and
ovaries coiled

Cloaca

Coiled testes,
and vas deferens
ejaculatory duct

Anus

2 spicules

15–20 × 2–4 mm

Papilla

30–35 cm × 4–6 mm

OVA

Thick mamillated shell

Unembryonated
60 × 45 μ

Decorticated

Embryonated

Unfertilised

Life Cycle Stages

Eggs in faeces: Fertilised eggs containing an unsegmented ovum are passed with faeces (not infective at this stage).

↓

Development in soil: In 10–40 days' time a rhabditiform larva is formed depending upon humidity and temperature and this occurs in the soil (outside the human body). The mature egg contains a coiled up embryo capable of infecting man. Before hatching the larva undergoes moulting.

↓

Infection by ingestion and larva liberation: When ingested and on reaching the duodenum, the digestive juices weaken the shell and stimulate the enclosed larva to activity. The shell is split and a 250 μ long larva is released into the upper ileum.

↓

Migratory phase: The newly hatched larvae burrow their way through the mucous membrane of ileum and enter hepatic portal circulation, here they stay for 3–4 days and finally via the right heart get caught in pulmonary circulation, here they grow and become longer (up to 2 mm) and molt twice (on 5th day or 6th day and later on the 10th day). They break open the capillaries and reach the lung alveoli. This migratory phase consumes 10–15 days' time.

↓

Re-entry into GI tract: From lower respiratory tract they crawl up the bronchi, trachea, larynx and pharynx and get swallowed once again. Through the oesophagus, via the stomach, they again reach upper ileum (their normal habitat). Another molting occurs between the 25th and 29th day of infection.

↓

Sexual maturation and egg release: Once in the upper ileum, the larvae mature sexually in about 6–10 weeks' time. The gravid females start discharging eggs in the stool in about 2 months time from the time of infection. This cycle is then repeated.

The larvae in heavy infections may get caught in aberrant sites, e.g. brain, spinal cord, kidneys, etc; at most of these sites they get destroyed.

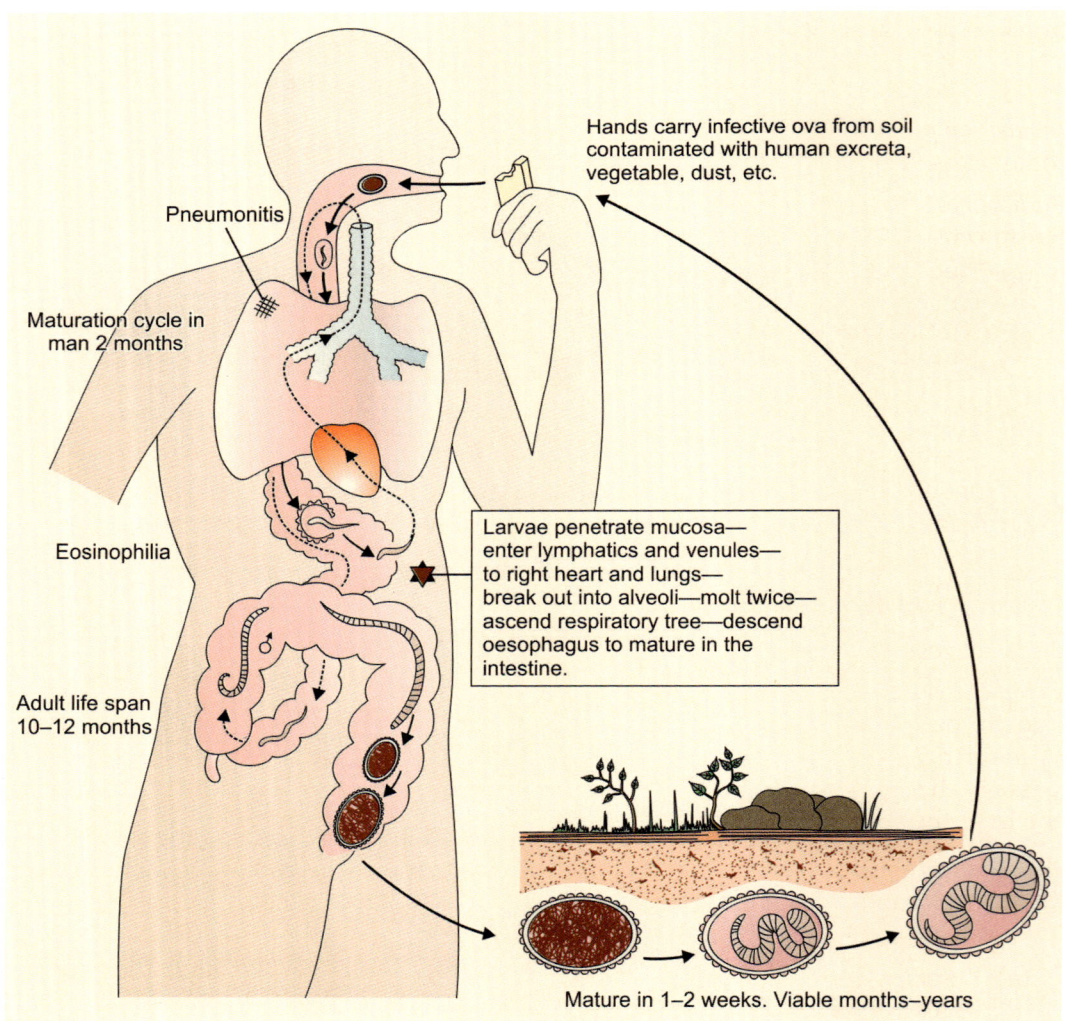

Hands carry infective ova from soil contaminated with human excreta, vegetable, dust, etc.

Pneumonitis

Maturation cycle in man 2 months

Eosinophilia

Adult life span 10–12 months

Larvae penetrate mucosa— enter lymphatics and venules— to right heart and lungs— break out into alveoli—molt twice— ascend respiratory tree—descend oesophagus to mature in the intestine.

Mature in 1–2 weeks. Viable months–years

Immunology: Migrating larvae may induce partial immunity. During moulting antigens are released and specific protective antibodies are produced. A severe allergic reaction (urticarial rashes and hypotension) occurs when larvae reach the ileum for the second time. At the time of tissue invasion there is eosinophilia in the peripheral blood.

Complement fixing and precipitating specific antibodies can be demonstrated in ascariasis. Hypersensitivity to ascaris can be determined by a skin test.

Pathology and Clinical Features

Symptoms related to migrating larvae

Pulmonary phase (Ascaris pneumonia or Loeffler's syndrome): Heavy infection may induce pneumonia symptoms such as fever, cough and dyspnoea. Sputum that is often blood tinged may reveal ascaris larvae. Urticarial rashes and moderate eosinophilia may also be observed.

Larvae in blood phase: Through blood the larvae may reach aberrant sites, e.g. heart, kidneys, brain and spinal cord. Specific symptoms related to these organs may appear. Stuck to the larvae, micro-organisms may also reach other sites from the intestine.

Symptoms related to adult worms

Incubation period: Average 60–75 days from the time of exposure for the mature female to lay eggs.

Pathogenesis: Most symptoms are related to their presence in the small intestine. Symptoms may occur due to:
  (a) **Mechanical effects:**
      (i) *A. lumbricoides* can cause intussusception,
      (ii) May penetrate through the intestinal ulcers,
      (iii) Numerous roundworms can actually cause intestinal obstruction (especially in young children).
  (b) **Toxic effects:** The body fluid of ascaris if absorbed can lead to typhoid-like symptoms and can also cause allergic manifestations such as urticaria, facial oedema, conjunctivitis and irritation in the upper respiratory tract.
  (c) **Spoliative effects:** The worm consumes proteins and vitamins which would have otherwise been absorbed for the patient. In children especially it may lead to protein-energy malnutrition. Hypovitaminosis A can cause night blindness. Antitryptic and antipeptic enzymes released by the worm protect it from the digestive action of hosts' enzymes.

Ectopic ascariasis: Mature worms can migrate through the stomach via the oesophagus to be vomitted out or may enter the respiratory passages to cause suffocation. Wandering ascaris may enter appendix to cause appendicitis. If they enter the biliary passage they may cause obstructive jaundice and if they happen to reach high up in the liver they may cause abscess too.

Laboratory Diagnosis

Direct evidences

  (a) **Demonstration of adult worms:** In the stool or vomitus. X-ray diagnosis— ingested barium emulsion appears as a string-like shadow on X-ray.

(b) **Demonstration of eggs:**
Stool: By direct microscopic examination or by concentration/floatation methods (unfertilised eggs do not float and if the patient has a single male, no eggs are seen).
Bile: Duodenal aspirate may reveal ascaris eggs.

Indirect evidences

(a) *Blood:* Eosinophilia is usually seen in the early phase, however, if seen in the intestinal phase, it should suggest associated toxocariasis or strongyloidiasis.

Treatment: Piperazine is good. However, tetramisole, pyrantel pamoate, bephenium hydroxynaphthoate, diethylcarbamazine (hetrazan), thiabendazole, mebendazole and albendazole can also be given.

Prophylaxis: Includes:
— Proper disposal of human excreta.
— Treatment of infected individuals.
— Observe good personal hygiene.

Anisakis Marina

Adult worm inhabits the intestine of larger sea mammals, while its larval stage is found in the flesh of various marine fishes (cod, salman and herring) and it leads to *Anisakiasis* or *herring worm disease* in man. It is found in Japan, Scandinavian region and Holland. The larvae liberated from digestion of fish flesh enter the gastric or intestinal mucosa to produce an eosinophilic granulomatous tumour resembling malignancy. The patient may complain of colicky abdominal pain or symptoms associated with intestinal obstruction. The diagnosis is established by demonstration of larvae in the surgically resected tissue. Complete life cycle of this parasite is still unknown. Indirect haemagglutination test with anisakis test is positive.

FILARIODEA

(Superfamily)

This includes nematodes residing in blood vessels, lymphatic system, connective tissues and serous cavities of man. Adult worms are large and slender (thread-like), varying in lengths from 2 to 10 cm; females are longer than the males.

The adult worm has a lipless mouth, a bulbless cylindrical oesophagus and a posteriorly atrophied intestine. Caudal alae are often missing and the copulatory spicules are dissimilar and unequal. Females are viviparous, giving birth to larvae called microfilariae. Needs two hosts to complete its life cycle—man and blood-sucking insects. Microfilaria completes its development in the insect host, giving rise to the infective form. The infected insect bites another man and transmits the infection. Species identification is made by studying the larvae, adult worms are rarely obtained.

Classification of Superfamily

The superfamily filarioidea is subdivided into 4 families. Of these acanthocheilonematidae encompasses the species parasitic to human beings. This family is subdivided as follows:

Subfamily	Genus	Species	Habitat of adultform	Microfilaria seen in
Acanthochei-lomantinae	Wuchereria	W. bancrofti	Lymphatics	Blood
	Brugia	B. malayi	Lymphatics	Blood
	Onchocerca	O. volvulus	Connective tissue	Skin
	Dipetatonema	D. perstans	Connective tissue	Blood
		D. streptocerca	Connective tissue	Skin
	Mansonella	M. ozzardi	Mesentery	Blood
Dirofilarinae	Dirofilaria	D. conjunctivas (D. repens and D. tenuis)	Connective tissue and eyelid	
		D. magalhaesi	Heart	
		D. immitis	Dog's heart	Blood
	Loa	L. loa	Connective tissue, conjunctiva	Blood

Differentiating Features of Adult Worms

Skin/Cuticle	Other features	Genus species
Smooth cuticle	Head with cuticular appendage	D. perstans
	Head without cuticular appendage	W. bancrofti, B. malayi
Cuticle not smooth	Possess minute warts	L. loa
	Possess annular and oblique thickening	O. volvulus

Differentiating Features of Microfilariae (Mf)

Location	Sheath features	Nuclei positions	Genus species
Blood	Sheathed and periodic	Nuclei up to tail tip	Mf. malayi, Mf. loa
		Tail tip free from nuclei	Mf. bancrofti
	Unsheathed and non-periodic	Nuclei up to tail tip	Mf. perstans
		Tail tip nuclei free	Mf. ozzardi
Skin	Unsheathed and non-periodic	Nuclei up to tail tip	Mf. streptocerca
		Tail tip nuclei-free	Mf. volvulus

Geographic Disposition

In India—expect *Mf. bancrofti* and *Mf. malayi.*
In Africa—expect *Mf. bancrofti, Mf. loa* and *Mf. perstans.*
In Latin America—expect *Mf. bancrofti, Mf. perstans* and *Mf. ozzardi.*
Two other species recognised are:
Wuchereria lewisi—found in Brazil.
B. malayi variant—found in East Timor.

Immunology: Viable adult worms and microfilariae do not evoke any significant host reaction. However, a profuse immune response is observed against killed adults and larvae. Man develops a significant resistance to superinfection, except in oncho-cerciasis. Both humoral and CMI mechanisms come into play against Wuchereriasis but these are effective against microfilariae only (so with advancing age the microfilarial density diminishes). A marked level of serum antibody seen in occult filariasis (tropical pulmonary eosinophilia) is associated with immune responses that develop against *W. bancrofti*, *B. malayi* or other animal strains and prevents microfilariae from reaching peripheral blood. Humoral antibodies associated with filarial infections are complement-fixing, haemagglutinating and fluorescent. Complement fixation test is done by employing antigen extracted from *D. immitis* (dog heartworm) and positive results are obtained in significant number of cases of loiasis and onchocerciasis, it is almost always found positive in occult filariasis. Cross sensitivity with CFT is also observed with other helminthic infections, e.g. strongyloidiasis, ascariasis and schistosomiasis. Intradermal injection of dead microfilarial forms evokes an immediate hypersensitivity type of humoral response as in Mazzotti's test for onchocerciasis and in wuchereriasis. A notable increase occurs in IgM in wuchereriasis and in IgE in onchocerciasis.

THE FILARIAL WORMS

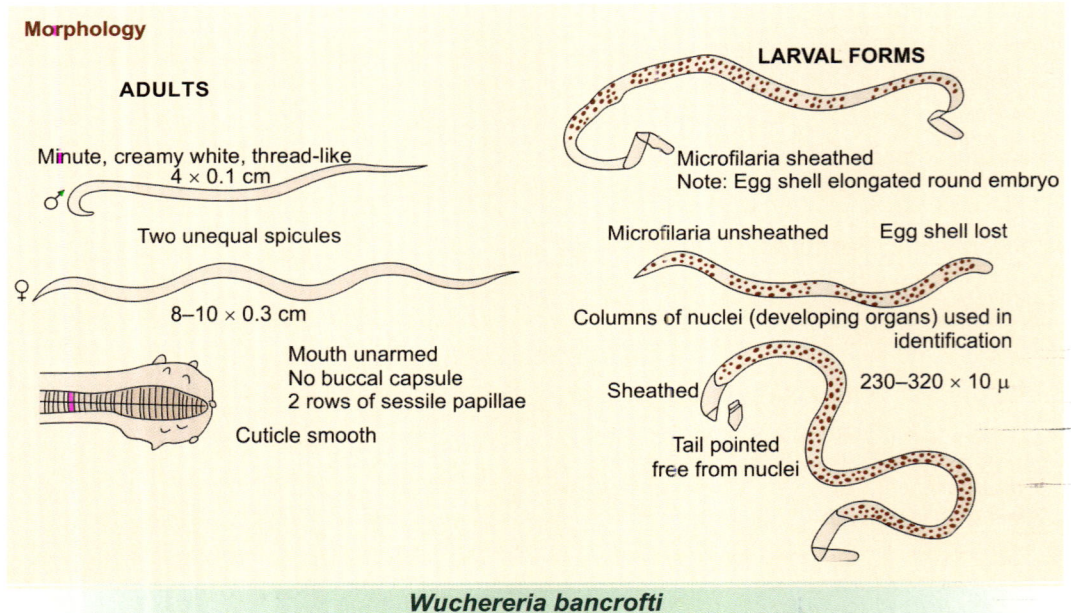

Morphology

ADULTS

LARVAL FORMS

Minute, creamy white, thread-like
4 × 0.1 cm

Microfilaria sheathed
Note: Egg shell elongated round embryo

Two unequal spicules

Microfilaria unsheathed   Egg shell lost

8–10 × 0.3 cm

Columns of nuclei (developing organs) used in identification

Mouth unarmed
No buccal capsule
2 rows of sessile papillae

Sheathed   230–320 × 10 µ

Cuticle smooth

Tail pointed
free from nuclei

Wuchereria bancrofti

In general like *W. bancrofti*
2 rows minute papillae round mouth   Sheathed

170–260 × 5–6 µ

Two discrete nuclei in tip of tail

Brugia malayi

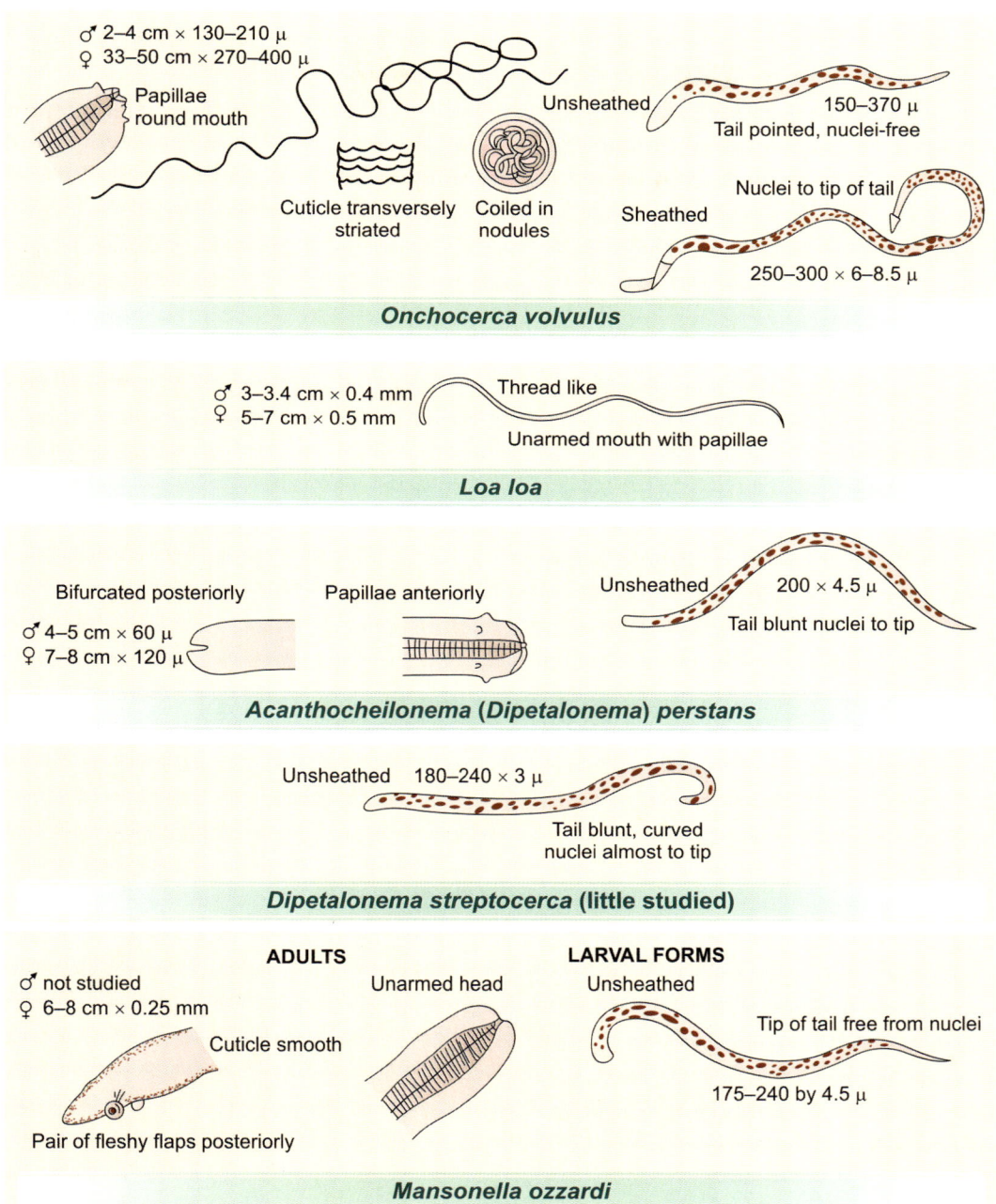

♂ 2–4 cm × 130–210 μ
♀ 33–50 cm × 270–400 μ

Papillae round mouth

Cuticle transversely striated

Coiled in nodules

Unsheathed
150–370 μ
Tail pointed, nuclei-free

Sheathed
Nuclei to tip of tail
250–300 × 6–8.5 μ

Onchocerca volvulus

♂ 3–3.4 cm × 0.4 mm
♀ 5–7 cm × 0.5 mm

Thread like

Unarmed mouth with papillae

Loa loa

Bifurcated posteriorly

♂ 4–5 cm × 60 μ
♀ 7–8 cm × 120 μ

Papillae anteriorly

Unsheathed 200 × 4.5 μ
Tail blunt nuclei to tip

Acanthocheilonema (Dipetalonema) perstans

Unsheathed 180–240 × 3 μ

Tail blunt, curved nuclei almost to tip

Dipetalonema streptocerca (little studied)

ADULTS

♂ not studied
♀ 6–8 cm × 0.25 mm

Cuticle smooth

Unarmed head

LARVAL FORMS

Unsheathed

Tip of tail free from nuclei

175–240 by 4.5 μ

Pair of fleshy flaps posteriorly

Mansonella ozzardi

Wuchereria bancrofti

(Bancroft's Filariasis, *Filaria bancrofti*)

Historical aspects

Demarguay (1863) found larvae in hydrocele fluid. Wucherer (1866) observed them in chylous urine. Lewis (1872) detected them in peripheral blood. Bancroft (1876) detected the adult females.

Geographical distribution

Mainly confined to tropical and subtropical regions. It is seen in India, West Indies, Southern China, Japan, West and Central Africa, South America and the Pacific Islands. In India it is observed chiefly along the coastal regions and along the banks of big rivers (except Indus and mainly along Ganges); it has also been reported from Kerala, Rajasthan, Punjab, Delhi and Uttar Pradesh.

Habitat

Adult worms are found in the lymphatic vessels and lymph nodes of man only. It is not observed in other animals.

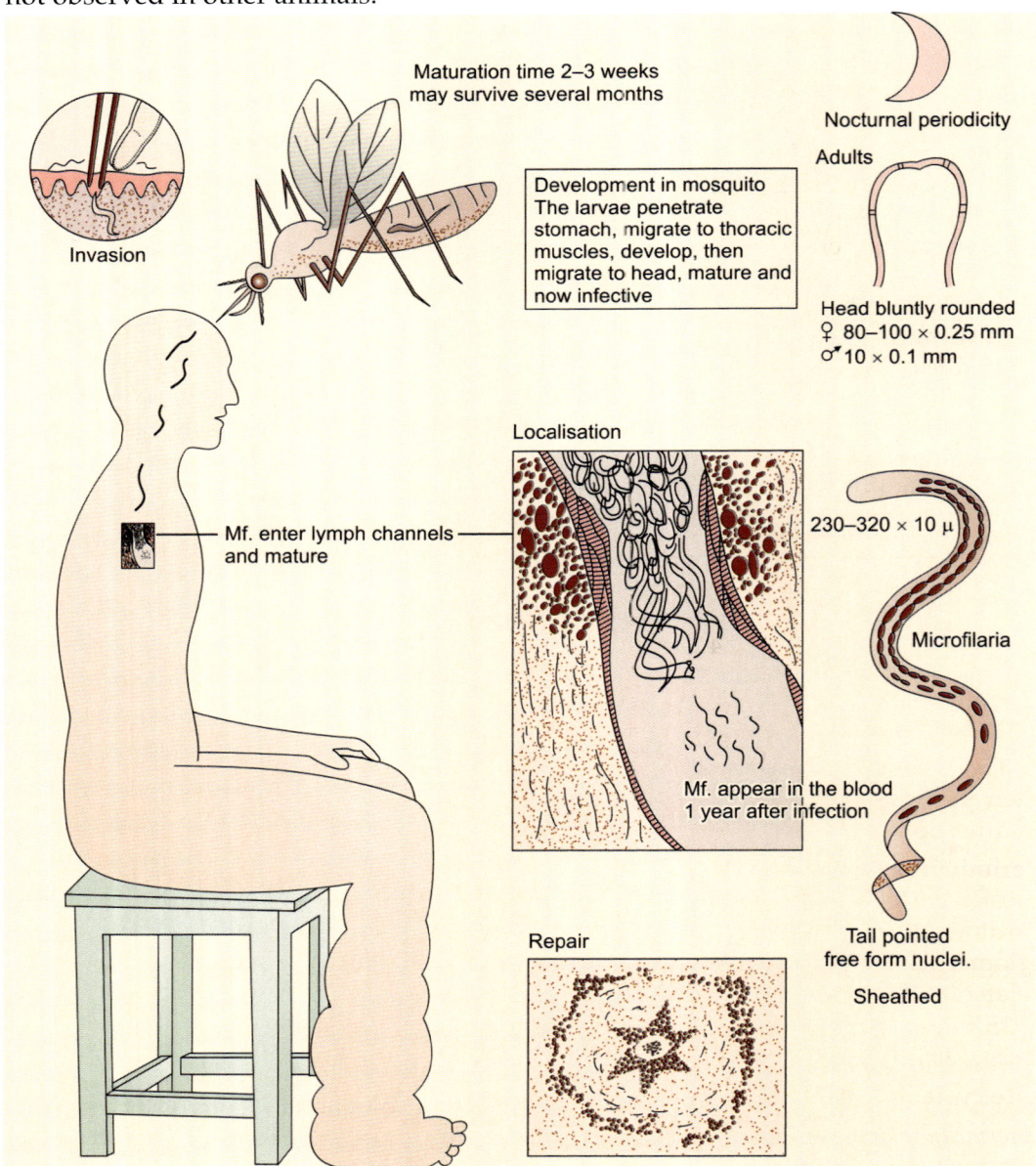

Maturation time 2–3 weeks may survive several months

Nocturnal periodicity

Invasion

Development in mosquito
The larvae penetrate stomach, migrate to thoracic muscles, develop, then migrate to head, mature and now infective

Adults

Head bluntly rounded
♀ 80–100 × 0.25 mm
♂ 10 × 0.1 mm

Localisation

Mf. enter lymph channels and mature

230–320 × 10 μ

Microfilaria

Mf. appear in the blood 1 year after infection

Repair

Tail pointed free form nuclei.

Sheathed

Morphology

Adult worm: Long thread-like transparent (creamy-white in colour quite often) nematodes. Are filiform in shape with both ends tapering, head-end terminates in a slight rounded swelling. *Males* measure 40 x 0.1 mm, their tail end is curved ventrally and contains two spicules of differing lengths. *Females* measure almost twice long and thick (80–100 × 0.25 mm), their tail-end is narrow and abruptly pointed. Females liberate active embryos, however, they actually are ovo-viviparous (the eggs contain well-formed embryos). The intercoiling between males and females is so much that they can only be separated with great difficulty (females usually outnumber males). The life span of an adult worm can be up to a decade. *Embryos* (Microfilariae = Mf.). Released from the lymph nodes they reach the lymphatic trunks and then into the general circulation. These larvae are actively motile either with or against the blood stream. Unstained, they are colourless with transparent bodies, blunt heads and somewhat pointed tails. They measure 230–320 × 10 μ. Stained after death they reveal underlying features.

(a) **Hyaline sheath:** Structureless sac best seen when it projects beyond the extremities of the Mf. Larva can actually move within its sheath. It represents the chorionic envelope of the egg; it remains as an investing membrane round the larva.

(b) **Cuticula:** Is lined by subcuticular cells visible only with vital stains.

(c) **Somatic cells/nuclei:** Extending from head to tail they appear as granules in the central axis of the body. Terminal 5% of the tip does not show any granules. This is a differentiating feature of *Mf. bancrofti*. The tiny squarish cephalic space at the anterior end is also devoid of granules. Vital stains also reveal a stylet. Granular line is broken at:

1. Nerve ring, an oblique space,
2. Anterior V-spot which represents the rudimentary excretory system, and
3. Posterior V-spot or tail spot that represents the anus or cloaca of the worms' alimentary canal.
   - G cells (few genital cells). While G cell 1 is situated a little in front, the G cells 2, 3 and 4 are just in front of the anal pore.
   - Central (internal) body of Manson (Innekorper of Fulleborn) extends between anterior V-spot till G cell 1. It represents the rudimentary alimentary canal.

These larval forms do not grow further in the human body. They are taken up by their proper intermediate mosquito host. If not sucked up by the mosquito they die in due course of time. These Mf. may live in the human body for up to 70 days or so.

Periodicity of Mf. bancrofti: The oriental Mf. show a nocturnal periodicity and appear mostly between 10 p.m. and 4 a.m. During daytime they reside in the capillaries of cardiorespiratory system (lungs, heart and big arteries such as the carotids) and kidneys (glomerular tufts). Exact reason for nocturnal periodicity is ill understood, it is perhaps related to the night feeding habit of their intermediate host, *Culex pipiens fatigans*.

In the pacific islands no such periodicity is observed, here, the intermediate host *Ades polynesienensis* feeds during the daytime also.

Life cycle: Needs two hosts: Man and mosquito. *Definitive host* is man.

Intermediate host is mosquito. A large number of species of mosquito belonging to the genus Culex, Aedes and Anopheles act as intermediate hosts for *W. bancrofti*.

DEVELOPMENTAL STAGES OF MF. IN MOSQUITO

Mf. ingested by the mosquito gather round the anterior end of its stomach. After casting off their sheaths they penetrate the gut wall in an hour or two and migrate to the thoracic muscles. Once in these muscles they rest and begin to grow.

↓

Within 2 days they become thicker, shorter and sausage-shaped with a short spiky tail and measure 125–250 × 10–17 μ. It is is the first stage larva possessing a rudimentary digestive tract.

↓

By third to seventh day the larva grows rapidly, moults (cuticle shedding) once or twice and comes to measure 220–330 × 15–30 μ (this is the second stage larva).

↓

On tenth or eleventh day the metamorphosis becomes complete—there is atrophy of tail and development of body cavity, digestive system and genitals. This third stage larva measures 1500–2000 × 18–23 μ and has 3 subterminal caudal papillae. Around fourteenth day it enters the proboscis sheath of the mosquito and is infective at this stage. One Mf. gives rise to only one larva in the proboscis sheath. When this mosquito takes the next blood meal it releases these mature infective larvae. Depending upon the environmental factors and species of mosquito, the development time in the mosquito can range between 10 and 20 days or more.

DEVELOPMENT IN MAN UP TO AN ADULT WORM

The third stage larvae are not released directly into circulation but are deposited on the skin near the site of puncture. These larvae either enter through the bite wound or penetrate on their own through the skin. Later they reach the lymphatic channels and settle down somewhere (inguinal, scrotal or abdominal lymphatics) and become sexually mature in 5–18 months' time. The male fertilises the female and the gravid female gives birth to larvae. The whole cycle is later repeated.

Pathology and Clinical Features

Wuchereriasis also called filariasis is primarily confined to involvement of lymphatic system and its effects.

Mode of infection: Inoculation, bite of a mosquito.

Transmitting agent: Female mosquitoes (Culex, Aedes or Anopheles).

In India and China : *Culex pipiens fatigans.*

In Pacific islands   : Melenesian Islands   : *Anopheles punctulatus.*

: Polynesian Islands   : *Aedes polyniensis.*

Infective form: Third stage larva of Mf. bancrofti.

Portal of entry: Skin.

Localisation site: Lymphatic system of upper or lower extremities depending upon site of bite. Commonly the inguino-scrotal region is involved.

Biological incubation period lasts from 1 to 1½ years. This is the time gap between inoculation of third stage larvae and subsequent parturition by fertilised females to produce Mf.

Pathogenesis: Adult worms living or dead are responsible for the signs and symptoms. Living Mf. produce no effects except in occult filariasis. Lymphangitis forms the basic classical lesion. In occult filariasis the Mf. are found not only in lymph nodes but also in lungs, liver and spleen.

Differences between classical and occult filariasis		
	Classical filariasis	*Occult filariasis*
Cause	Adults and developing worms	Microfilariae
Basic pathological lesion	Acute inflammation followed by an epithelioid granuloma surrounding the adult worm and fibrous scar	An eosinophilic granuloma (allergic or hypersensitivity reaction)
Organs involved	Lymphatic system (Lymph nodes and vessels)	Lymphatic system, liver, lungs and spleen
Therapy	No therapy available	Responds to diethylcarbamazine
Immunological test	CFT not so sensitive	CFT highly sensitive

Metabolites of growing larvae (in unsuitable hosts or immigrants) may produce urticarial rashes and lymphoedema. The symptoms may appear within 3½ months after exposure. Peripheral blood reveals no Mf. but biopsy of the regional lymph node might show presence of mature/immature adult Wuchereria.

Lymphangitis: Its causes are:

Mechanical irritation caused by worm motion within.

Metabolite liberation by growing larvae and release of toxic fluid by fertilised females during parturition.

Toxic products' absorption while the dead worms are being disintegrate.

Bacterial infection (though not certain). Streptococci as secondary invaders may supplement the wuchereriae in development of the classical lesion.

Lymphatic obstruction: Its causes are:

Mechanical obstruction by dead worms lying in the lumen.

Obliterative endolymphangitis: Endothelial proliferation and inflammatory thickening of walls of lymphatic vessels.

Fibrosis (excessive) of lymph vessels by repeated attacks of lymphangitis. Fibrosis of afferent lymph nodes draining a particular region.

Sequelae of lymphatic obstruction

Lymph varix—varicosity of lymph vessels.

Elephantiasis—hypertrophy of affected part/s.

Immunity and Wuchereriasis: *Role of RE system:* The worm derives its nutrition from lymph and any factor causing its obstruction also leads to its death. In initial stages there is an eosinophilic reaction to metabolites and body fluid of growing larvae and parturiting females respectively. In strongly reacting individuals, these excite a local allergic reaction, lymphangitis and lymphadenitis—all these tend to strangulate the worm. Consequently there is lymphoedema that provides nutrition to the worm. The littoral cells and the endothelial cells of the lymphatic channels subsequently undergo proliferation. *When the worm dies or undergoes degeneration:* R.E. system comes into play. The tissue surrounding the worm undergoes necrosis. Dead worm gets fragmented and may ultimately be calcified. The area then is invaded by tissue macrophages and may show giant cells too, eosinophilic infiltration gradually disappears. Finally filroblasts arrive to wall off the dead parasite—a hyalinised scar tissue is formed. Other organs possessing RE system cells are not involved actively in Wuchererial infections, however, they do take part disposing the microfilariae.

Occult filariasis (*Meyers-Kouwenaar syndrome*): There is marked eosinophilia (30–80%) with an absolute eosinophil count usually going beyond 3,000/cu. mm, generalised lymphadenopathy, hepatosplenomegaly, pulmonary symptoms (cough and wheeze) but no Mf. are seen in the peripheral blood. The adult worm produces Mf. continuously but they never reach the peripheral blood as they are destroyed in the tissues. This is on account of an unusual reaction to the filarial antigen by the host. *Evidences supporting a filarical aetiology:*
   (a) Filarial complement—fixing antibody titre is high,
   (b) Microfilaricidal drug diethylcarbamazine brings about a rapid response, and
   (c) The syndrome has been largely reported from filarial regions or belts.

Tropical pulmonary eosinophilia (eosinophilic lung or Weingarten's syndrome): This is a part of occult filariasis and is characterised by low fever, weight loss, paroxysmal cough with scanty sputum (may be blood-tinged), non-expiratory dyspnoea and splenomegaly. Chest X-ray exhibits prominent bronchovascular markings or diffuse miliary mottling in the lungs.

Classical Filariasis (*W. bancrofti*) Pathogenic Lesions

   A. **Inflammation:** Periodic attacks of fever with lymphangitis and lymphadenitis (not necessarily due to presence of worms in lymph nodes but may be a reaction to metabolites of worms located elsewhere).
   B. **Lymphatics' dilatation:** Lymphangiovarix.
   C. **Rupture of lymphangiovarix:**
   Lymphorrhagia: Lymph scrotum, lymphocele, lymphuria. *Chylorrhagia* (Obstruction in chyle-bearing vessels, thoracic duct)—chylocele, chyluria or haematochyluria, chylothorax, chylous diarrhoea, chylous ascites.
   D. **Skin and connective tissue hyperplasia:** Elephantiasis or solid oedema of various parts.
   E. **Secondary bacterial infection** (with *Streptococcus pyogenes* or *Staphylococcus aureus*): Septic lymphangitis, abscess and septicaemia.

Lymphangitis: Parts most commonly involved are the lymphatics of the testicle and epididymis (epididymo-orchitis), lymphatics of spermatic cord (funiculitis), abdominal lymphatics (retroperitoneal lymphangitis) and the lymphatics of the upper and lower extremities. The most favoured site for adults of *W. bancrofti* however is the globus major of epididymis. The involved lymphatic vessels appear as red congested streaks through the overlying skin. On touching—they appear as painful cord-like swellings. Involvement of retroperitoneal lymphatics may create an acute abdomen-like symptoms. The Wuchererial lymphangitis recurs once every month, perhaps related to a particular lunar phase.

Lymphadenitis: It may precede or accompany an attack of lymphangitis. Usually seen in the groin or axilla. Appear as soft and lobulated masses and are usually free from the overlying skin. They are nontender/painful in the absence of acute inflammation.

Filarial fever: Filarial lymphagitis is often accompanied by a rise in temperature (103° to 104°F) which may continue for several days. The temperature falls by crisis and profuse sweating. Peripheral blood shows transient leucocytosis.

Hydrocele: Recurrent Wuchererial orchitis and epididymitis attacks predispose to hydrocele, it may coexist with elephantiasis of scrotum. Mf. may be seen in the hydrocele fluid in which they sooner or later die. Wall of the sac is thickened and adult Wuchereriae (living/dead/calcified) may be seen in the Wuchererial granulation tissue. Spermatic cord lymphatic vessels are also thickened, causing lymphatic varicoceles (funicular lymphangio-varices). Hydrocele occurs from obstruction of para-aortic lymph nodes that interfere with lymph drainage from tunica vaginalis, epididymis and spermatic cord.

Elephantiasis: Affected part shows tumour-like solidity. This is the end result of a prolonged and continuous (for years) Wuchererial infection. These attacks cause fibrotic constriction of all the afferent lymphatics draining the region. Their blockage leads to exudation of the protein rich lymph—this, in turn, causes hypertrophy and hyperplasia—chiefly involving connective tissue. So elephantiasis of legs results from obstruction of inguinal or iliac lymph nodes while that of scrotum follows obstruction of superficial inguinal lymph nodes. *Grossly* the skin appears rough, fissured and papillomatous. The associated hair too become rough and sparse. The thickened, dense and fibrous skin cuts with difficulty. The subcutaneous tissues show a blubbery appearance in which the dilated and thickened lymphatics and veins are visible. The underlying musculature and bones show no changes. *Microscopically* Wuchererial granulation tissue consists of hyperplastic connective tissue infiltrated by eosinophils, plasma cells, monocytes and giant cells around a degenerating, dead or calcified parasite. Lymphatic vessels exhibit obliterative endolymphangitis with occlusion by thrombi. *Peripheral smear* usually does not show Mf. either on account of death of adult worms or their failure to reach the systemic circulation due to lymphatic obstruction.

Chyluria: It is the escape of chyle through the urine; due to rupture of varicose chyle vessels through the mucous membrane of urinary tract. Urine appears milky white owing to the fat particles (that dissolve in ether, chloroform or xylene), albumin (precipitates on boiling) and fibrinogen (forms a coagulum). Microscopic examination of urinary sediment may reveal Mf. and a few red blood cells.

Filarial manifestations: Geographical variations

1. **Chyluria:** Seen predominantly in China, Japan and South India but rare in Africa and Pacific Islands.
2. **Hydrocele:** Is prevalent in East Africa, Japan and China but less so in India and the Pacific Islands.
3. **Elephantiasis of leg and scrotum:** Common in China, India and Pacific Islands but rare in West Africa.

Clinical presentation of classical filariasis

1. **Asymptomatic cases**—light infections may pass unnoticed.
2. **Symptomatic filariasis**—may be divided into:
   A. *Inflammatory phase*—characterised by lymphangitis and lymphadenitis. Lasts for a few days and subsides but recurs at irregular intervals for a period of weeks or months.

B. *Obstructive phase*—characterised by varicose lymph vessels, lymphadenitis (groin and axilla), lymph scrotum, hydrocele, chyluria and elephantiasis of various parts. These are observed at sites where inflammatory reactions have occurred earlier. The obstructive lesion may take up to 20 years to develop and manifest.

Diagnosis can be divided into direct and indirect evidences.

Direct evidences

A. **Demonstration of Mf.**— Sheathed Mf. having tail-tip free from nuclei may be seen in:
- peripheral blood.
- chylous urine.
- exudate of lymph varix.
- hydrocele fluid.

One may use a thin film, thick film or a concentration technique for showing Mf. in peripheral blood.

Microfilariae may not be observed in peripheral blood under the following circumstances:

(a) In cases of elephantiasis on account of lymphatic obstruction.
(b) After an attack of lymphangitis due to death of an adult worm.
(c) During early allergic manifestations.
(d) In occult filariasis.

B. **Demonstration of adult worms:**
(a) In lymph node biopsy (usually not necessary for diagnosis).
(b) Calcified worm demonstration by X-ray.

Indirect evidences (serological/allergic tests)

A. **Allergic tests:**
(i) Eosinophilia (5–15%) on peripheral smear, (ii) Intradermal test—an immediate hypersensitivity test. Formation of weal more than 2 cm after half an hour.

B. **Serological/Immunological techniques:**
(i) Complement fixation test,
(ii) ELISA test—very specific and sensitive,
(iii) Fluorescent antibody test available but not found to be satisfactory.
(iv) PCR is available in tertiary labs

Treatment: Drugs are subdivided into those acting on:
(i) Adult worms—Mel. W, an arsenical preparation, found to be useful.
(ii) Microfilariae—Diethylcarbamazine (Hetrazan).
(iii) Infective larvae and immature adult worms—para-melaminyl phenyl stibonate (MSb).

Prophylaxis: Includes:
(i) Destruction of mosquitoes,
(ii) Self-protection from mosquito bites,
(iii) Biotechnology methods—releasing fish that eat mosquito larvae—Guppy variety currently being used,
(iv) Treatment of carriers by using Hetrazan.

Brugia malayi

(Malayan Filaria)

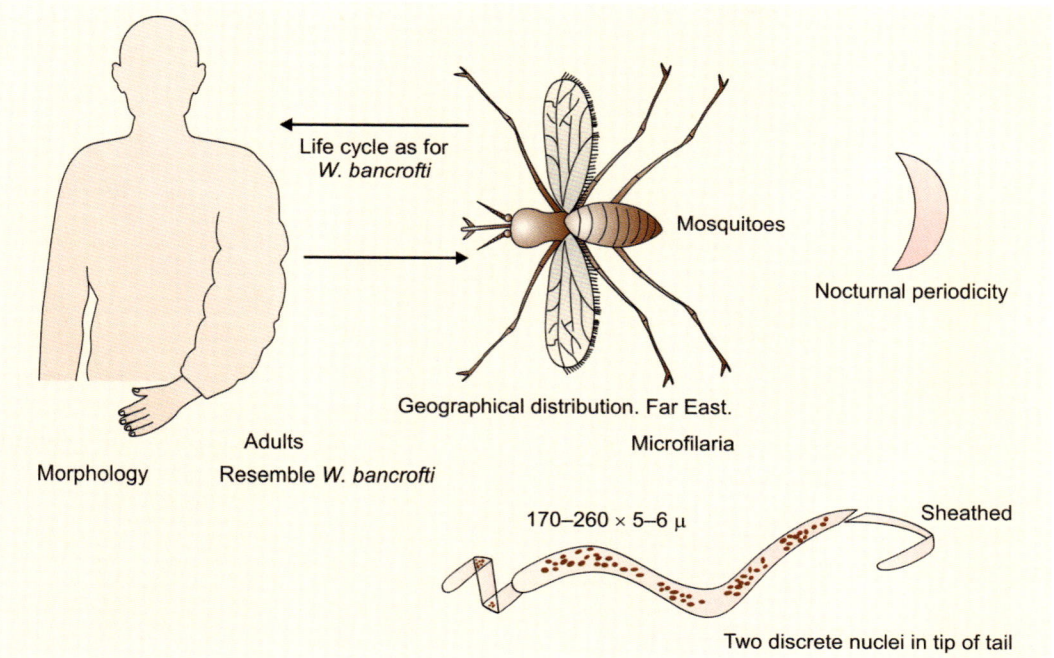

Life cycle as for W. bancrofti

Mosquitoes

Nocturnal periodicity

Geographical distribution. Far East.

Adults

Microfilaria

Resemble W. bancrofti

Morphology

170–260 × 5–6 μ

Sheathed

Two discrete nuclei in tip of tail

Pathology as for *W. bancrofti*

Laboratory diagnosis as for *W. bancrofti*

Geographical distribution: India (chiefly reported from Kerala, Orissa, Madhya Pradesh and Assam), Indonesia, Borneo, Thailand, Vietnam, Malaysia, Burma, Southern China, Korea, Japan (Koshima Island).

Habitat and morphology: As for *W. bancrofti*—adult females are identical in both but adult males differ in minor details. Mf appears in peripheral blood at nighttime (sometimes subperiodic, may appear during daytime too). *Mf. malayi* is enveloped in sheath and differs from *Mf. bancrofti* in the following aspects:
   (i) Is smaller, 170–260 × 5–6 μ, lies folded with head close to tail.
  (ii) Possesses secondary kinks and bends, instead of smooth curves.
 (iii) Has two stylets at anterior end.
  (iv) Cephalic space is larger.
   (v) Has blurred nuclei therefore counting is difficult. Tail tip shows 2 nuclei

Life cycle: As for *W. bancrofti*.
   Intermediate hosts in India are different.

Genus	Species
Mansonia	Indiana/annulifera/uniformis
Anopheles	barbirostris

Culex is not the intermediate host. Larval development is completed in 6–8 days. Domestic animals, cats and dogs may act as reservoirs of infection.

Pathology: As for *W.bancrofti,* however, Malayan filariasis is characterised by absence of chyluria and scrotal swellings are rare.

Diagnosis, treatment and prophylaxis: As for *W. bancrofti.*

Loa loa

(The eye worm)

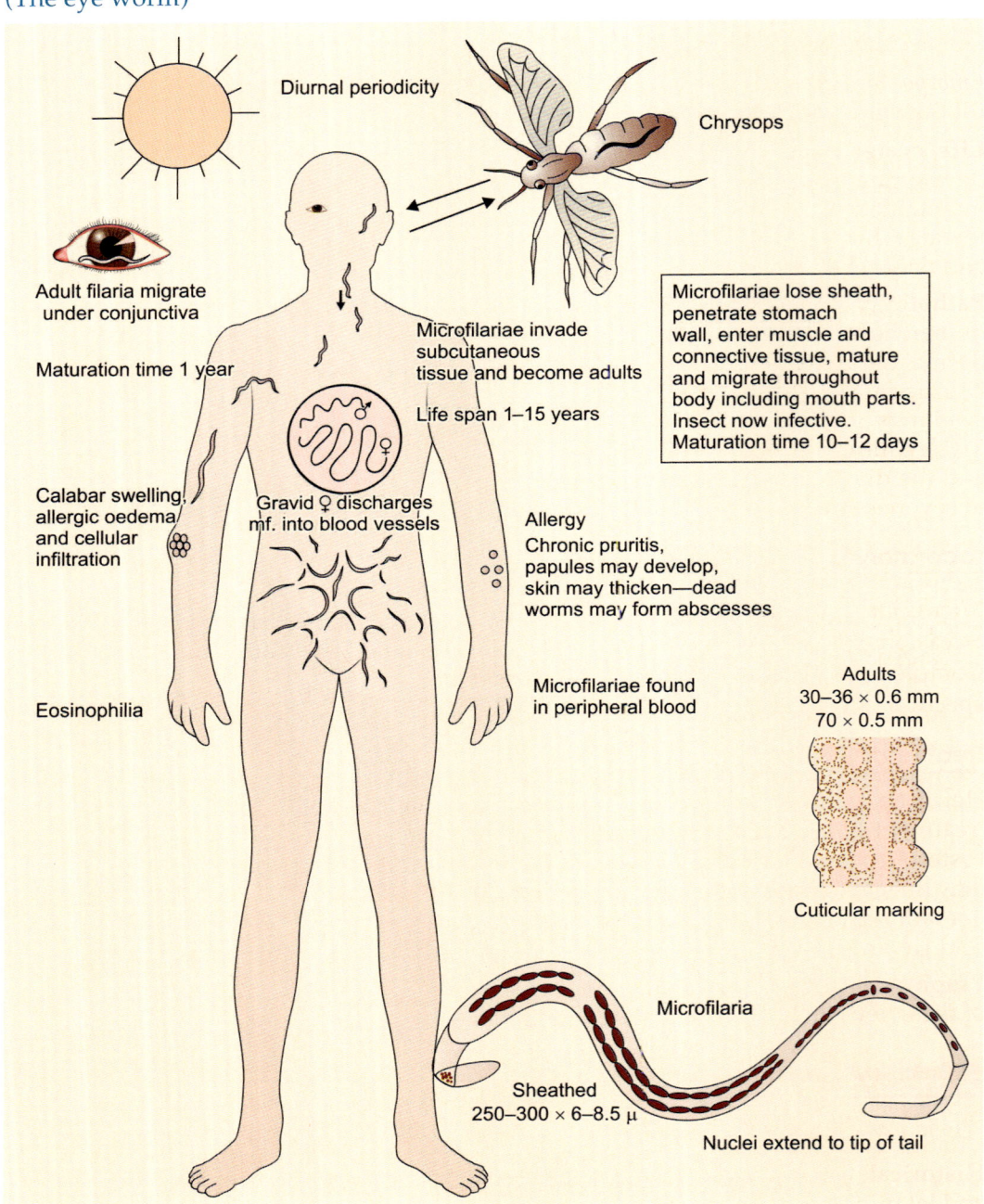

Diurnal periodicity

Chrysops

Adult filaria migrate under conjunctiva

Maturation time 1 year

Microfilariae invade subcutaneous tissue and become adults

Life span 1–15 years

Microfilariae lose sheath, penetrate stomach wall, enter muscle and connective tissue, mature and migrate throughout body including mouth parts. Insect now infective. Maturation time 10–12 days

Calabar swelling, allergic oedema and cellular infiltration

Gravid ♀ discharges mf. into blood vessels

Allergy
Chronic pruritis, papules may develop, skin may thicken—dead worms may form abscesses

Eosinophilia

Microfilariae found in peripheral blood

Adults
30–36 × 0.6 mm
70 × 0.5 mm

Cuticular marking

Microfilaria

Sheathed
250–300 × 6–8.5 µ

Nuclei extend to tip of tail

Historical: First identified by Cobbold in 1864 and later described by Castellani and Chalmers 1913. Loa is West African name for this worm.

Habitat: Subcutaneous connective tissues of man, often in the subconjunctival tissue of the eye.

Morphology

Adult worm: Cuticle shows microscopic excrescences (cuticular bosses) that vary in number and placement in the two sexes. Males measure 30–36 x 0.6 mm while the females measure 70 × 0.5 mm. Average life span of an adult is about 15 years.

Embryo: Measure 250–300 × 6–8.5 μ. It is sheath enveloped and the nuclei extend right till the tail-tip. These are found in peripheral blood by daytime.

Life cycle: Needs two hosts—man and Chrysops (Mango or deer flies). Larval development follows the same course of development as for other larvae. *Loa loa* is maintained in nature by interhuman transmission. Infection being transmitted by female Chrysops—*C. silacea* and *C. dimidiata,* these are day-biters, canopy dwellers and only the females suck blood.

Pathology: It causes loiasis. Incubation period is about 3–4 years. After entering the human host it rapidly migrates to various parts of the body through the subcutaneous dermal tissues and exhibits a special predilection for creeping in and around the eyes. During migratory phase it causes oedema of subcutaneous tissues known as Calabar swellings 'fugitive swellings'. These are allergic reactions and vanish within 2–3 days. Mf. are mostly found during this swelling phase (i.e. in the first 4 years of infection) and the diagnosis is based upon history of such swellings associated with moderate to severe eosinophilia (30–80%).

Laboratory Diagnosis

Microfilariae in blood.
Occasionally adult seen under conjunctiva or by biopsy of swelling.
Complement fixation or intradermal tests with dirofilarial antigen (group, not species, specific).

Treatment

Hetrazan is most effective. Sometimes violent allergic reactions may occur with treatment but these can be managed by concurrently using antiallergics and corticosteroids. Heavy infection cases when treated with Hetrazan (diethylcarbamazine) may develop nephrotic syndrome or meningoencephalitis (because of toxic products' liberation on worm death)—these patients must always be treated under corticosteroid cover.

Prophylaxis: Includes personal protection from bites of infected flies and elimination of flies themselves.

Onchocerca Volvulus

(The convoluted Filaria)

Historical: Onchocerca means hooked tail. It was first described by Leuckart in 1893 and later in 1910 by Railliet and Henry. It is commonly known as the blinding worm.

Geographical distribution: Africa, Central America (Guatemala, Mexico, Venezuela and surrounding countries), it has also been reported from the Southern Arabic nations.

Habitat: The adult worm resides in the connective tissues of man.

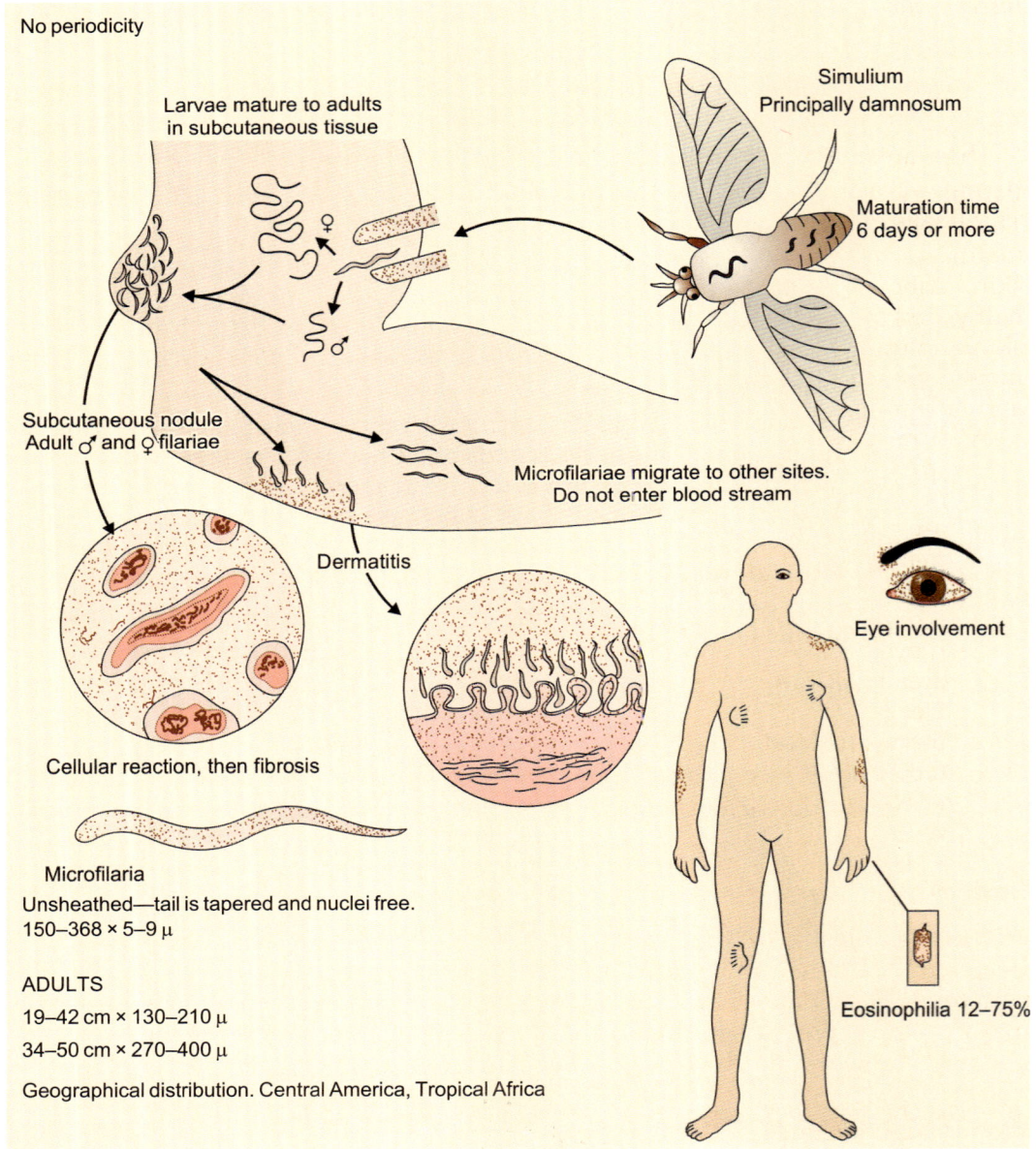

No periodicity

Larvae mature to adults in subcutaneous tissue

Simulium
Principally damnosum

Maturation time 6 days or more

Subcutaneous nodule
Adult ♂ and ♀ filariae

Microfilariae migrate to other sites.
Do not enter blood stream

Dermatitis

Eye involvement

Cellular reaction, then fibrosis

Microfilaria
Unsheathed—tail is tapered and nuclei free.
150–368 × 5–9 µ

ADULTS
19–42 cm × 130–210 µ
34–50 cm × 270–400 µ

Geographical distribution. Central America, Tropical Africa

Eosinophilia 12–75%

Morphology

Adult worm: The cuticle is raised in well-marked annular and oblique thickenings (more marked in females). Males measure 19–42 cm × 30–210 µ and females measure 34–50 cm × 270–400 µ. Gravid females may survive up to 15 years. *Microfilariae* are found in the skin are unsheathed and nonperiodic. Nuclear column does not extend till the tapered tail tip. They measure 150–368 × 5–9 µ.

Life cycle: Definitive host—man. Intermediate host—day biting female 'black fly' of genus Simulium. Development phase in the fly is identical to that of *Mf. bancrofti,* however, it takes only 6 days to complete that cycle.

Insect vectors: In Africa — *S. damnosum*
                                    — *S. navei*
                 In America — *S. onchraceum* (Mexico and Guatemala)
                                    — *S. metallicum* (Venezuela)

These are day-biting small flies (1–5 mm long) and their females are blood suckers.

Pathology: Infection is transmitted by the bite of an infected female simulium. The infective larvae stay localised and grow in the skin into adult worms. Once matured, the gravid females release unsheathed motile Mf which migrate in the skin, subcutaneous tissues and eyes until they die (may survive up to two and a half years) or they may be sucked up by Simulium. The pathological changes in the skin and eyes occur due to hypersensitivity reaction to the dead or dying Mf. The incubation period is about 12 months. Lesions can be subdivided into subcutaneous and ocular lesions.

A. **Subcutaneous nodules (onchocercomas):** Size may vary from few millimeters to 6 cm. Maximum size may be reached in several years' time. Average number of nodules is 3 to 6, however, they can be single to multiple too. In Africa they are predominantly located in the trunk and limbs, whereas in America they are mainly found over the head especially over the scalp. This variation is due to preferred locations of the fly to bite. The adults die within these nodules only. Nodules are raised, painless and non-suppurating. On biopsy, microscopically, they reveal a concentric fibrous tissue mass enveloping a honeycombed central area containing the adult worms of both sexes seen in an intertwined fashion. Dead worms may get calcified (dystrophic calcification) and may evoke a foreign body giant cell reaction. Peripheral smear reveals marked eosinophilia. Other complications that may occur are:
   • Hydrocele or lymph scrotum development.
   • Elephantiasis of legs and scrotum.
   • Hanging groin (in African form), the atrophied elasticityless skin in the groin region hangs in a fold containing enlarged/sclerosed femoral or inguinal lymph nodes. The skin exhibits lichenification and mottled depigmentation (leopard skin).

B. **Ocular lesions (caused by Mf):** Seen especially where head lesions are present. The Mf may be observed moving about in the substantia propria of the cornea and also in the anterior chamber of the eye. They cause conjunctivitis, opacities and pannus in the anterior quadrant of cornea. Subsequent complications include iridocyditis, secondary glaucoma and papillitis (optic atrophy) to end in total blindness.

Diagnosis

Detection of adults in excised nodules.
Presence of Mf in shavings of skin.
Eye examination by slit lamp.
Nodule puncturing leads to severe allergic reaction.
Peripheral smear shows marked eosinophilia.

Mazzotti's skin test—On giving 50–100 mg Hetrazan and subsequent appearance of pruritic papular rash in 24 hours indicates a positive test, implying presence of cutaneous Mf. The reaction occurs due to dead Mf. of *O. volvulus* killed by the drug.

Fluorescent antibody test—Mf. of *O. volvulus* are used as antigens. Sera from patients having onchocerciasis react positively.

Treatment: Specific drugs include hetrazan and suramin. The nodules can be excised and enucleated. Excision helps in reduction of ocular complications.

Prophylaxis: Measures directed against the insect host—the Simulium.

OTHER FILARIAL WORMS

Microfilariae of other species may be found in the blood and tissues. These worms appear to be non-pathogenic and differentiation of microfilariae from Wuchereria and Brugia necessary.

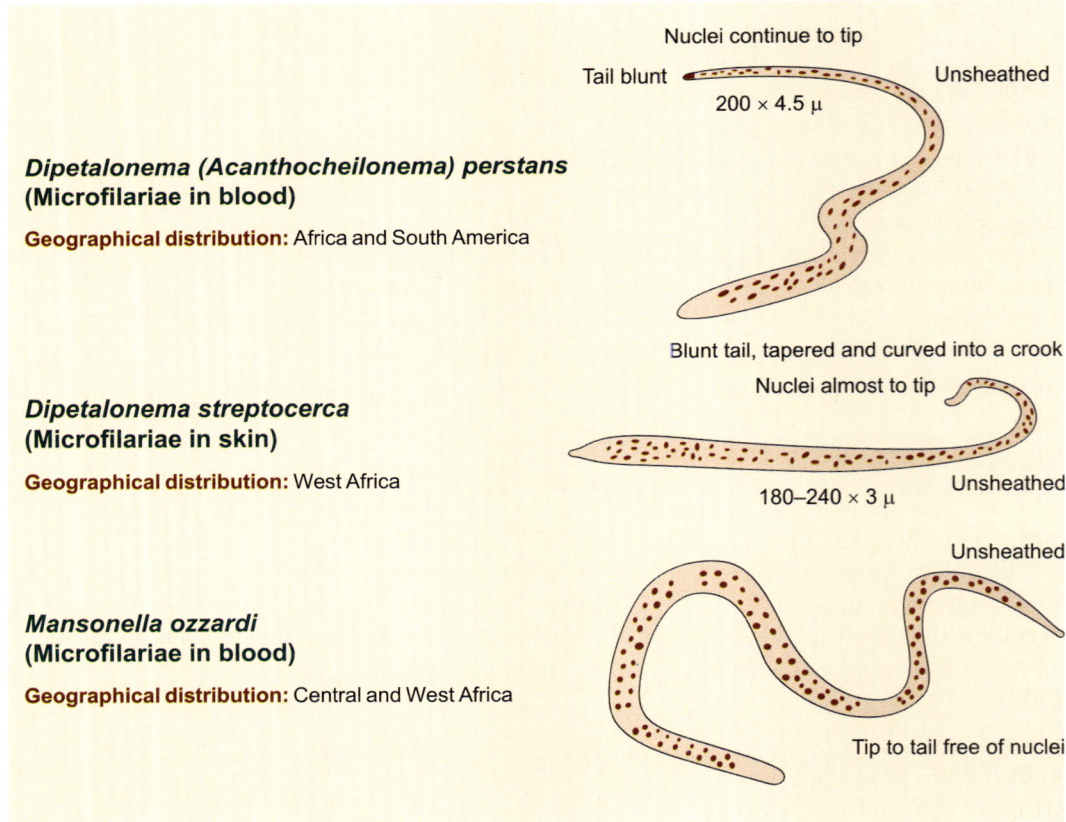

Dipetalonema (Acanthocheilonema) perstans (Microfilariae in blood)

Geographical distribution: Africa and South America

Nuclei continue to tip
Tail blunt
Unsheathed
200 × 4.5 μ

Dipetalonema streptocerca (Microfilariae in skin)

Geographical distribution: West Africa

Blunt tail, tapered and curved into a crook
Nuclei almost to tip
Unsheathed
180–240 × 3 μ

Mansonella ozzardi (Microfilariae in blood)

Geographical distribution: Central and West Africa

Unsheathed
Tip to tail free of nuclei

DIROFILARIASIS OF HUMAN BEINGS

Animal Dirofilaria may reach adulthood in man without producing microfilariae. Included in this are:

1. *Dirofilaria immitis:* A dog parasite, lives in cardiac chamber. It is the usual source of antigen (group-specific) for intradermal and complement fixation tests for

filarial infections in man. Causes subcutaneous nodules and coin lesions in lung. It can also cause eosinophilic meningitis in man.

2. *Dirofilaria conjunctivae:* It is a natural parasite of animals. It lives encysted in subcutaneous tissues. Has more or less a worldwide distribution. Other species being *D. repens* and *D. tennis.* Both cause subcutaneous nodules and abscesses (in eyelids and palpebral conjunctiva also).

DRACUNCULOIDEA

(Superfamily)

These are long cord-like worms, mouth is a simple opening surrounded by circumoral papillae. Have a rudimentary oesophagus and intestine. Vulva is seen in the middle of the body but it atrophies before the worm matures. Females are viviparous and much larger than the males. Larvae are classical rhabditoid. Need two hosts to complete their life cycle with Cyclops being the intermediate host.

Dracunculus medinensis

(The Guinea worm)

Historical: It has been known since the ancient times. It is also known as Guineaworm, Serpent worm, Dragon worm or Medina worm. Galen at about 200 AD named it 'dracontiasis'. The Arabian physician Avicenna in eleventh century named it, Vena Medina. Bible describes it as 'fiery serpent'.

Geographical distribution: India, Pakistan, Burma, Iraq, Iran, Saudi Arabia, South-Eastern states (new countries) of erstwhile USSR., Africa (East, West and Central), West Indies and South America. The states afflicted in India are those on the Western boundary—Punjab, Rajasthan, Madhya Pradesh, Gujarat, Maharashtra and South India. It has not yet been observed in Eastern states.

Habitat: Adult females reside in the subcutaneous tissues, mainly in the legs, arms and back.

Male: Male worms have not been recovered from man (rare case reported). It measures 12–29 × 0.4 mm.

Female: Very long, filiform and measures 70–120 cm × 0.9–2.7 mm. The cylindrical smooth body is milky-white in colour. Posterior extremity is tapering and bent like a hook. They are viviparous and discharge embryos in successive batches for up to 3 weeks till the uterus empties completely. Body fluid is toxic and causes blisters if it escapes into the tissues. Life span of a female is about a year and that of a male 6 months or less.

Embryos: Are coiled with rounded heads and long slender tapering tails. They measure 500–700 × 15–25 μ. Embryos are set free at the time of parturition when the affected part is submerged in water. Further development occurs in Cyclops. If not taken up by a Cyclops, they die within a weeks' time.

Life cycle: Needs 2 hosts—man and cyclops. *Definitive host*—man. It harbors the adults. *Intermediate host*—Cyclops, in which the embryos undergo developmental changes before becoming infective to man. Worldwide, *Mesocyclops leuekarti* acts as the intermediate host (including India). Other vectors described are *Mesocyclops hyalinus, Thermocyclops vermifer, Encyclops serrulatus* and *Tropocyclops multivolor.*

Morphology

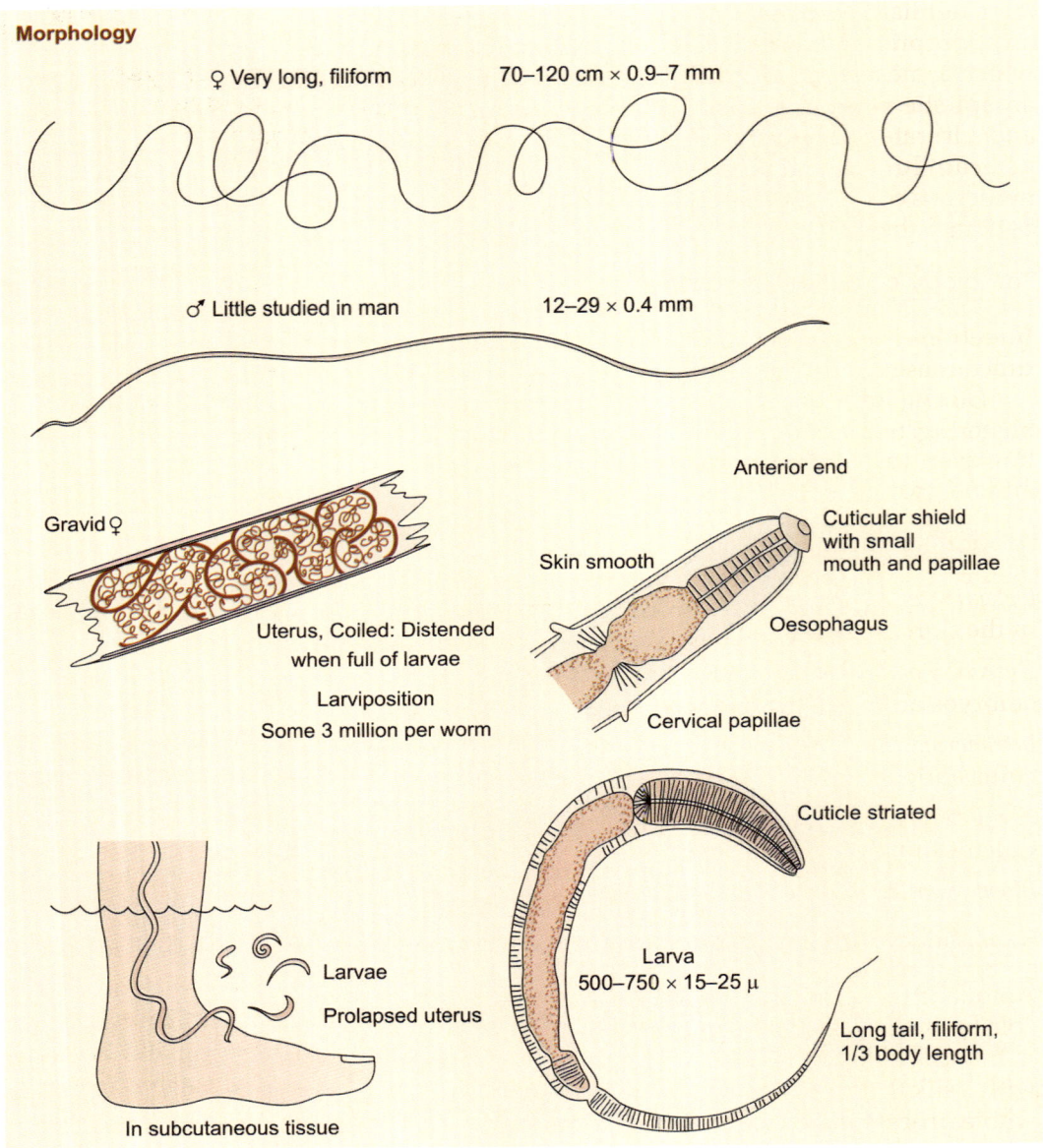

♀ Very long, filiform   70–120 cm × 0.9–7 mm

♂ Little studied in man   12–29 × 0.4 mm

Gravid ♀

Uterus, Coiled: Distended
when full of larvae

Larviposition
Some 3 million per worm

Anterior end

Skin smooth

Cuticular shield
with small
mouth and papillae

Oesophagus

Cervical papillae

Larvae

Prolapsed uterus

In subcutaneous tissue

Cuticle striated

Larva
500–750 × 15–25 µ

Long tail, filiform,
1/3 body length

Development within the cyclop: Each cyclops can ingest up to 15–20 guinea worm embroys. Normal life span of cyclops is about 90 days, however, the infected ones barely survive beyond 42 days (heavier the infection, lesser the life span). Within 6 hours the embryos pass through the gut wall and reach the body cavity where they metamorphose and increase in size up to 1 mm. Under favourable circumstances they complete their development in a fortnight.

Development within a human host: The infected cyclops containing infective larvae is ingested by man along with water. Once in the stomach, the cyclops is digested by gastric juice and the larvae are released. They pass through the gut wall to reach the retroperitoneal connective tissues where they grow till sexual maturity. Males die after fertilising the females and disappear within 6 months after injection. To select an appropriate site for discharging embryos in water. It selects only those sites of skin which come into contact with water regularly—the extremities and back. On reaching an apt site it releases a toxin that produces a blister which subsequently ruptures and ulcerates. When this region is dipped into water the gravid female protrudes its head through the ulcer and causes a reflex discharge of a milky fluid containing numerous coiled embryos. The whole cycle is then repeated. Incubation period is about 8–12 months.

Pathology and Clinical Features

Infection is termed guinea worm disease, dracunculosis, dracunculiasis or dracontiasis.

During parturition, the toxin released brings about allergic reactions (itching) and blistering. Secondary bacterial infection may follow at the site of ulceration. Initially, however, the blister fluid is sterile, yellowish and contains monocytes, eosinophils and neutrophils.

Laboratory Diagnosis

Detection of adult worms: It is possible when the female worm appears at the surface of the skin.

Detection of embryos: The affected part may be bathed in water to induce discharge of embryos and the fluid exuded may be examined microscopically.

Intradermal test: Positive test is indicated when the intradermal injection of dracunculus antigen produces a wheal in 24 hours.

X-ray examination: Following their death, the worms either get calcified or are absorbed. Calcification can be detected by radiography.

Blood examination: Reveals eosinophilia.

Treatment

Ambilhar (nitrothiazole) has given excellent results. Thiabendazole and metronidazole have also been used for treating dracontiasis.

In India the worm is also extracted mechanically. When the head shows up, it is tied with a silk thread to a matchstick. Inch by inch it is rolled onto the stick everyday. The whole process may take 15–20 days.

Prophylaxis: Aim is to break the man-cyclops-man cycle. This can be done by:
— Prevention of pollution of drinking water by an infected individual
— Chemical treatment of water for eradication of cyclops
— Drinking strained, filtered or boiled water.

SPIRUROIDEA

(Superfamily)

Gnathostoma spinigerum: About 3 cm long adults are normally found in the gastric walls of canine and feline animals (the definitive hosts—dogs, cats, tigers, etc). The eggs (oval with unipolar mucous plug) are evacuated via the faeces into water where they embryonate and hatch. The larvae produced are taken up by Cyclops (the first intermediate host) and are metamorphosed into second stage larvae. These are consumed by a fish, frog or snake (the second intermediate host) and develops into third stage larvae in the flesh of these animals. The definitive hosts (may be man too) get infected by consuming the third stage larvae in the second intermediate host and then develop into adult worms in about 7 months in the stomach wall.

When man consumes ill-cooked flesh of second intermediate host he gets infected by third stage larvae of *G. spinigerum* but the larvae are unable to reach adulthood. The immature third stage larvae resemble adults morphologically. They migrate through subcutaneous tissues and cause cutaneous larva migrans. They are also known to invade eyes and brain. The diagnosis is established by finding immature worm in the lesion and by an intradermal skin test with the larval or adult antigen. No effective chemotherapy is available, therefore, surgery is the only alternative for their removal. Infection can be prevented by sterilising the infected second intermediate host by boiling or immersing in strong vinegar (acetic acid) for about 6 hours. Gnasthotomiasis is commonest in Thailand but has also been reported from Vietnam, Malaysia and India too.

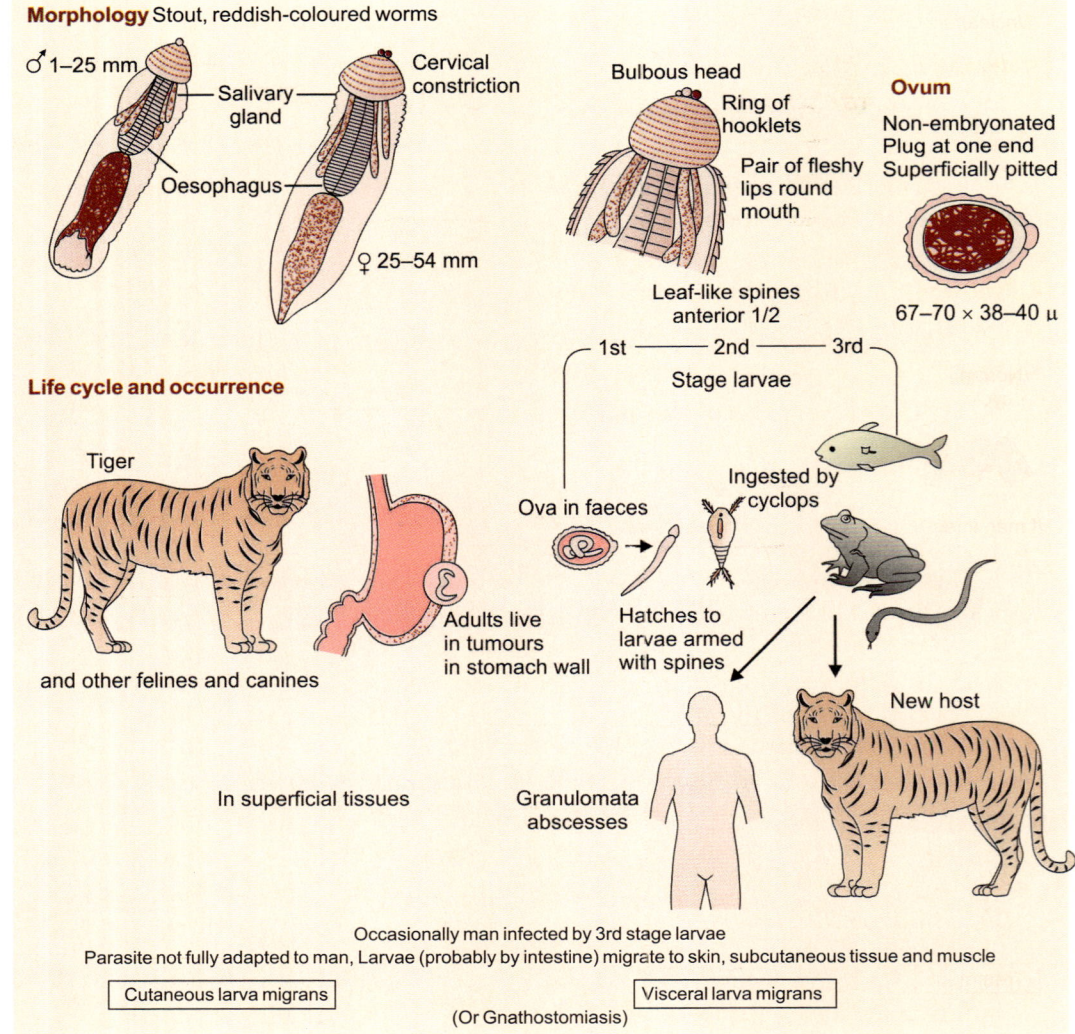

Morphology Stout, reddish-coloured worms

♂ 1–25 mm
Salivary gland
Cervical constriction
Oesophagus
♀ 25–54 mm

Bulbous head
Ring of hooklets
Pair of fleshy lips round mouth
Leaf-like spines anterior 1/2

Ovum
Non-embryonated
Plug at one end
Superficially pitted
67–70 × 38–40 μ

1st ——— 2nd ——— 3rd
Stage larvae

Life cycle and occurrence

Tiger
and other felines and canines

In superficial tissues

Adults live in tumours in stomach wall

Ova in faeces
Hatches to larvae armed with spines

Ingested by cyclops

New host

Granulomata abscesses

Occasionally man infected by 3rd stage larvae
Parasite not fully adapted to man, Larvae (probably by intestine) migrate to skin, subcutaneous tissue and muscle

Cutaneous larva migrans   Visceral larva migrans

(Or Gnasthotomiasis)

LARVA MIGRANS

When certain nematode larvae enter an unnatural host, man, are unable to complete their life cycle and get lodged either in the subcutaneous tissue or in the viscera and the corresponding conditions are labelled as cutaneous larva migrans (creeping eruption) and visceral larva migrans respectively.

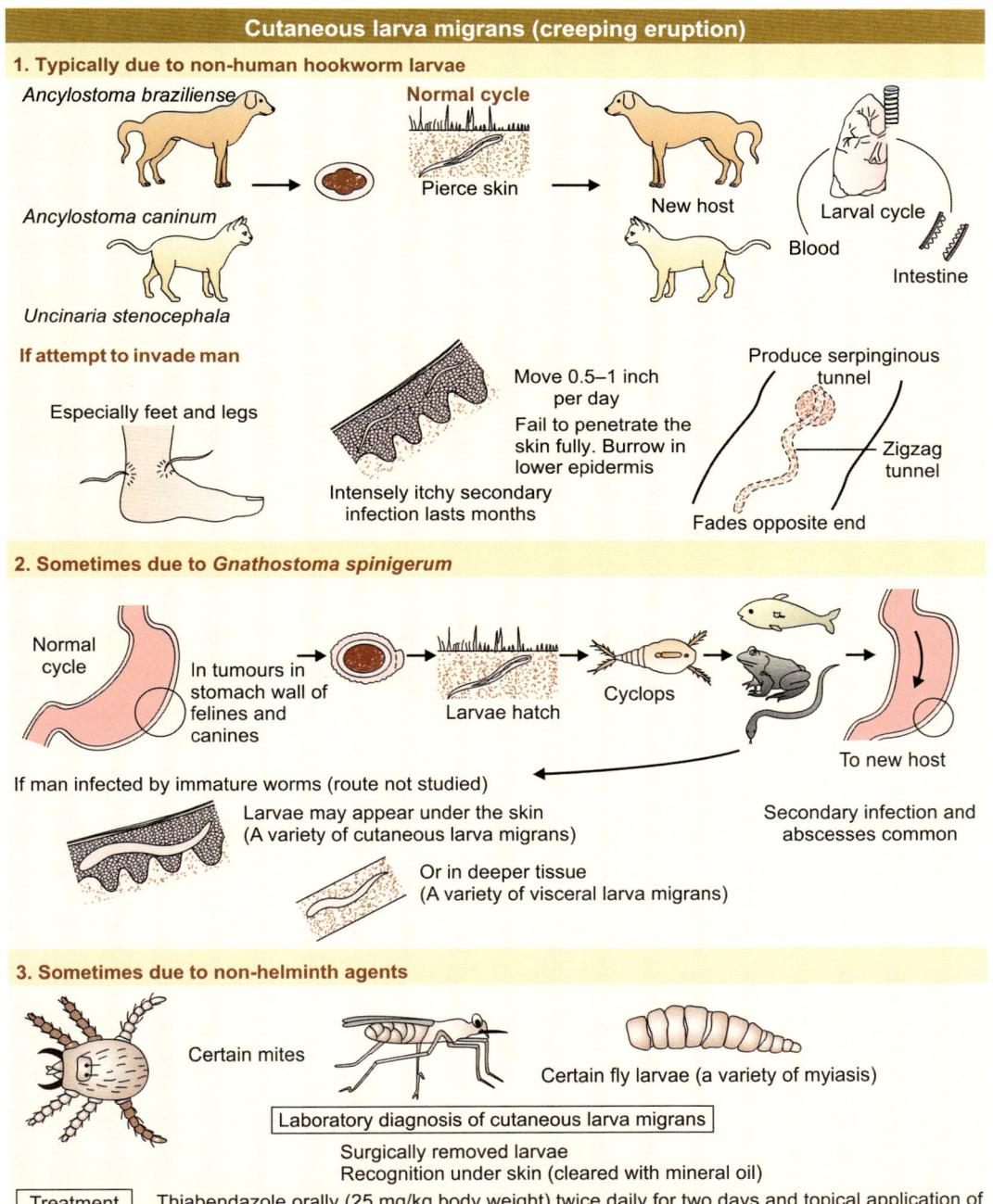

Cutaneous larva migrans (creeping eruption)

1. Typically due to non-human hookworm larvae

Ancylostoma braziliense

Ancylostoma caninum

Uncinaria stenocephala

Normal cycle

Pierce skin

New host

Larval cycle

Blood

Intestine

If attempt to invade man

Especially feet and legs

Move 0.5–1 inch per day

Fail to penetrate the skin fully. Burrow in lower epidermis

Intensely itchy secondary infection lasts months

Produce serpinginous tunnel

Zigzag tunnel

Fades opposite end

2. Sometimes due to *Gnathostoma spinigerum*

Normal cycle

In tumours in stomach wall of felines and canines

Larvae hatch

Cyclops

To new host

If man infected by immature worms (route not studied)

Larvae may appear under the skin
(A variety of cutaneous larva migrans)

Or in deeper tissue
(A variety of visceral larva migrans)

Secondary infection and abscesses common

3. Sometimes due to non-helminth agents

Certain mites

Certain fly larvae (a variety of myiasis)

Laboratory diagnosis of cutaneous larva migrans

Surgically removed larvae
Recognition under skin (cleared with mineral oil)

Treatment | Thiabendazole orally (25 mg/kg body weight) twice daily for two days and topical application of 15% thiabendazole powder in cream form (hydrosoluable)

VISCERAL LARVA MIGRANS

Definition

Infection by   1. Larvae of non-human nematodes attempting to invade man fail to complete normal life cycle.
2. Larvae of human nematodes getting lost in ectopic sites

Aetiology

Suggested classification

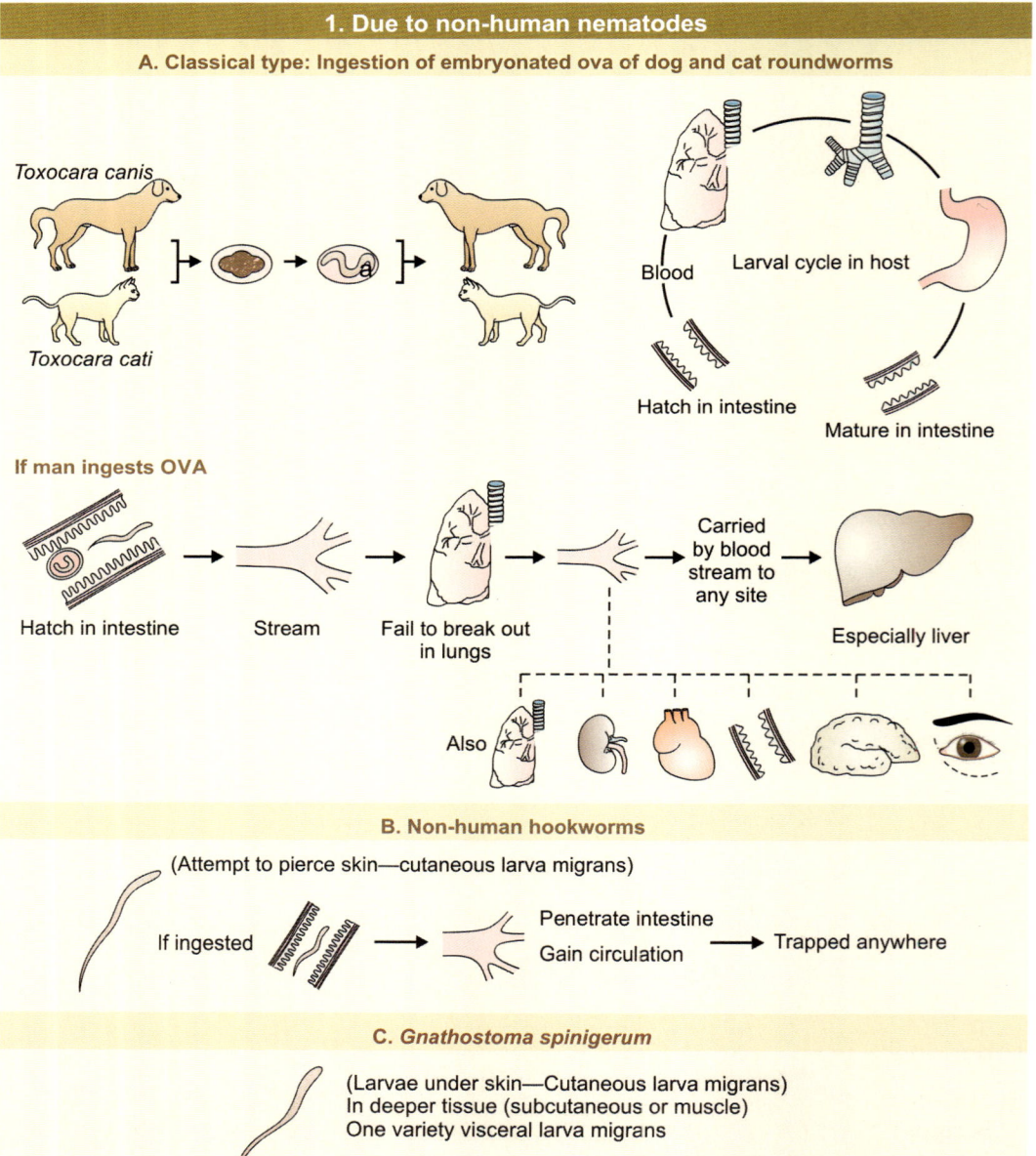

1. Due to non-human nematodes

A. Classical type: Ingestion of embryonated ova of dog and cat roundworms

Toxocara canis

Toxocara cati

Blood   Larval cycle in host

Hatch in intestine

Mature in intestine

If man ingests OVA

Hatch in intestine   Stream   Fail to break out in lungs   Carried by blood stream to any site   Especially liver

Also

B. Non-human hookworms

(Attempt to pierce skin—cutaneous larva migrans)

If ingested   Penetrate intestine   Trapped anywhere
Gain circulation

C. Gnathostoma spinigerum

(Larvae under skin—Cutaneous larva migrans)
In deeper tissue (subcutaneous or muscle)
One variety visceral larva migrans

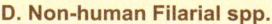

D. Non-human Filarial spp.

Microfilaria are possible cause of tropical eosinophilia
Serum gives—CFT for filaria
Spp. incriminated Dirofilaria immitis (The dog filaria)
    Brugia pahangi ⎫
    Brugia patai ⎬ Parasites of dogs and cats

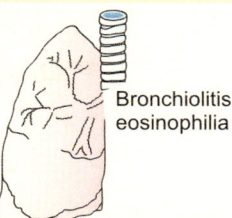

Bronchiolitis
eosinophilia

2. Due to human nematodes

A larvae of ascaris lumbricoides (in heavy infections) strongyloides stercoralis (in Alto and hyperinfections)

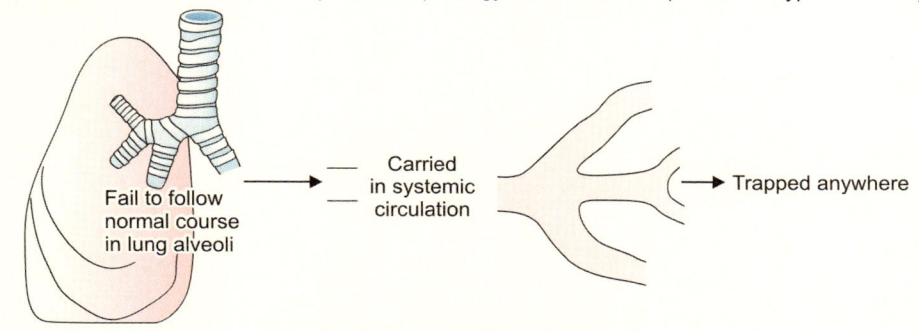

Fail to follow
normal course
in lung alveoli

Carried
in systemic
circulation

Trapped anywhere

B. Microfilaria of *Brugia malayi* can cause a syndrome like trophical eosinophilia

Pathology

1. Larva trapped in tissue

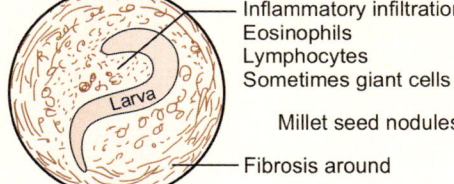

Larva

Inflammatory infiltration
Eosinophils
Lymphocytes
Sometimes giant cells

Millet seed nodules

Fibrosis around

May be nothing untoward
May be allergy (eosinophilia)
May be organ dysfunction

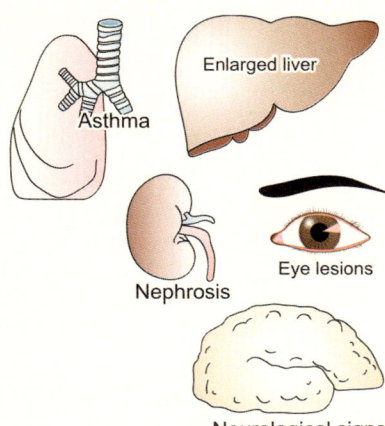

Enlarged liver

Asthma

Nephrosis

Eye lesions

Neurological signs

2. Tropical eosinophilia

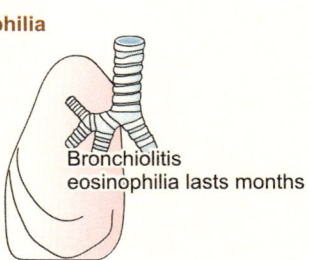

Bronchiolitis
eosinophilia lasts months

Laboratory Diagnosis of Visceral Larva Migrans

- Histology of biopsy specimens
- Serological in some cases (e.g. complement fixation test in tropical eosinophilia)
- Intradermal tests in some cases (e.g. toxocara)

Details of *T. canis* and *T. cati*—that cause visceral larva migrans

Toxocara canis (the dog roundworm)

Morphology

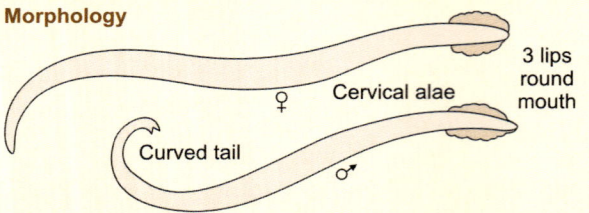

3 lips
round
mouth

Cervical alae

♀

Curved tail

♂

Specific papillary arrangement

Ovum

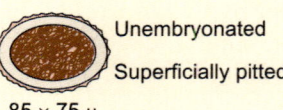

Unembryonated

Superficially pitted

85 × 75 μ

Life cycle

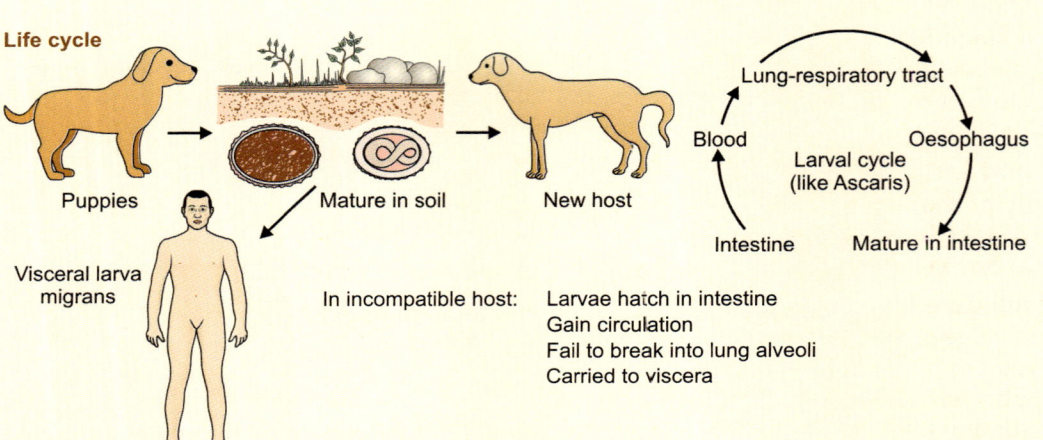

Puppies

Mature in soil

New host

Lung-respiratory tract

Blood

Oesophagus

Larval cycle
(like Ascaris)

Intestine

Mature in intestine

Visceral larva
migrans

In incompatible host: Larvae hatch in intestine
Gain circulation
Fail to break into lung alveoli
Carried to viscera

Toxocara cati (the cat roundworm)

Morphology

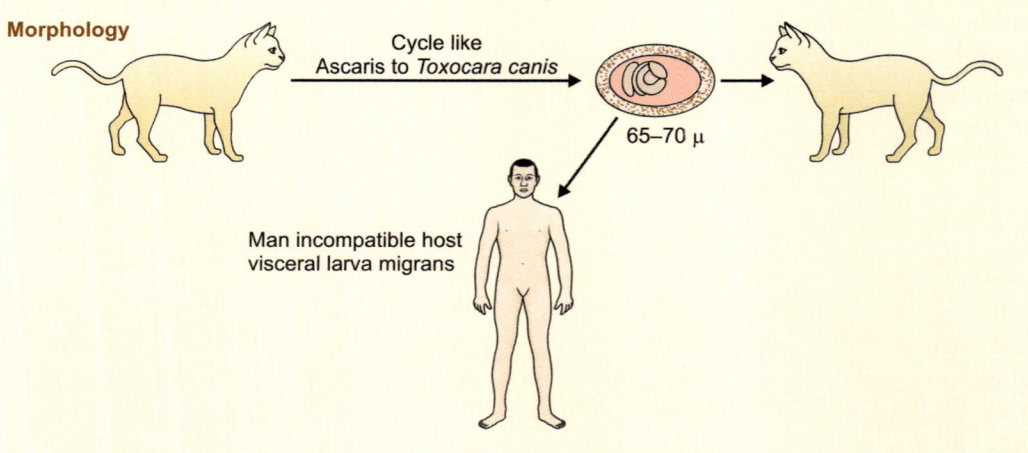

Cycle like
Ascaris to *Toxocara canis*

65–70 μ

Man incompatible host
visceral larva migrans

EOSINOPHILIC MENINGOENCEPHALITIS

Angiostrongylus cantonensis

(The rat lungworm)

Eosinophilic meningoencephalitis is caused by *A. cantonensis* prevalent in the Pacific Islands and South-East Asia. It was first demonstrated in Formosa in 1944 by Nomura (and later by Lin in 1945) from the CSF of a patient.

A. cantonensis needs molluscs as the intermediate hosts and rat as the final or definitive host. Both, male and female adults reside in the two main branches of the pulmonary artery of the rat. The gravid female lays eggs that are carried by the bloodstream into the smaller pulmonary vessels where they are lodged as emboli. In 6 days the eggs are embryonated. The adult worms measure from 17 to 25 mm in length.

First stage larvae: Measuring 0.27–0.3 x 0.015–0.016 mm, they are released from the eggs, breakthrough the alveolar walls, migrate up to the trachea and larynx to be swallowed back into the alimentary canal. Evacuated with the faeces into fresh water or sea, they can survive for six or three days respectively.

Second and third stage larvae: Snails and lugs (molluscs) take up the first stage larvae orally or the larvae penetrate their cuticle. They undergo two moultings and become third stage larvae in about two weeks time (measuring 0.5 x 0.25 mm) and can survive up to one year in the molluscs.

Development in definitive host: Rat gets infected by eating the mollusc infected with third stage larvae or by drinking water contaminated with such larvae. The third stage larvae pass through the stomach or intestine to the portal circulation and then via the hepatic vein are passively transferred to the lungs. Ultimately they enter the systemic circulation to be lodged in the central nervous system. Two additional moultings occur in the brain within a fortnight and they are converted into adult worms. They emerge on the brain surface and remain in the subarachnoid space for about 2 weeks time. The worms at this stage measure 11–12 mm. They then enter the cranial venules and then via the right ventricle travel to the main trunks of the pulmonary artery. Maturing in about a week, they start laying eggs which need about 6 days' time to hatch in the lung capillaries.

Human infection: Occurs by:
1. Ingestion of raw vegetables containing third stage larvae of *A. cantonensis* or by ingestion of tissues of improperly cooked infected intermediate host and carrier or paratenic hosts.
2. Drinking water contaminated with the infected larvae.

As in rat, the third stage larvae reach the brain, but cannot proceed any further and die, exciting an inflammatory reaction in the brain and meninges. The eosinophilic response in CSF occurs to their metabolic products or dead parasites. In the Pacific Islands the disease is of short duration and terminates spontaneously; only a few cases develop residual paralysis (often facial palsy). No immunity is known to develop.

In the Pacific Islands anyone who develops the brain syndrome (headache, neck rigidity and paraesthesia in limbs) along with peripheral eosinophilia and CSF showing eosinophils should be suspected as a case of angiostrongyliasis. Other parasites that may evoke a similar syndrome are cerebral gnasthostomiasis, cerebral cysticercosis, cerebral echinococcosis, cerebral schistosomiasis, trichinelliasis, cerebral paragonimiasis, dirofilariasis and toxocariasis.

OTHER NEMATODES OF LESSER IMPORTANCE

Gongylonema pulchrum (The scutate threadworm)

Morphology

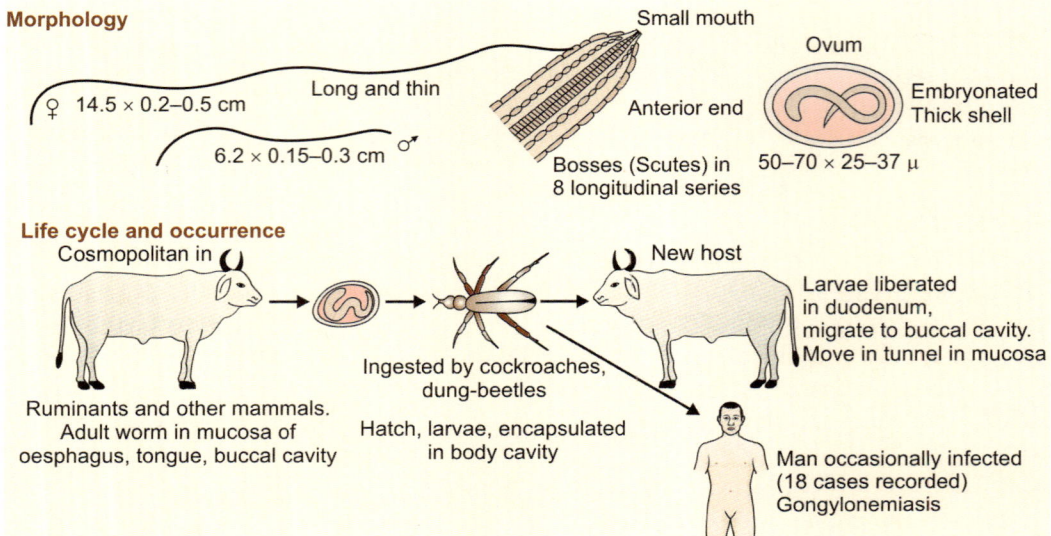

Small mouth

♀ 14.5 × 0.2–0.5 cm   Long and thin

6.2 × 0.15–0.3 cm ♂

Anterior end

Bosses (Scutes) in 8 longitudinal series

Ovum

Embryonated Thick shell

50–70 × 25–37 µ

Life cycle and occurrence

Cosmopolitan in

New host

Larvae liberated in duodenum, migrate to buccal cavity. Move in tunnel in mucosa

Ingested by cockroaches, dung-beetles

Hatch, larvae, encapsulated in body cavity

Ruminants and other mammals. Adult worm in mucosa of oesphagus, tongue, buccal cavity

Man occasionally infected (18 cases recorded) Gongylonemiasis

Physaloptera caucasica

Morphology

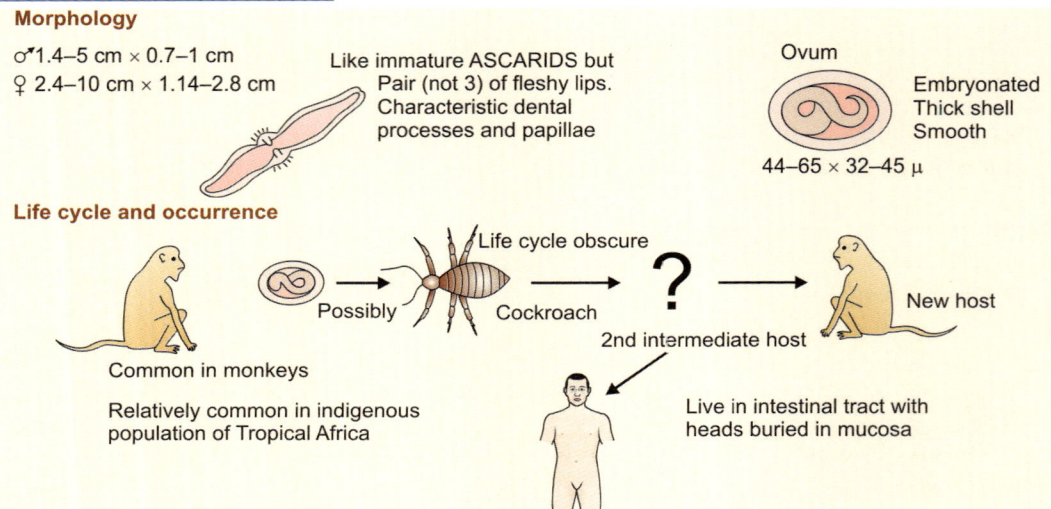

♂1.4–5 cm × 0.7–1 cm
♀ 2.4–10 cm × 1.14–2.8 cm

Like immature ASCARIDS but Pair (not 3) of fleshy lips. Characteristic dental processes and papillae

Ovum

Embryonated Thick shell Smooth

44–65 × 32–45 µ

Life cycle and occurrence

Life cycle obscure

Possibly   Cockroach

2nd intermediate host

New host

Common in monkeys

Relatively common in indigenous population of Tropical Africa

Live in intestinal tract with heads buried in mucosa

Thelazia callipaeda (The oriental eye worm)

Morphology: Thread-like, 5–17 mm, long
Characteristic oephalic papillae

Occurrence

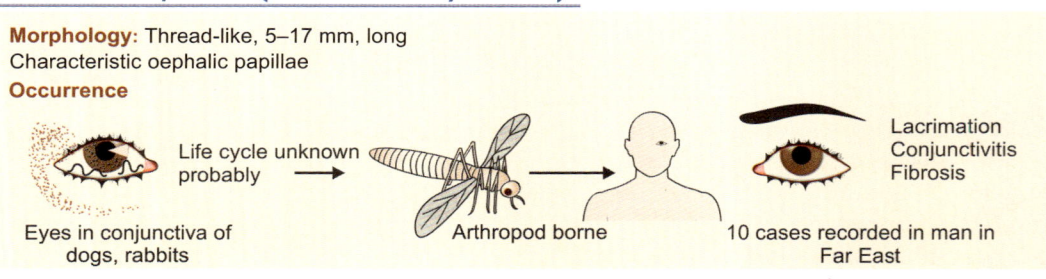

Life cycle unknown probably

Arthropod borne

Lacrimation Conjunctivitis Fibrosis

Eyes in conjunctiva of dogs, rabbits

10 cases recorded in man in Far East

MISCELLANEOUS WORMS

Phylum nematophora (Gordiid worms or hair snakes)

Class   Gordiacea. Elongated, wiry worms 10– 50 cm long. Digestive tract atrophied.

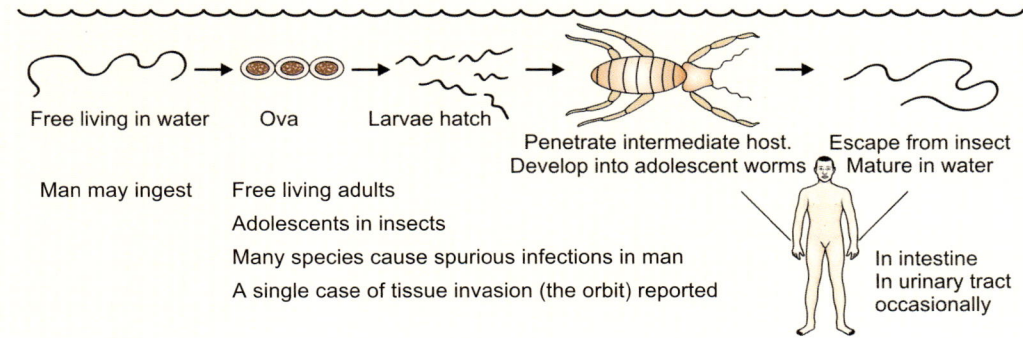

Free living in water   Ova   Larvae hatch

Penetrate intermediate host.   Escape from insect
Develop into adolescent worms   Mature in water

Man may ingest   Free living adults
Adolescents in insects
Many species cause spurious infections in man
A single case of tissue invasion (the orbit) reported

In intestine
In urinary tract
occasionally

Phylum acanthocephala (Thorny headed worms)

Morphology   Possess proboscis armed with spines
♂ 5–10 cm ♀ 20–65 cm in length

Life Cycle

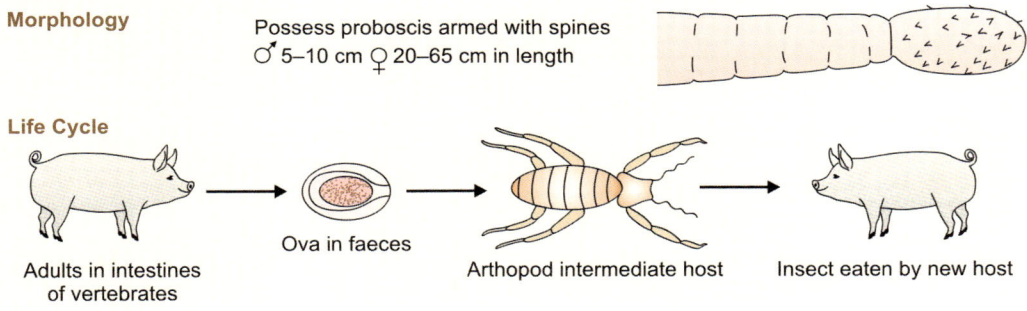

Ova in faeces

Adults in intestines
of vertebrates

Arthopod intermediate host   Insect eaten by new host

Species

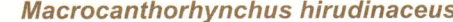

Macrocanthorhynchus hirudinaceus

Ovum

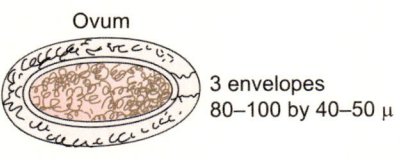

3 envelopes
80–100 by 40–50 μ

Cosmopolitan in pigs
A few spurious infections reported in man

Moniliformis moniliformis

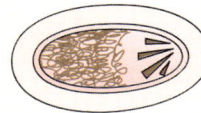

3 envelopes
spinose embryo
85–118 by 40–52 μ

Found in rats

Solitary human infections reported in man in Italy.
Sudan and British Honduras

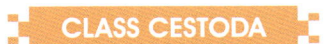

CLASS CESTODA

Basic Classification of Metazoans

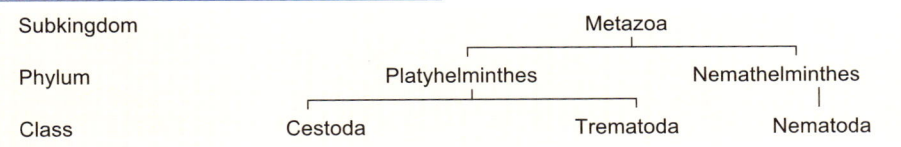

Subkingdom		Metazoa	
Phylum		Platyhelminthes	Nemathelminthes
Class	Cestoda	Trematoda	Nematoda

General features of Cestodes

A. Cestodes (most) are long, segmented and tape-like, therefore, called tapeworms. They are flattened dorsoventrally.
B. Vary in length from a few mm to several metres.
C. Adult worms reside in intestinal tract of man and animal.
D. Heads possess suckers (slit-like or cup-like), may sometimes have hooks that assist in attachment.
E. Adult worm is divided into 3 regions:
  (i) Head or scolex,
  (ii) Neck, and
  (iii) Strobila (body/trunk) consisting of series of segments or proglottides.
F. Sexes are not separate (each worm is a hemaphrodite).
G. Do not have any body cavity.
H. Alimentary canal is totally lacking.
I. Excretory and nervous systems are present.
J. The reproductive system is highly developed and complete in each segment. As per maturity of reproductive organs three types of segments of the strobila can be identified from front backwards.

Immature—male and female organs undifferentiated.
Mature—male and female organs identifiable (male organs differentiate first).
Gravid—uteri filled with eggs (other organs atrophy or disappear).

CESTODA

(Tapeworms)

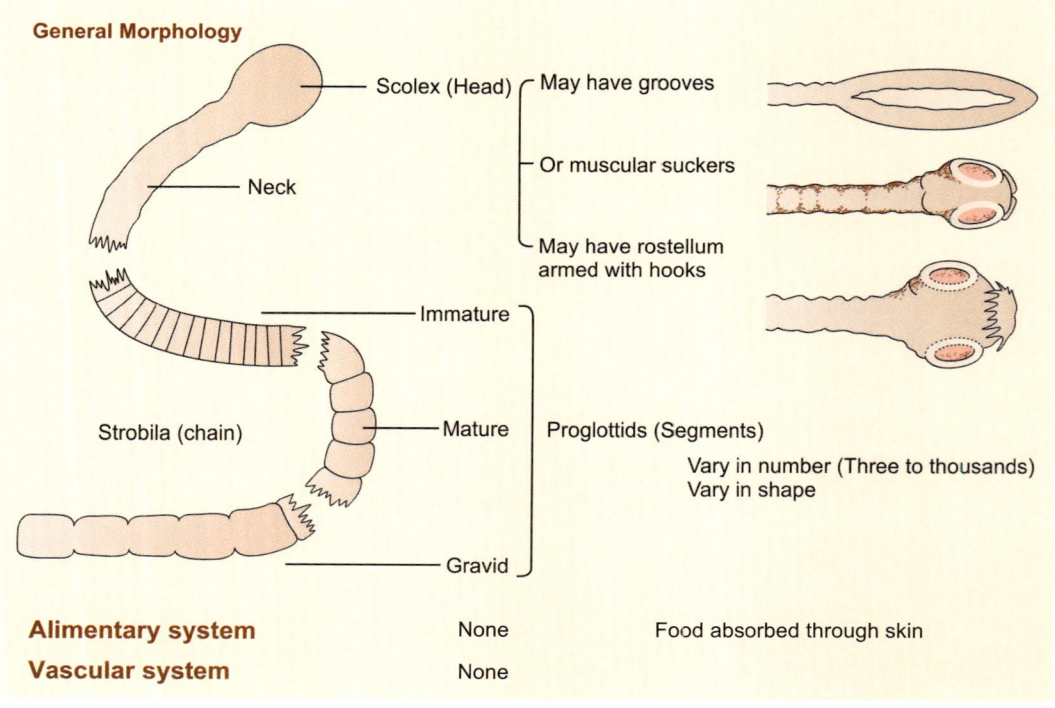

General Morphology

Scolex (Head) — May have grooves
Or muscular suckers
May have rostellum armed with hooks

Neck

Immature
Mature
Gravid

Strobila (chain)

Proglottids (Segments)
Vary in number (Three to thousands)
Vary in shape

Alimentary system	None	Food absorbed through skin
Vascular system	None	

Excretory System

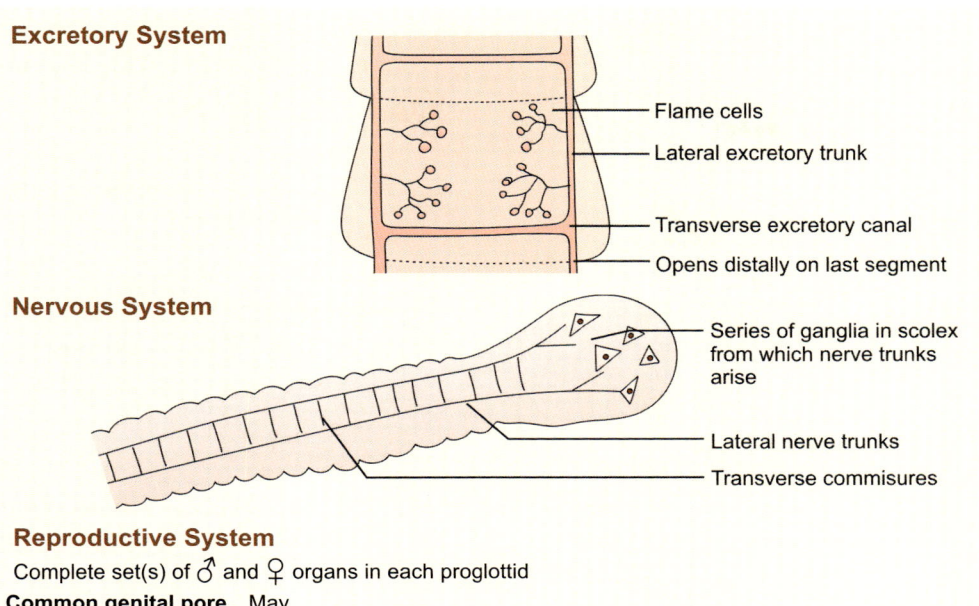

Flame cells
Lateral excretory trunk

Transverse excretory canal
Opens distally on last segment

Nervous System

Series of ganglia in scolex from which nerve trunks arise

Lateral nerve trunks
Transverse commisures

Reproductive System

Complete set(s) of ♂ and ♀ organs in each proglottid

Common genital pore May open

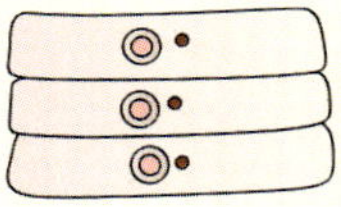

Or ventral surface (with uterine pore) as in Dibothriocephalus

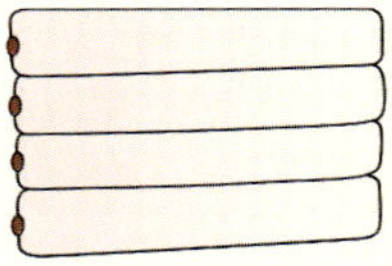

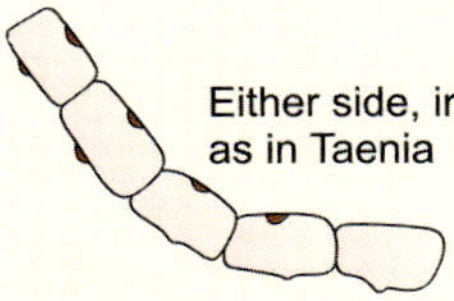

Either side, irregularly, as in Taenia

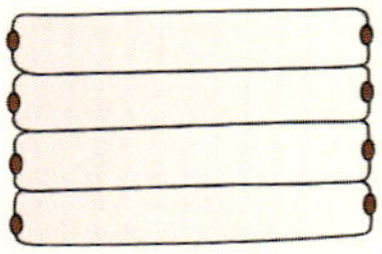

On same lateral margin of each segment, as in Hymenolepis

One on each side as in Dipligonoporus

Testes May be

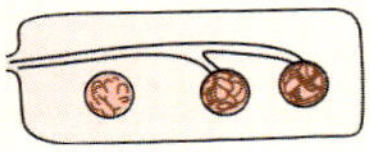

Few and large as in Hymenolepis

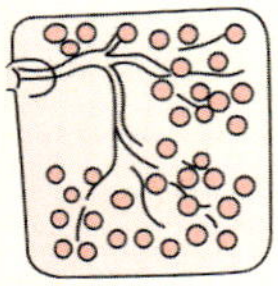

Numerous (500 or more) and small as in Taenia. Dibothriocephalus

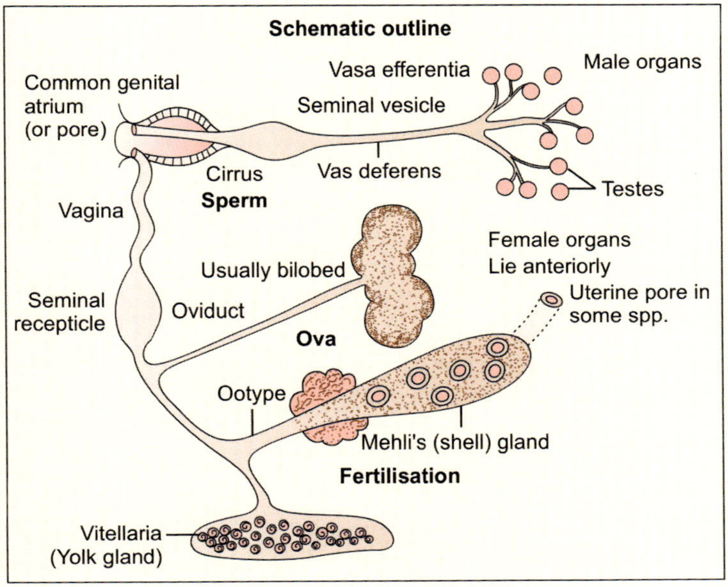

Schematic outline

Common genital atrium (or pore)

Vasa efferentia   Male organs
Seminal vesicle

Cirrus   Vas deferens
Sperm

Vagina

Testes

Usually bilobed

Female organs
Lie anteriorly

Uterine pore in some spp.

Seminal recepticle   Oviduct

Ova

Ootype

Mehli's (shell) gland

Fertilisation

Vitellaria (Yolk gland)

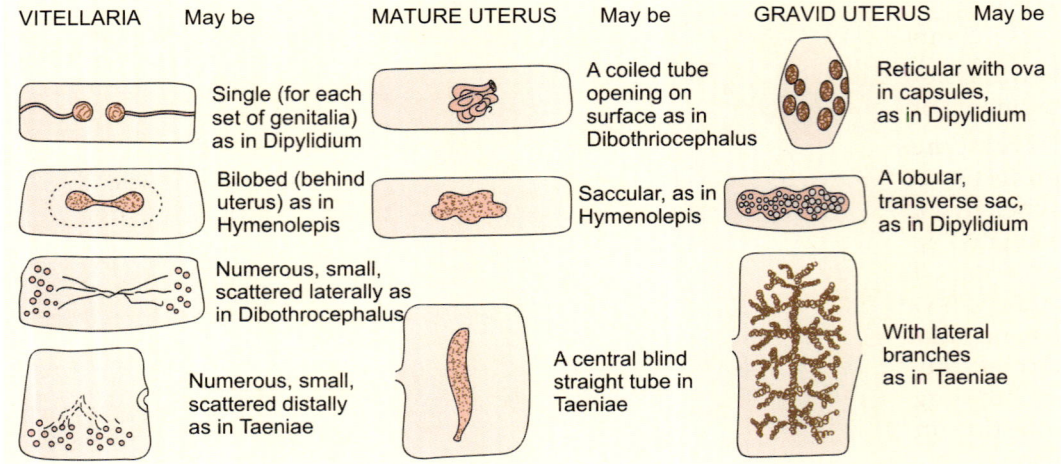

Reproductive System

Male genital system: Lies dorsally and matures earlier than female genital system. It comprises:

(i) **Testes:** Are usually multiple follicles, excepting in dwarf tapeworm (*H. nana*) and are scattered throughout the parenchyma. They are connected by vasa efferentia (appears as minute tubes) with the vas deferens.

(ii) **Vas deferens:** Is a thick, convoluted (usually) tube. It begins in the middle of each segment and in cyclophyllidea, passes to the lateral margin to open in the genital atrium (the common genital pore). At the beginning point it may be enlarged for the purpose of storage of sperms and is known as the seminal vesicle. In pseudophyllidea it ascends upwards as a convoluted tube to open in the genital pore.

(iii) **Cirrus sac:** At the terminal end it shows a sac that contains a coiled-up muscular organ called the cirrus (or the penis). The cirrus and the vagina both open into a common cup-shaped chamber (the common genital pore) either on the lateral border, as in cyclophyllidea or on the mid ventral surface, as in pseudophyllidea.

Female genital system: Lies on the ventral surface. Consists of:

(i) **Ovary:** Single or paired. Usually a bilobed organ lying behind the equatorial plane of each segment. It discharges into a minute oviduct that connects the spermatic duct with the ootype.

(ii) **Vagina:** Extending from genital pore to the ootype, it is meant for entrance of sperms. At its inner end it contains an elongated chamber (the terminal receptacle) for sperm storage, it is followed by a constricted tubule (the spermatic duct).

(iii) **Uterus:** Is a straight tube arising from ootype and when gravid, gets filled with eggs. In pseudophyllidea it is open but in cyclophyllidea it remains as a blind sac.

(iv) **Ootype:** Is the egg fertilising chamber. It is situated posteriorly in the middle of each segment,

(v) **Vitelline glands:** May remain as a single mass lying behind the ovary, as in cyclophyllidea, or scattered diffusely in the segment as in pseudophyllidea.

(vi) **Mehli's gland (shell glands):** Is a tiny organ surrounding the ootype. It is composed of many unicellular glands which open separately into the ootype.

Fertilisation: Takes place between the segments. Fertilisation may occur between segments of same worm (self-fertilisation) or another worm (cross-fertilisation).

Development of eggs: Eggs are formed in the ootype where they are provided a protective covering. In pseudophyllidea the egg is operculated, has a single covering. When first laid it does not contain an embryo. The membrane covering the embryo has a ciliated epithelium. In cyclophyllidea the egg is not operculated and possesses two coverings. The outer cover is called the egg-shell and the inner one surrounding the embryo is called the embryophore. The egg when first laid, contains an embryo which has no ciliated epithelium. The formed embryo is a six-hooked (hexacanth) sphere, termed the oncosphere. Yolk-material lies in the space between the embryophore and the egg-shell. In some cases the egg shell is lost during its passage through the intestine, in these cases the embryophore becomes thick and radially striated for the protection of the embryo within.

Larval development: Two types of development are seen.
In pseudophyllidea—Solid larval forms are seen which are called procercoid and plerocercoid.

In cyclophyllidea—Larval forms are transformed into bladders (bladder-worm).

Classification	Morphological	Differences
Pseudophyllidea		**Cyclophyllidea**
2 sucking grooves	Scolex	4 muscular suckers
Centre of segment	Genital pore	Margin(s) of segment
Centre of segment	Uterine pore	None, Uterus ends blindly
Coiled	Uterus	Sac-like Branched Contains egg capsules
Operculate immature	Ova	Non-operculate mature

Contd.

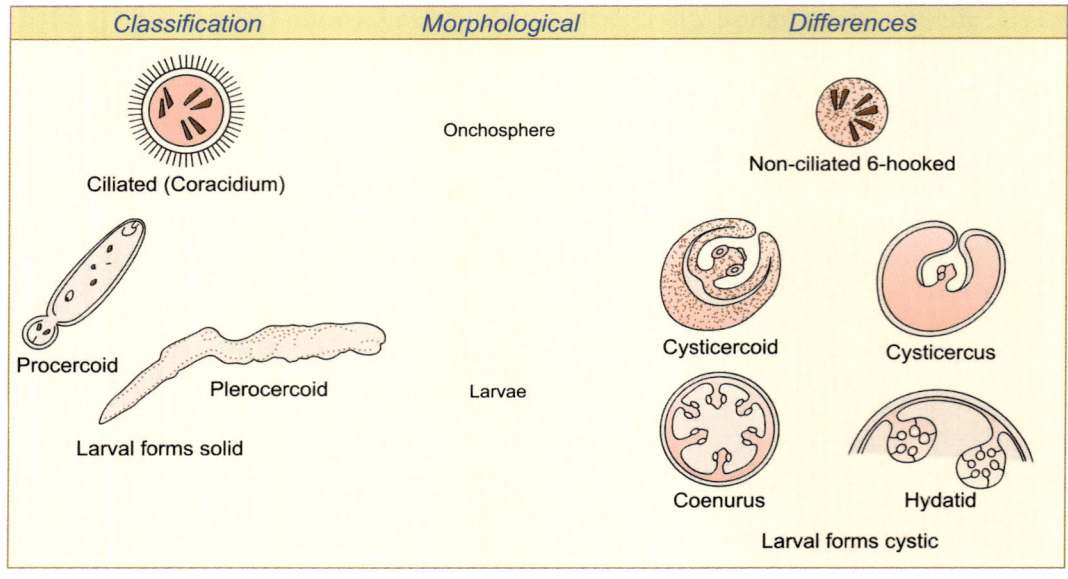

Classification	Morphological	Differences

Ciliated (Coracidium)

Onchosphere

Non-ciliated 6-hooked

Procercoid

Plerocercoid

Larvae

Larval forms solid

Cysticercoid

Cysticercus

Coenurus

Hydatid

Larval forms cystic

Life cycle in general

1. No intermediate host required as in *Hymenolepis nana*

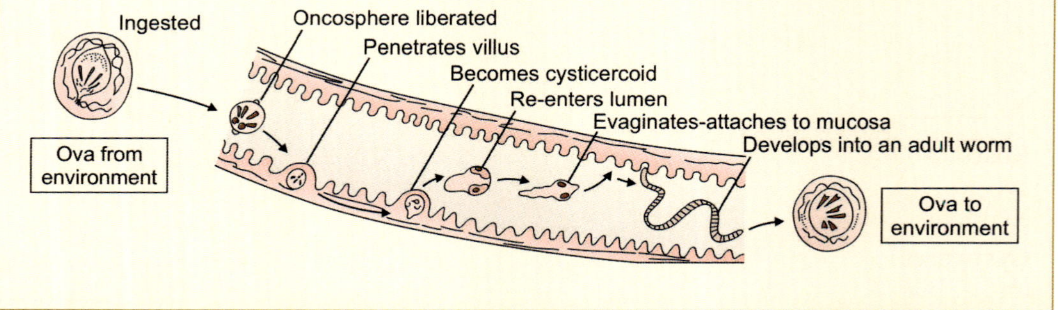

Ingested

Oncosphere liberated
Penetrates villus
Becomes cysticercoid
Re-enters lumen
Evaginates-attaches to mucosa
Develops into an adult worm

Ova from environment

Ova to environment

2. Intermediate host(s) required as in all other species of Cestoda

A. Immature ova mature and hatch in water as in Pseudophyllidea

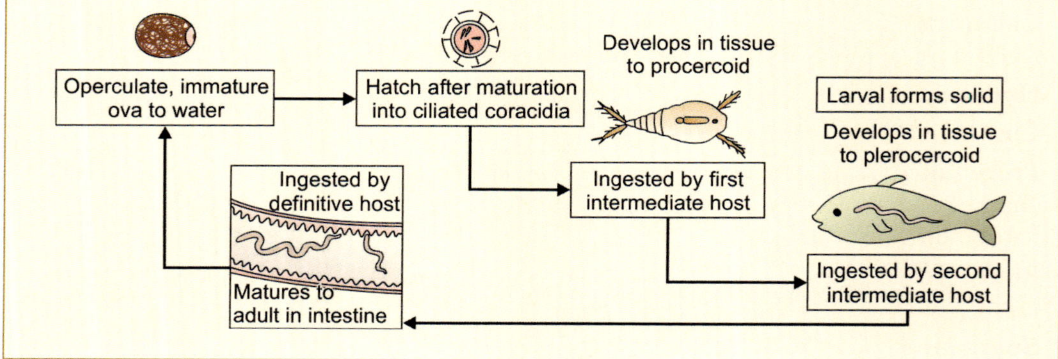

Operculate, immature ova to water

Hatch after maturation into ciliated coracidia

Develops in tissue to procercoid

Larval forms solid

Develops in tissue to plerocercoid

Ingested by definitive host

Ingested by first intermediate host

Ingested by second intermediate host

Matures to adult in intestine

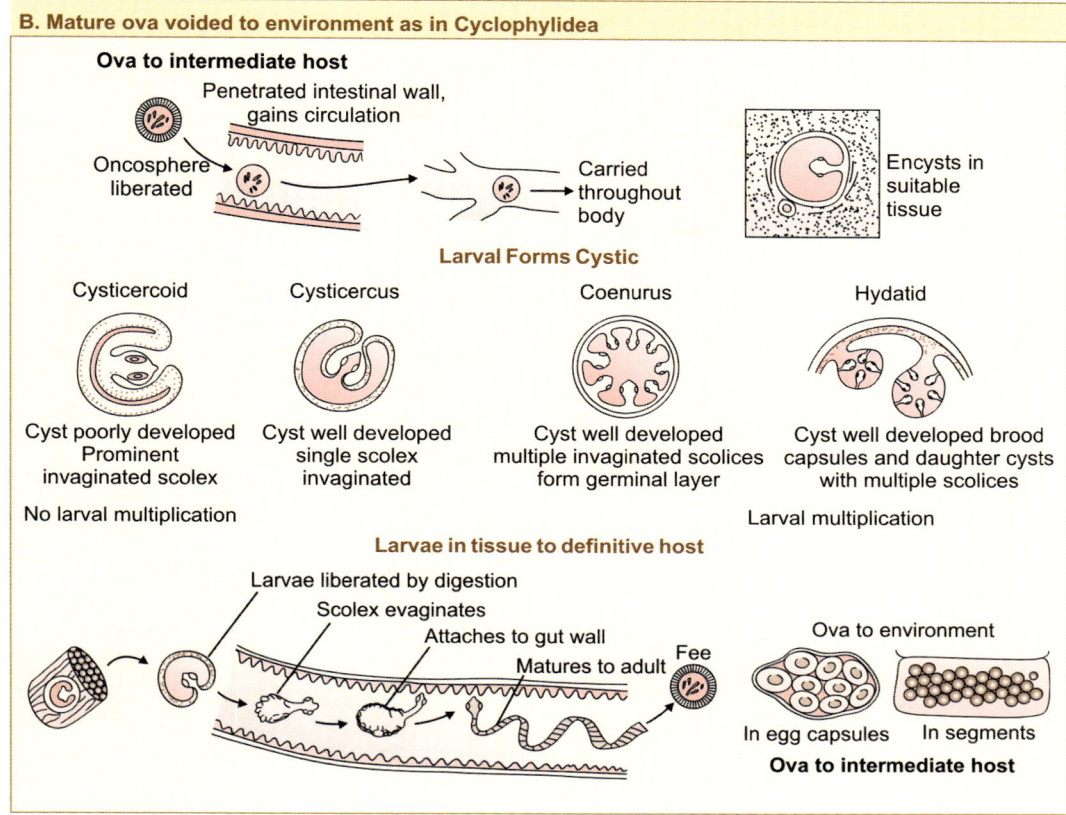

B. Mature ova voided to environment as in Cyclophylidea

Ova to intermediate host

Oncosphere liberated — Penetrated intestinal wall, gains circulation — Carried throughout body — Encysts in suitable tissue

Larval Forms Cystic

Cysticercoid | Cysticercus | Coenurus | Hydatid

Cyst poorly developed Prominent invaginated scolex | Cyst well developed single scolex invaginated | Cyst well developed multiple invaginated scolices form germinal layer | Cyst well developed brood capsules and daughter cysts with multiple scolices

No larval multiplication | Larval multiplication

Larvae in tissue to definitive host

Larvae liberated by digestion
Scolex evaginates
Attaches to gut wall
Matures to adult — Fee

Ova to environment

In egg capsules   In segments

Ova to intermediate host

Other Important Terms Employed to Describe Cestodes

Rostelluni: Is a beak-like projection on the head which carries booklets in the armed species. It may stay invaginated between the suckers. The rostellar booklets shape is characteristic in each family.

Cysticercus: Is the resting stage of the larva in the intermediate host where it develops into a 'bladder-worm'. It consists of a hollow vesicle with the invaginated scolex on its wall and a central cavity containing a little fluid.

Cysticercoid: A small bladder containing the invaginated 'head' proximally and a solid, elongated portion as a caudal appendage.

Coenurus: A larval stage in the form of 'bladder-worm' containing many invaginated scolices.

Hydatid cyst: Is the larval stage of Echinococcus.

Coracidiuni: Is the ciliated oncosphere of Diphyllobothrium.

Procercoid: Is the first larval stage of Diphyllobothrium found in cyclops. It is spindle-shaped solid body with cephalic invagination and a caudal spherical appendage (cercomer) containing embryonal booklets.

Plerocercoid: Is the second larval stage of Diphyllobothrium. The caudal appendage is solid, elongated and the head is invaginated in the neck.

Sparganum: Is the plerocercoid larva infecting man.

CLASSIFICATION OF CESTODES

Based on Habitat

I. Pseudophyllidean cestodes—have false or slit-like grooves.
  - A. Adult worm in intestine — *Diphyllolothrium latum* (fish tapeworm).
  - B. Larval stages in man   — *Sparganum mansoni*
    - — *Sparganum proliferum*

II. Cyclophyllidean cestodes—have cup-like and round suckers.
  - A. Adult worms in intestine:

Genus Taenia	— *T. saginata* (beef tapeworm)
	— *T. solium* (pork tapeworm)
Genus Hymenolepis	— *H. nana* (dwarf tapeworm)
	— *H. diminuta* (rat tapeworm)
Genus Dipylidium	— *D. caninum* (double-pored dog tapeworm)

  - B. Larval stages in man:

Genus Echinococcus	— *E.granulosus* (dog tapeworm).
Hydatid cyst.	— *E. multilocularis.*
	— *Genus Taenia*—Cysticercus cellulosae of *T. solium*.
Genus multiceps	— Coenurus cerebalis of *M. multiceps*.
	— Coenurus glomeratus of *M. glomeratus*.

Order	Superfamily	Family	Genus	Species	Definitie host	Interme-diate host	Stage found in man
Pseudo-phyllidea	Bothrioce-phaloidea	Diphllobo-thriidae	Diphyl-lobo thrium	D. latum	Man, dog, cat	Cyclops and fish	Adult worm
				D. mansoni	Dog, cat	Frog, snake and man	Larval stage
Cyclophy-yllidea	Taenioidea	Taenlidae	Taenla	T. saginata	Man	Cow,	Adult worm
				T. solium	Man	pig, man	Adult, rarely larvae
			Echino-coccus	E. granu-losus	Dog, wolf, jackal	Sheep, cattle, man, pig	Larval stage
				E. multilo-locularis	Fox, dog, wolf, dingo	Field mouse, man	Larval stage
			Multiceps	M. multiceps	Dog	Sheep, goat, cattle, man	Larval stage
		Hymeno-lepidae	Hyme-nolepis	H. nana	Man, rat	Not needed	Adult and larval stages in intestine
		Dilepi-didae	Dipyli-dium	H. diminuta	Rat (man)	Rat flea	Adult worm
				D. caninum	Dog, cat (man)	Dog flea	Adult worm

Diphyllobothrium latum

(Fish tapeworm, Broad tapeworm)

Historical: First reported by Linnaeus in 1758 and later by Luhe in 1910.

Geographical distribution: America, Japan, Central Africa and Central Europe. Not yet reported from India.

Habitat: Adult worm resides in the small intestine of man; also in dog, cat, fox and other fish-eating mammals.

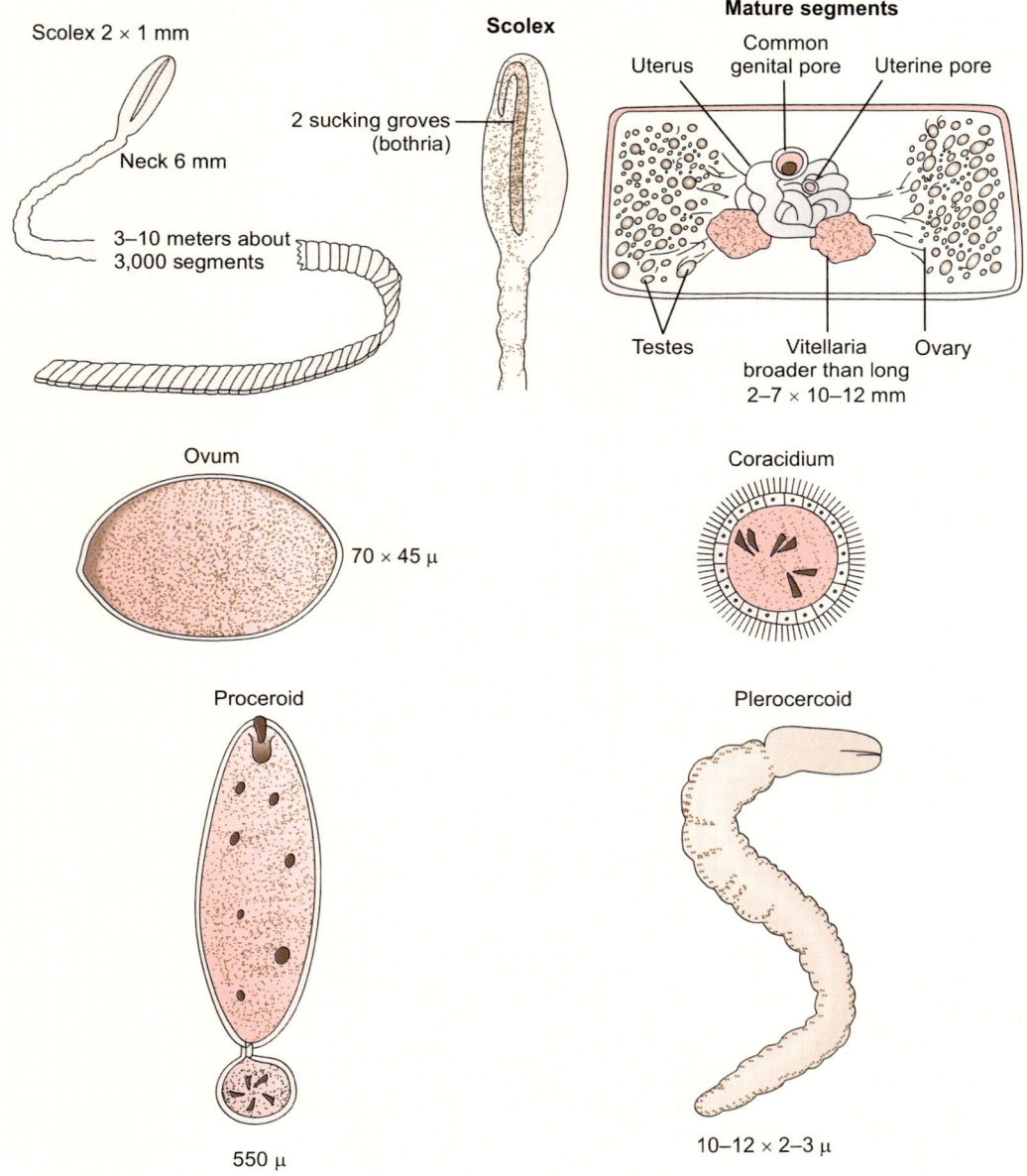

Morphology

Adult worm

The adult worm is yellowish-grey with dark central streak caused by the egg filled uteri. It measures 3–10 metres in length and can survive up to 13 years or so. The *scolex* is elongated and spoon-shaped and measures 2×1 mm. It bears two slit-like grooves (bothria) situated on the dorsal and ventral surfaces respectively. There are no rostellum and no booklets too. *Neck* is thin, unsegmented and is much longer than the head. *Proglottides* (segments) are up to 3,000 in number. Their breadth is more than length, 2–7 × 10–12 mm. They are practically filled with male and female reproductive organs. The terminal segments being egg-free and shrunken are empty. Later the dried-up segments break off in chains and are evacuated with faeces. There are three genital pores consisting of the openings of vas deferens, vagina and uterus. The ovary is bilobed, uterus is large and remains coiled in the centre of each segment in the form of a rosette.

Eggs: Are passed out in large numbers. They are oval, brown (bile stained), measure 70 × 45 μ, contain abundant yolk granules and an unsegmented ovum. They have an inconspicuous operculum at one end with a small knob at the other. It does not float on the saturated solution of common salt. The eggs are not infective to man. One egg gives rise to a single larva only.

Larval stages: Are first passed in water and then in respective intermediate hosts. Larval development has three stages.

First stage larva is called *coracidium*; it develops from egg in water.

Second stage larva is labelled as *procercoid* and is found within cyclops (the first intermediate host).

Third stage larva is known as *plerocercoid* and is found in freshwater fish (the second intermediate host).

Life cycle: Life cycle is passed through one definitive host and two intermediate hosts. *Definitive hosts* can be man, dog, cat and the adults are found in their intestines. The *intermediate hosts* are first, cyclops and second, a freshwater fish.

Development of Egg in Water and Release of Coracidium: Evacuated with faeces, the eggs reach water and within 2 weeks a *coracidium forms* which is ingested by cyclops. Coracidium is ciliated embryo with 3 pairs of hooklets.

↓

Larval development inside cyclops: In the cyclops it loses its cilia and the supporting cubical cells. After penetrating through the intestinal wall it comes to lie in the body cavity and in 3 weeks it is transformed into an elongated solid body with a caudal spherical appendage containing the six (now vestigeal) hooks. It is now known as the *procercoid larva.* This cyclops is then consumed by a fresh-water fish.

↓

Larval development inside fish: In the fish's intestine, the procercoid larva frees itself, passes through the gut wall and comes to lie in liver, muscles or the mesenteric fat. In less than 3 weeks it changes to a *plerocercoid larva* or *sparganum.* Now the spherical caudal appendage is missing and the anterior end shows a depression (representing the inverted head of the future adult worm). The larva is whitish, somewhat flattened and marked by irregular unsegmented wrinkles.

Infection of man and development to adulthood: With consumption of uncooked or ill-cooked fish, the plerocercoid larva too is ingested and in the human intestine it develops into an adult worm. On attaining maturity in 5–6 weeks, it starts discharging eggs that are passed out with the faeces. The cycle is then repeated.

Pathology: Diphyllobothriasis causes gastrointestinal disturbances and macrocytic anaemia. There is an early eosinophilia too. The worm may interfere with intrinsic factor (on account of unsaturated fatty-acids liberated by it) or may consume the vitamin B_{12} present in the food eaten by the host.

Diagnosis: Established by microscopic stool examination of stool and looking for the characteristic operculated eggs. Gross examination may sometimes reveal the segments passed with the stool.

Treatment: Mepacrine, dichlorophen and niclosamide can be used.

Prophylaxis: Includes the undermentioned methods:
— Prevention of contamination of water.
— Personal prophylaxis—Cook all fish etc. very well before eating.
— Do not feed the other definitive hosts (dogs and cats) offals of fish.

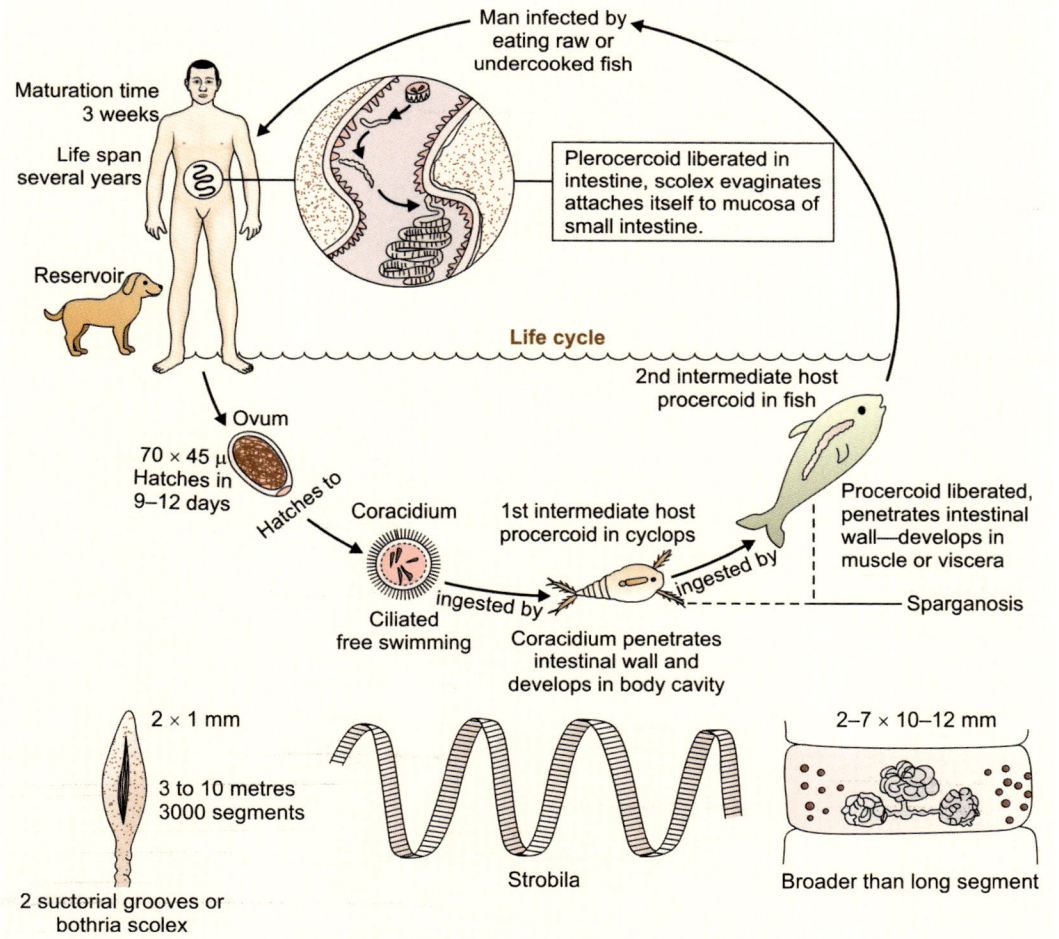

Life cycle

SPARGANUM

The term sparganum was introduced to label Diphyllobothrioid larvae of unknown parentage and whose development was advanced enough to be grouped under a specific Genus.

Larval forms of Pseudophyllidea in man

Sparganosis

The extra-intestinal presence in human body of larvae of non-human tapeworms of the genus Diphyllobothrium.

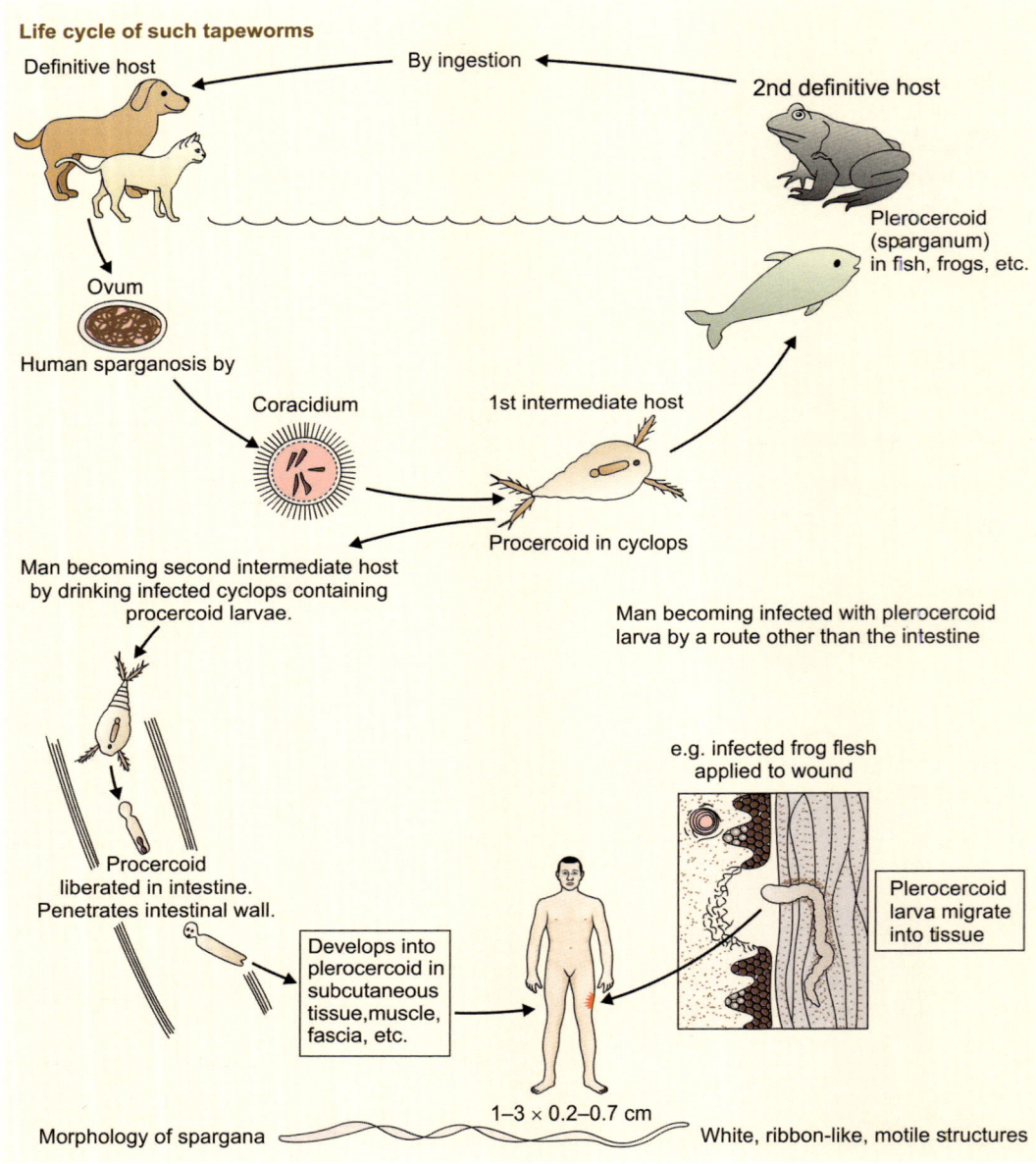

Life cycle of such tapeworms

Definitive host — By ingestion — 2nd definitive host

Plerocercoid (sparganum) in fish, frogs, etc.

Ovum

Human sparganosis by

Coracidium   1st intermediate host

Procercoid in cyclops

Man becoming second intermediate host by drinking infected cyclops containing procercoid larvae.

Man becoming infected with plerocercoid larva by a route other than the intestine

e.g. infected frog flesh applied to wound

Procercoid liberated in intestine. Penetrates intestinal wall.

Plerocercoid larva migrate into tissue

Develops into plerocercoid in subcutaneous tissue, muscle, fascia, etc.

1–3 × 0.2–0.7 cm

Morphology of spargana   White, ribbon-like, motile structures

Types of Spargana At least 2

1. *Sparganum mansoni* Plerococercoid stage of *Dibothriocephalus mansonoides* (dog and cat tapeworm)
Does not proliferate in human tissues
2. *Sparganum proliferans* Plerocercoid stage of tapeworms the adults of which are unknown
This larva proliferates in human tissues.

Geographical Distribution Far East, occasionally elsewhere

Pathology	**Living Larvae**	Painful, oedematous reaction
	Dead Larvae	Intense local inflammatory reaction
		Numerous eosinophils
		Sometimes abscess formation.
		Ocular sparganosis (in soft tissues near eye)
		Severe damage may result
	Proliferating larvae	Thousands may develop in same host

Laboratory Diagnosis Of the disease—examination of biopsy material.
Of the sparganum—determined by feeding recovered
larvae
to cats and dogs and studying resulting adult form.

Another Rarely Confronted Pseudophyllidean

Diplogonoporus grandis

Morphology

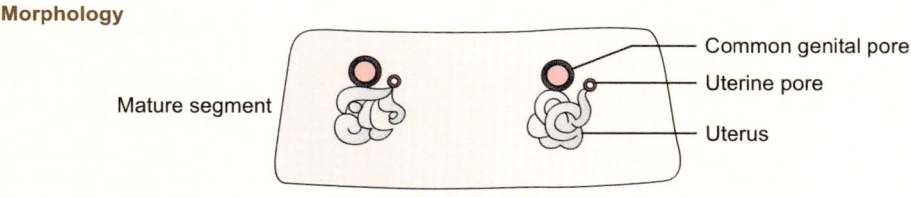

Common genital pore
Uterine pore
Uterus
Mature segment
Genitalia twinned

Life cycle

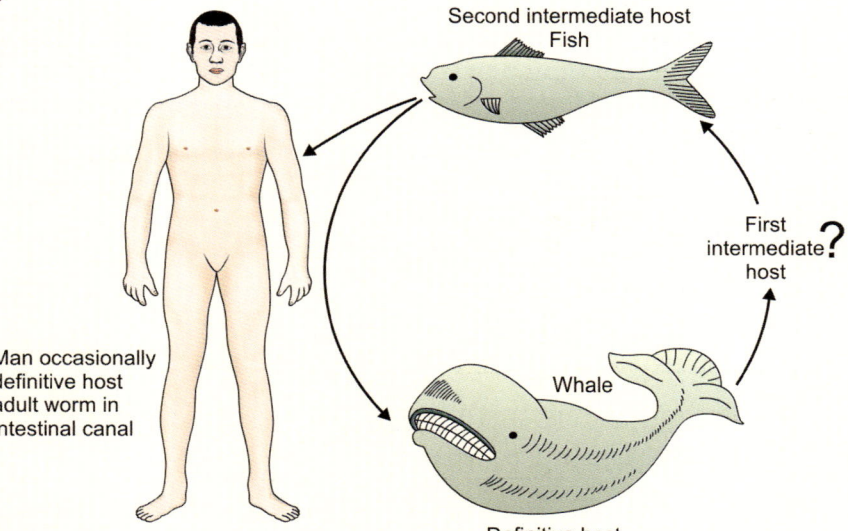

Second intermediate host
Fish

First intermediate ? host

Man occasionally definitive host adult worm in intestinal canal

Whale

Definitive host

Occurrence: Reported 6 times in Japanese patients, causing intestinal upset.

CYCLOPHYLLIDEAN TAPEWORMS OF MAN

General Characters of Cyclophyllidean Cestodes

1. May be small or large worms consisting of chains of segments.
2. Head is quadrate with a cup-like round sucker at each of the four angles. The centre may show an apical rostellum with booklets.
3. Vitelline glands are huddled into a single mass behind the ovary near the posterior margin of each segment.
4. Common genital pore is marginal (on the lateral side of each segment).
5. They lack a uterine opening for the exit of eggs from the gravid uterus. Eggs escape only by rupture of the mature segment. In dilepdidae and taeniidae the ripe segments are detached from the main body.
6. Eggs have no operculum and can further develop only in an intermediate host. Eggs are fully embryonated when detached from the segment. The oncosphere is never a ciliated embryo.
7. Only one intermediate host is needed for larval development.

Larval Development of Cyclophyllidean Cestodes

A. **Cysticercoid:** Entire larva is solid except for the proximal portion which is vesicular containing the invaginated scolex. This is typical of tapeworms where the intermediate hosts are insects (exception being *H. nana* where the cysticercoid stage of the larval development is passed in a vertebrate hosts either in man or in rat).

B. **Cysticercus (Bladder worm):** The entire larva is converted into a bladder form from which the scolex or head of the future adult worm sprouts. Cysticerci can be divided as:

  (i) **True cysticercus:** Consists of a bladder with one scolex (as in *T. saginata* and *T. solium*). Scolex remains invaginated within the cyst-wall and can be seen with naked eyes as a milky-white spot about the size of a pin-head.

  (ii) **Coenurus:** A bladder with multiple scolices as in multiceps.

  (iii) **Echinococcus (Hydatid):** A bladder that multiplies by budding and forms many daughter and granddaughter bladders. On the cyst-wall brood capsules are produced, inside which lie the scolices, as in *Echinococcus granulosus*.

Each scolex can produce one adult worm from larval cysts swallowed by the definitive host.

CYCLOPHYLLIDEAN TAPEWORMS OF MAN

CLASSIFICATION	A. Of common or important occurrence			
FAMILY	Hymenolepididae	Taenidae		
GENUS	Hymenolepis	Taenia	Echinococcus	Multiceps
SPECIES	*H. nana* Adult and larval stages in man	*T. solium* Adult, sometimes larval stages in man	*E. granulosus* Larval stage only in man	*M. multiceps* Larval stage only in man
	H. diminuta Adult stage in man	*T. saginata* Adult stage in man	*E. multiocularis* Larval stage in man	And related spec. Larval stage in man

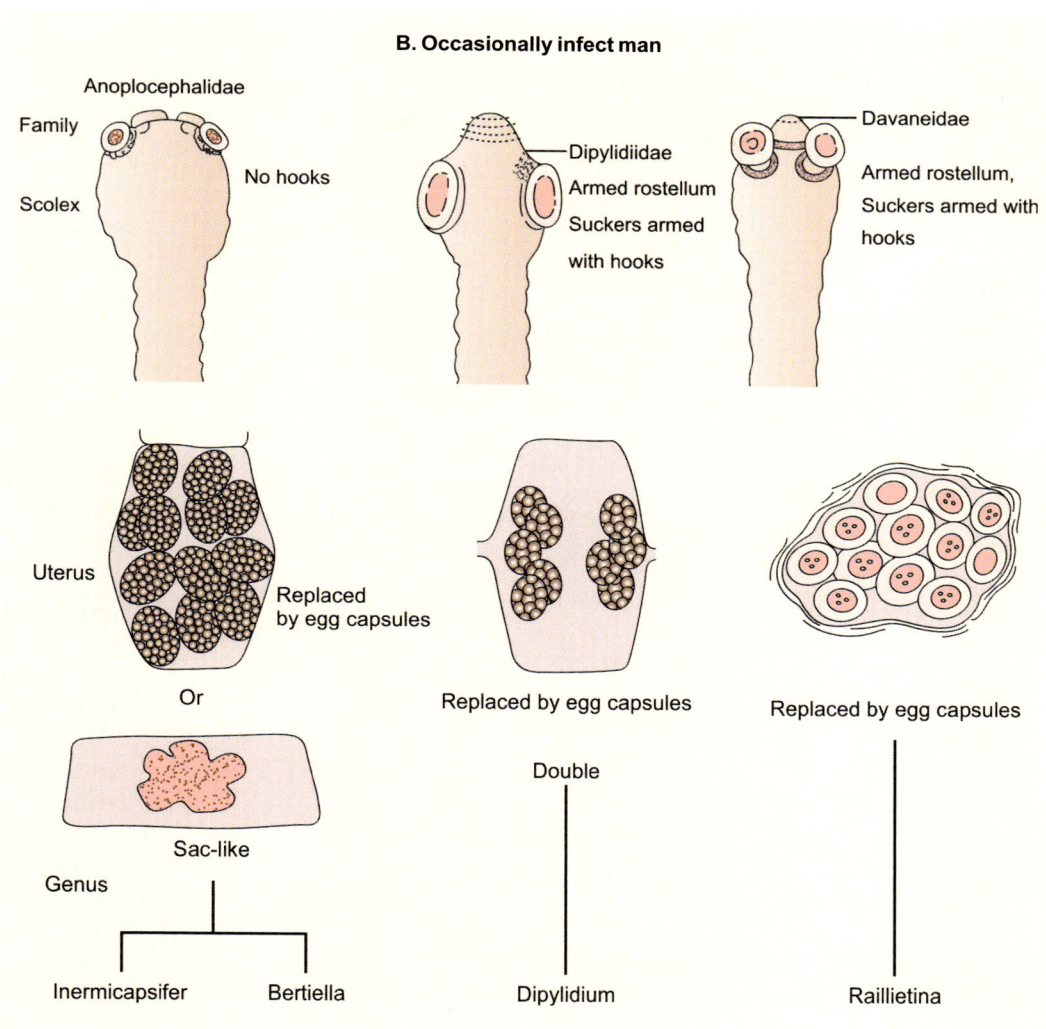

B. Occasionally infect man

Family — Anoplocephalidae

Scolex — No hooks

Dipylidiidae — Armed rostellum, Suckers armed with hooks

Davaneidae — Armed rostellum, Suckers armed with hooks

Uterus — Replaced by egg capsules

Or

Sac-like

Replaced by egg capsules

Double

Replaced by egg capsules

Genus

Inermicapsifer   Bertiella   Dipylidium   Raillietina

Taenidae (Family), Taenia (Genus)

Taenia saginata and Taenia solium		
Feature/Heading	Taenia saginata	Taenia solium
First described by	Goeze in 1782	First described by Linnaeus in 1758
Common name	Beef tapeworm or the unarmed tapeworm of man	Pork tapeworm or the armed tapeworm of man
Geographical distribution	Worldwide. In India seen amongst the beef-eaters (especially the muslim community)	Worldwide. Commonly seen amongst pork-eaters (Jews and Muslims rarely infected)
Habitat	Small intestine (upper jejunum) of man. It moves against the direction of peristaltic movement.	Small intestine (upper jejunum) of man

Contd.

Taenia saginata and Taenia solium (Contd.)		
Feature/Heading	Taenia saginata	Taenia solium
Morphology		
Adult worm	Whitish, semitransparent, 5–10 metres long	Measures 2–3 metres in length
Scolex	Measures 1–2 mm, is quadrate, has 4 circular suckers. Has no rostellum or any hooklets	Measures 1 mm, is globular and has 4 circular suckers. It has a rostellum that is armed with a double row of alternating large and small hooklets
Neck	Fairly long and narrow (0.5 mm wide), it is quite fragile	Neck is short, about 5–10 mm in length
Proglottides	Number varies from 1000–2000. The common genital pore is situated marginally near the posterior end of each segment and alternates irregularly between ihe left and right margins. Vagina is provided with a sphincter muscle. The gravid uterus consists of a central longitudinal stem with 15–30 lateral branches on each side, these too then subdivide leaving no space in between. The gravid segments are expelled singly. The free gravid proglottid while crawling out of the anal orifice oviposits in the perianal skin. The gravid segment measures 16–20 × 5–7 mm	Number of segments is from 800 to 1000. Common genital pore is marginal, thick-lipped and is situated near the middle of lateral margin of each segment, alternating irregularly between the left and the right margins. Vaginal opening does not have any sphincter. The gravid uterus consists of a median longitudinal stem with 7–12 compound lateral branches on each side. The gravid segment are expelled passively in chains of 5–6 together and not singly.
Life span	Adult worm may live for 10 years or more	Adult worm may live for up to 25 years
Eggs	Eggs are liberated by rupture of the ripe segment	
	Eggs are spherical and brown being bile-stained	Features of T. solium eggs are identical to those of T. saginata
	Measures 31–43 µ in diameter	
	The thin, outer transparent shell, when observed, represents the remnant of the yolk mass; it brings about clumping of eggs.	
	The inner embryophore is brown, thick-walled and radially striated.	
	Contain an oncosphere 14–20 µ in diameter with 3 pairs of hooklets	
	Does not float on saturated solution of common salt	
	Eggs are resistant, may retain viability for 8 weeks	
	They are infective only to cattle	Eggs are infective to pigs as well as man

Taenia solium (The pork tapeworm) | *Taenia saginata* (The beef tapeworm)

Morphology

Rostellum
2 rows of hooks
1 mm

No rostellum
No hooklets

5–10 mm neck

3 metres
800–1000 segments

Mature segments (similar each species)

5–10 metres
1000–2000 segments

Common genital pore
Lateral, irregularly on either side

Testes, lateral, small

Uterus,
simple tube

Ovary,
bilobed

Vitellaria,
scattered,
dorsal

Roughly square

Gravid segment

Gravid segment

Ovum (similar each species)

31–43 μ

Longer than broad
7–12 lateral uterine branches
12 × 6 mm

Longer than broad, 15–30
lateral uterine branches
16–20 × 5–7 mm

Cysticercus (larval form)

Invaginated
scolex

Cyst well
developed

Cysticercus bovis
Never found in man

Cysticercus cellulosae
Occasionally found in man

Life cycle of *T. saginata*

It needs two hosts. Definitive host—man. Intermediate host—cattle.

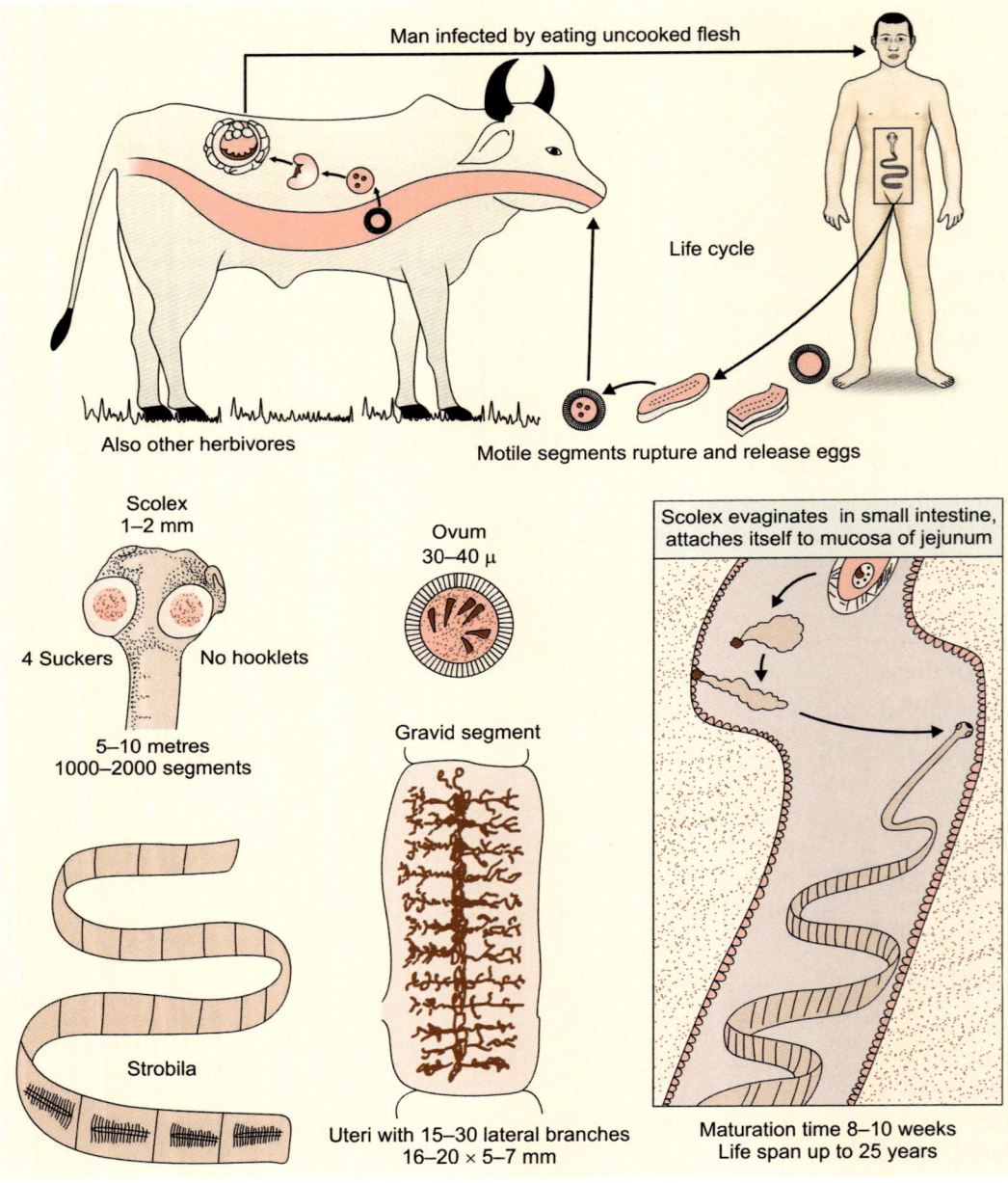

Man infected by eating uncooked flesh

Life cycle

Also other herbivores

Motile segments rupture and release eggs

Scolex
1–2 mm

4 Suckers   No hooklets

5–10 metres
1000–2000 segments

Ovum
30–40 μ

Scolex evaginates in small intestine, attaches itself to mucosa of jejunum

Gravid segment

Strobila

Uteri with 15–30 lateral branches
16–20 × 5–7 mm

Maturation time 8–10 weeks
Life span up to 25 years

Adult worm resides in small intestine of man. Gravid segments containing the eggs are passed out with faeces. Cows or Buffalos swallow these while grazing. On reaching their (intermediate hosts) intestine, the radially striated walls of the eggs rupture liberating the oncosphere. These penetrate the gut wall and enter into portal vessels or mesenteric lymphatics to reach the systemic circulation from where they ultimately come to lie in the muscular tissues for further development. The commonly selected muscles are those of the tongue, neck, shoulder and ham (sometimes, the cardiac muscle may also be involved). The oncospheres lose their hooks, cells in the centre are liquified and after about 8 days each oncosphere forms a vesicle that gradually increases in size and contains at its bottom, the larva, (the scolex of the future worm)—known as *cysticercus*. About 60–70 days are required for oncospheres to metamorphose into cysticercus stage. Humans are infected by consuming under-cooked infected beef containing the cysticerci. Within man, inside the intestine, the scolex on coming in contact with bile, exvaginates and attaches to the gut-wall by means of its suckers and develops into an adult worm by gradual strobilisation. It takes 2–3 months to mature and start producing eggs that are passed along with the faeces while still present in the gravid segments.

Life cycle of *T. solium*: Is essentially similar to that of *T. saginata*, however, the inter-mediate host is the pig. Man is infected after consuming undercooked pork containing the cysticerci.

Larval development of T. saginata and T. solium

Cysticercus bovis: Is the larval stage of *T. saginata* developing in the muscles of cow or buffalo. It measures 5–10 × 3–4 mm and contains the unarmed scolex invaginated on one side. It can survive up to 8 months in the cattle flesh and can develop further only after being eaten by man. *Cysticercus bovis* is not found in man.

Cysticercus cellulosae: Is the larval stage of *T. solium* developing in the muscles of the pig. A mature cyst is opalescent ellipsoidal measuring 5 × 8–10 mm. The longitudinal axis of the cyst lies parallel to that of the muscle fibre. It contains a dense milky-white spot at the side where the scolex with its hooks and suckers remains invaginated. The cyst fluid is rich in salt and albuminous material. In the pig muscles it can survive for up to 8 months and can develop further only after it is ingested by man. *Cysticercus cellulosae* has also been found in man.

Pathology: Adult worms residing in the intestine do not usually produce any symptoms. They may, however, occasionally cause abdominal discomfort, chronic indigestion, anaemia and diarrhoea alternating with constipation. Patient may notice segments in his stool.

Larval stages of *T. saginata* are not seen in man.

Cysticercus cellulosae: Man gets infected the same way as does the pig-—through drinking contaminated water or by eating uncooked raw vegetables contaminated with eggs. Man may have auto-infection or by reverse peristaltic movements of the intestine the gravid segments may be thrown back into the stomach (this amounts to like ingesting a thousand eggs). Cysticerci are usually numerous but on occasions a single one may be encountered. Effects produced by cysticerci depend upon the organ they are localised in. Usually they are found in subcutaneous tissues and muscles causing palpable nodules but involvement of brain produces severe consequences including epilepsy. In the eye, the Cysticercus can be visualised by ophthalmoscopy. Cysticerci ultimately get calcified.

Life cycle of *Taenia solium*

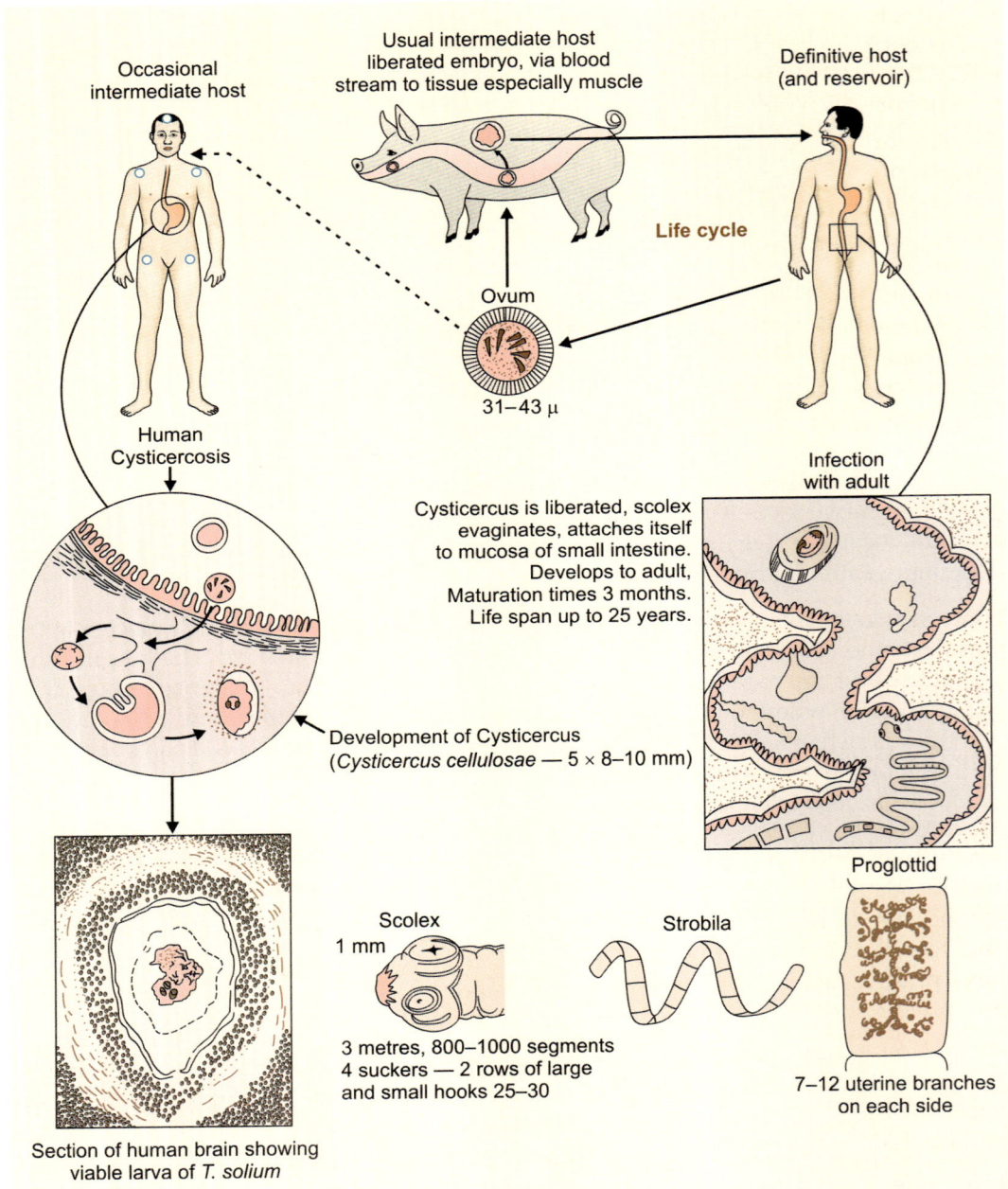

Occasional intermediate host

Usual intermediate host
liberated embryo, via blood
stream to tissue especially muscle

Definitive host
(and reservoir)

Life cycle

Ovum

31–43 μ

Human
Cysticercosis

Infection
with adult

Cysticercus is liberated, scolex
evaginates, attaches itself
to mucosa of small intestine.
Develops to adult,
Maturation times 3 months.
Life span up to 25 years.

Development of Cysticercus
(*Cysticercus cellulosae* — 5 × 8–10 mm)

Proglottid

Scolex
1 mm

Strobila

3 metres, 800–1000 segments
4 suckers — 2 rows of large
and small hooks 25–30

7–12 uterine branches
on each side

Section of human brain showing
viable larva of *T. solium*

Diagnosis

Stool examination—Grossly look for segments or if obtained after purgation, one may look for scolices too. Microscopically one may search for eggs. Perianal NIH swab may be used for demonstrating eggs of *T. saginata*. Species differentiation can only be done by carefully examining the head and the gravid segment.

Diagnosis of cysticercosis

- Biopsy study of the subcutaneous nodule.
- X-rays to reveal calcified cysticerci.
- Eosinophilia in peripheral smear.
- Positive indirect haemagglutination test using antigen from pig's cysticerci.
- A history of intestinal taeniasis is useful.

Treatment: Mepacrine, dichlorophen, yomesan or the newer generation broad spectrum anthelmintics like albandazole can be used. For cerebral cysticercosis hetrazan may be used.

Prophylaxis: Measures include:
- Individual prophylaxis, avoiding consumption of raw or undercooked meat of the intermediate hosts.
- Adequate scrutiny of meat at slaughterhouses.
- Proper sewage disposal and effective treatment of infected individual to prevent infection of intermediate hosts.
- Those harboring adult worms should take extra precautions regarding their personal hygiene.

Echinococcus granulosus

(Dog tapeworm, Hydatid worm)

Historical: Adult worm was discovered by Hartmann in 1965 while the larval form was first made known by Goeze in 1782.

Geographic distribution: Worldwide. Commonly found in sheep and cattle-raising regions and is more prevalent in temperate climates than tropical environment.

Habitat: Man harbours the larval form while the adult worm is found in the small intestine of dog and other canines.

Morphology: Adult worm is a small tapeworm measuring 3–8 mm in length. It has a scolex, neck and strobilla consisting of 3–4 segments. The scolex shows four suckers and 30–36 hooks in two rows. Neck is short and thick. The first segment is immature, second is mature while the third (and fourth where present) is gravid. *Egg:* Is ovoid and resembles other taenia eggs, it measures $25–32 \times 30–37$ μ. The egg contains a hexacanth embryo with 3 pairs of hooks. The egg is infective to man, cattle, sheep and other herbivores.

Larval form: Found within the hydatid cyst developing inside the intermediate hosts. It represents the scolex of the future adult worm and remains invaginated within a vesicular body. After entering the definitive host, the scolex complete with suckers and hookles, exvaginates and develops into an adult worm.

Life cycle: To complete the life cycle, the worm needs 2 hosts.

Definitive hosts: Dog, wolf, jackal and fox (dog being the ideal host). The worm resides in the small intestine of these animals and discharges numerous eggs that come out with the faeces.

Intermediate hosts: Sheep, pig, cattle, goat, horse and man. Larval stage gives rise to hydatid cyst. Sheep appears to be the ideal or optimum host.

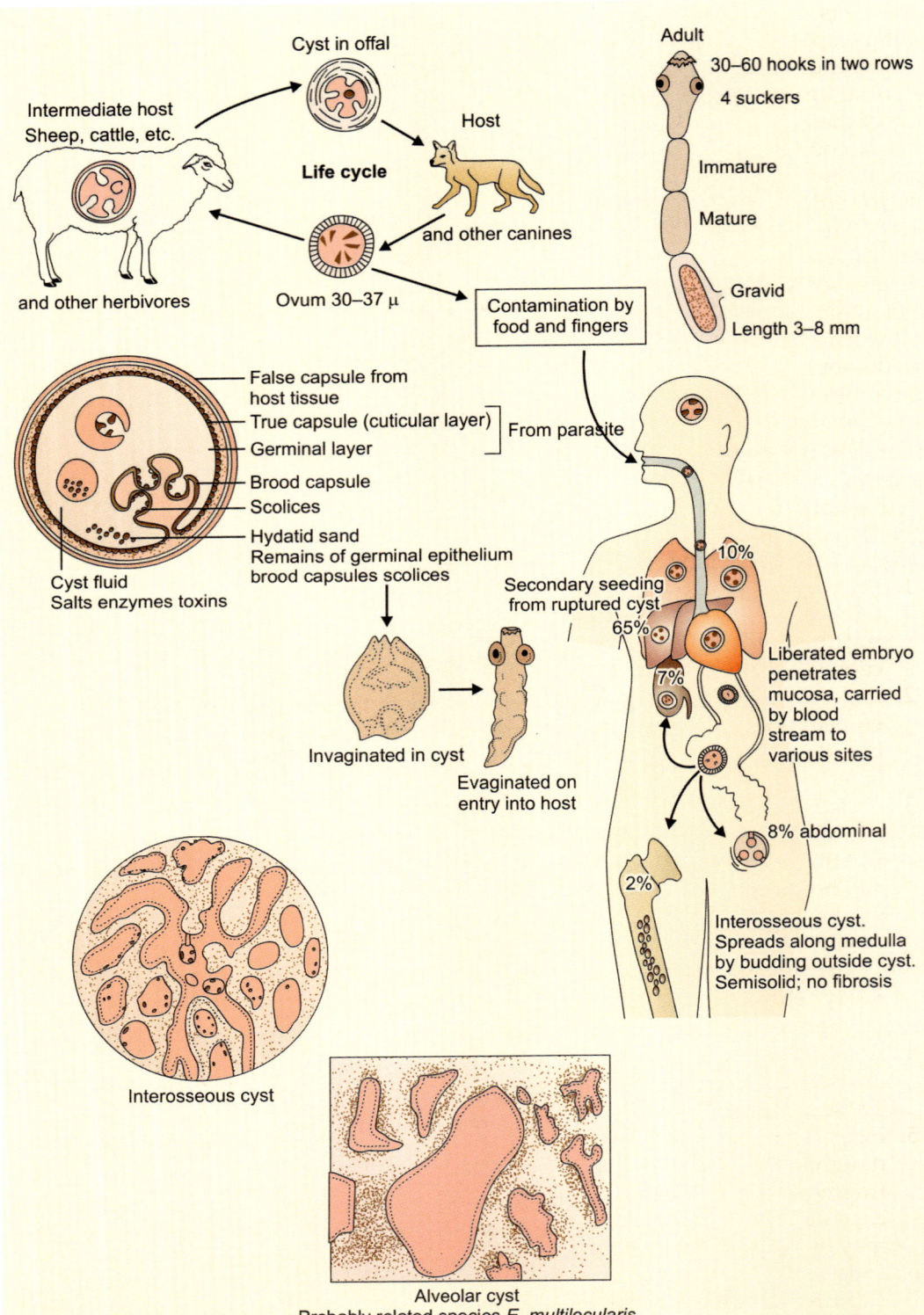

Cyst in offal

Intermediate host
Sheep, cattle, etc.

Host

Life cycle

and other canines

and other herbivores

Ovum 30–37 μ

Contamination by
food and fingers

Adult
30–60 hooks in two rows
4 suckers

Immature

Mature

Gravid
Length 3–8 mm

False capsule from
host tissue
True capsule (cuticular layer)
Germinal layer
Brood capsule
Scolices
Hydatid sand
Remains of germinal epithelium
brood capsules scolices

From parasite

Cyst fluid
Salts enzymes toxins

Secondary seeding
from ruptured cyst

10%

65%

7%

Liberated embryo
penetrates
mucosa, carried
by blood
stream to
various sites

Invaginated in cyst

Evaginated on
entry into host

8% abdominal

2%

Interosseous cyst.
Spreads along medulla
by budding outside cyst.
Semisolid; no fibrosis

Interosseous cyst

Alveolar cyst
Probably related species *E. multilocularis*

The eggs discharged with faeces are swallowed by intermediate hosts, and also by man (especially children) who handle infected dogs. The embryos are hatched in the duodenum. Within 8 hours, the embryos pass through the intestinal wall to enter the portal vein radicles and are carried to the liver (this is the first filtering organ). Some of them may pass through the hepatic capillaries to enter the pulmonary circulation (second filtering organ). Few embryos may even pass through the pulmonary capillaries to reach systemic circulation to be lodged in various organs. Wherever the embryo settles, it forms a hydatid cyst, the young larva is transformed into a hollow bladder. From the inner surface develop several brood capsules with scolices. Consequently a hydatid cyst developing from a single egg (oncosphere) may contain several thousand scolices. A mature fully developed scolex is the end-product and represents full biological development. These fertile hydatids if ingested by a dog develop into adult worms in 6–7 weeks, time in the intestine. However, this hardly happens, as the dogs do not have access to the hydatid cysts present in human viscera, therefore, the cycle comes to a dead end. The natural cycle is hence carried on by dog and sheep. Life span of an adult worm is about 6 months, that of larval stage is many years.

Pathology: The adult worms in the dogs do not cause any noticeable effects at all. The larval stage in man causes hydatid disease. Individuals very closely involved with dogs often get the disease (usually) during childhood while the manifestations appear later in adult life.

Pathogenesis of hydatid cyst: The cyst-wall secreted by the embryo consists of 2 layers:

1. *Ectocyst—outer cuticular layer:* Is a laminated hyaline membrane up to 1 mm thick. Grossly it appears like the white of a hard-boiled egg. When incised or ruptured it curls on itself and exposes the inner layer that contains the brood capsules and daughter cysts.

2. *Endocyst—inner germinal layer:* Is cellular and consists of a number of nuclei embedded in a protoplasmic mass. It is 22–25 μ in thickness. It gives rise to brood capsules with scolices, secretes the hydatid fluid and forms the outer layer.

3. *Hydatid fluid:*
   - Straw coloured, odourless, clear fluid.
   - Mildly acidic (pH = 6.7) and of low specific gravity 1.005 to 1.010.
   - Chemically it is found to contain sodium chloride, sodium sulphate, sodium phosphate and sodium and calcium salts of succinic acids.
   - Fluid is antigenic and highly toxic, when absorbed it gives rise to anaphylactic symptoms.
   - Hydatid sand is a granular deposit found settled at the bottom. It consists of liberated brood capsules, free scolices and loose hooklets.

4. *Acephalocysts (without heads):* Sometimes brood capsules are developed without any scolices; these cysts are sterile or noninfective and are called acephalocysts. These are usually found in cattle.

5. *Endogenous daughter cysts:* After many years (especially in human beings), the daughter cysts develop inside the mother cyst and may arise from the detached fragment of germinal layer or from regressive changes of the young brood capsule and scolex bud. The daughter cysts are identical to mother cysts and may even produce granddaughter cysts within.

6. *Exogenous cyst:* In bone hydatid, the growth continues outwardly and the cyst ruptures resulting in formation of exogenous cysts. [The percentage involvement of various organs is given in the figure presented earlier.]

Development of Brood Capsules and Scolices

Brood capsules arise from germinal layer. Initially spherical, it becomes vacuolated and gets transformed into a vesicle. 5–20 scolices develop inside and a fully grown scolex represents the future head of the adult worm with suckers and a circle of hooklets invaginated inside the scolex. Immature to fully mature scolices may be found in the same brood capsule, they may remain attached to inner membrane or be free as hydatid sand in the hydatid fluid.

Host's reaction: Surrounding the embryo there is infiltration by monocytes, tissue macrophages, giant cells and eosinophilis. Many embryos are thus destroyed by phagocytic activity of these cells, few, however, escape destruction and develop into hydatid cysts. In time, the cellular reaction disappears to replaced by fibroblasts and neovascularisation—this is the walling off attempt by the human body and this layer is designated as the *pericyst*. In older cysts, the pericyst may get sclerosed or even calcified and subsequently the parasite within may die or degenerate because of lack of nutrition.

Hydatid cyst in man grows to just 4 cm diameter at the end of first year and the brood capsules and scolices begin to appear.

Clinical: Signs and symptoms are dependent upon the location of the cyst.

When superficial it produces a visible swelling.

In most cases, they are silent (symptomless) and are discovered only at autopsy or when they evoke pressure effects (pressure symptoms too are location/site related).

Ruptured cyst may give rise to anaphylactic symptoms and formation of localised or generalised secondary echinococcosis.

Laboratory Diagnosis

1. *Casoni's reaction (Introduced by Casoni in 1911):* Intradermal injection of 0.2 ml of a fresh sterile hydatid fluid (by using a seitz filter) produces a large wheal (5 cm in diameter) within half an hour, in all positive cases. It shows multiple pseudopodia and fades in an hour or so. For control, sterile normal saline (0.2 ml) is similarly injected (by using a separate needle and syringe) on the other arm. Hydatid fluid from human cases or from animals is used as an antigen.
2. *Peripheral blood* smear shows moderate eosinophilia.
3. *Serological tests*—Precipitin reaction and CFT done with hydatid antigen are also found to be positive. Other tests available are haemagglutination test, flocculation and ELISA tests. Indirect fluorescent antibody test is very useful and immunoelectrophoresis technique is also very well accepted.
4. PCR test also available. Very sensitive and very specific
5. *Exploratory cyst puncture or fine needle aspiration* reveals scolices or hooklets in fluid. This is, however, a dangerous procedure (to be avoided).
6. *X-ray/imaging techniques:* Useful for cysts in lungs and liver. X-ray, ultrasound, CAT scan or MRI scanning may reveal the cyst. X-ray of a bone cyst shows a mottled bony appearance.

Treatment: No specific drug known so far. Prophylaxis: Measures include:
— Prevention of infection of dogs and their regular deworming.
— Personal prophylaxis, especially for dog handlers. Laboratory personnel should be careful, while examining dog's faeces.

Echinococcus multilocularis

(Alveolar or Multilocular hydatid disease)

First described by Leuckart in 1863 and then by Vogel in 1955. The *definitive hosts* are dogs, foxes and wolves and the *intermediate hosts* (those harboring larval forms) are mice and tundra wolves.

Geographical distribution: Chiefly Russia, Siberia, Bavaria, the Tyrol and North America (especially Canada and Alaska). Organ most commonly involved is liver and causes central necrosis and cavitation in it. Cavity contains a little or no fluid. The outer hyaline layer is inconspicuous while the germinal layer is hyperplastic and thrown into folds. There is often a persistent cellular reaction of eosinophils and endothelial cells in the surrounding tissues. The multilocular cysts have a tendency to proliferate and are mostly sterile.

Life cycle of Echinococcus multilocularis

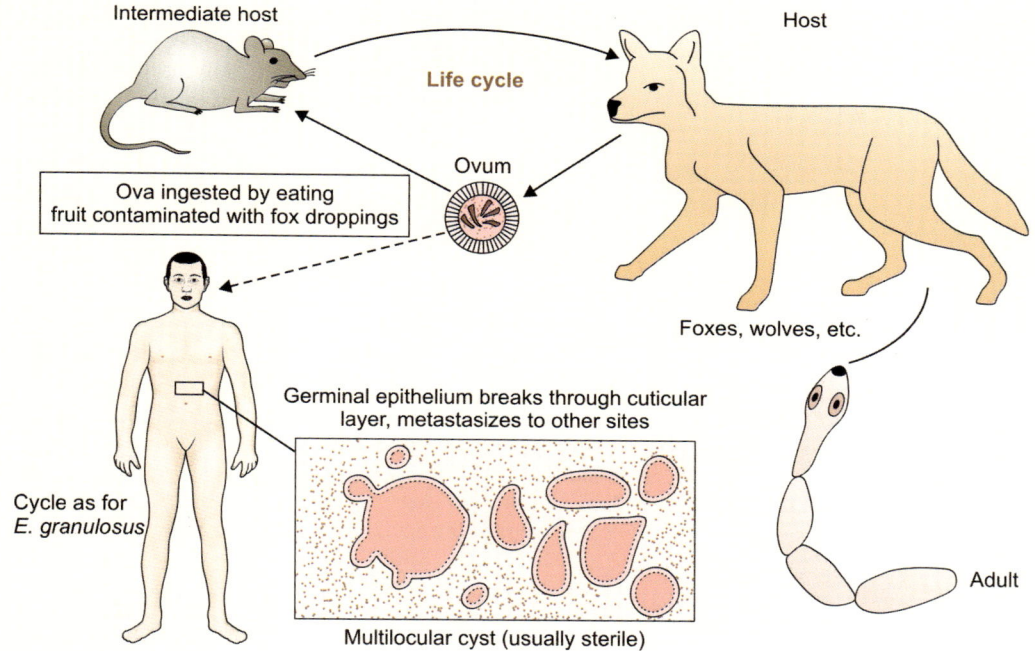

Multilocular cyst (usually sterile)

Pathology of hydatid disease

1. **Unilocular cysts:**
   (a) Surrounding inflammatory reaction and fibrosis. After years may die, shrink, calcify.
   (b) General allergy—eosinophilia, asthma, etc.
   (c) Pressure effects—local tissue damage.
                    obstruction of natural channels.
   (d) Leakage or rupture—allergy accentuated
                        anaphylactic shock sometimes
                        secondary implantation (e.g. peritoneal)
   (e) Secondary infection with abscess formation.

2. **Osseus cysts:**
   (a) No fibrosis (some cellular infiltration).
   (b) Bone destruction sometimes leading to
   (c) Spontaneous fracture.
3. **Alveolar cysts:**
   (a) Local pressure effects.
   (b) Allergy.
   (c) Germinal epithelium acts like a neoplasm with local infiltration or distant metastases.

HYMENOLEPIDIDAE (FAMILY) HYMENOLEPIS (GENUS)

Hymen * Membrane, Lepis = shell.

Each mature segment has three testes, the uterus is sac-like and transverse. Individual segment is broader than length. Eggs possess two membranes, the outer one is thin and transparent. Larval stage is cysticercoid.

Feature	Hymenolepis nana	Hymenolepis diminuta
Historical	First described by Siebold in 1852 and later by Blanchard 1891	First described by Rudolphi in 1819 and later by Blanchard in 1891.
Geographic distribution	Worldwide	Worldwide
Habitat	Adult worm in distal ileum of man. Also found in rats and mice	Adult stage in rats and mice and occasionally in man. Larval stage (cysticercoid) in fleas. Human beings are infected accidentally by swallowing infected fleas.
Adult worm	One of the smallest cestodes infecting man, measuring 2 cm x 0.5–0.9 mm. Have about 200 segments	Is a common parasite of rats and mice. Measures 30–60 cm x 4 mm. Possess 800–1000 segments.
Scolex	Globular, has 4 suckers, is provided with a short retractile rostellum armed with a single row of 20–30 hooks. Rostellum stays invaginated and rostellar hooklets are shaped like tuning forks. Neck is long. Head measures 0.3 mm	Head measures 0.2–0.4 mm. It has no hooks.
Proglottides	Mature segment measures 0.22 x 0.85 mm. Genital pores are marginal and are situated on the same side. Uterus is transverse sac with tabulated walls while there are 3 testes	Mature segment measures 0.75 × 2.5 mm. Other features are identical to H. nana segments.
Eggs	Are liberated with faeces by gradual disintegration of the terminal segments • Are spherical or oval measuring 45 × 35 μ • Outer membrane is thin and colourless and the inner embryophore encloses an oncosphere with three pairs of lancet-shaped hooklets. • The space between the two membranes is filled with yolk granules and polar filaments, It floats on saturated solution of common salt	Are liberated with faeces by gradual disintegration of terminal gravid segments Outer shell is yellowish, inner embryophore has two knob-like thickenings. There are no polar filaments.

Hymenolepis nana

Hymenolepis diminuta

Morphology

Hymenolepis nana

Single row
20–30 hooks
0.3 mm

2 cm × 0.5–0.9 mm
Some 200 segments

Mature segment

Common
genital
pore
lateral
same side

Testes
(3)

Vitelleria — Sac-like uterus

Broader than long
0.22 × 0.85 mm

Ovum

Polar points but no filaments 6

Filaments between membranes

6 hooked oncosphere 45 × 35 μ

Hymenolepis diminuta

No hooks
0.2–0.4 mm

30–60 cm × 4 mm
800–1,000 segments

Mature segment

Common
genital
pore
lateral
same side

Testes
further
apart

Broader than long
0.75 × 2.5 mm

Ovum

Polar thickening either end

Hooked oncosphere 70 × 60 μ

Hymenolepis nana

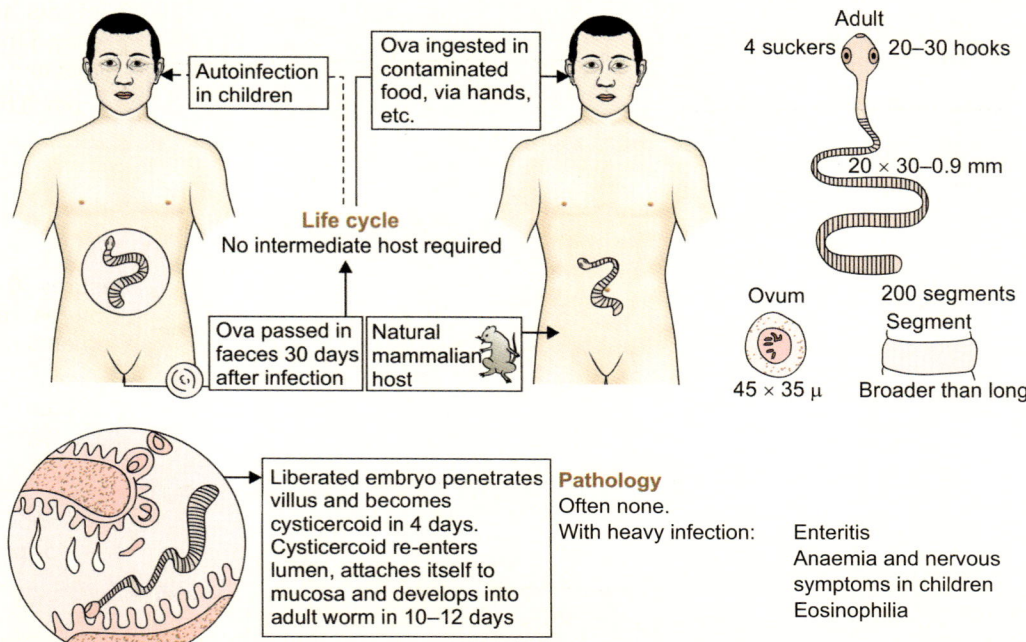

Autoinfection
in children

Ova ingested in
contaminated
food, via hands,
etc.

Life cycle
No intermediate host required

Ova passed in
faeces 30 days
after infection

Natural
mammalian
host

Adult

4 suckers — 20–30 hooks

20 × 30–0.9 mm

Ovum

200 segments

Segment

45 × 35 μ   Broader than long

Liberated embryo penetrates
villus and becomes
cysticercoid in 4 days.
Cysticercoid re-enters
lumen, attaches itself to
mucosa and develops into
adult worm in 10–12 days

Pathology
Often none.
With heavy infection:

Enteritis
Anaemia and nervous
symptoms in children
Eosinophilia

Laboratory diagnosis: Ova in faeces

Hymenolepis diminuta intermediate host

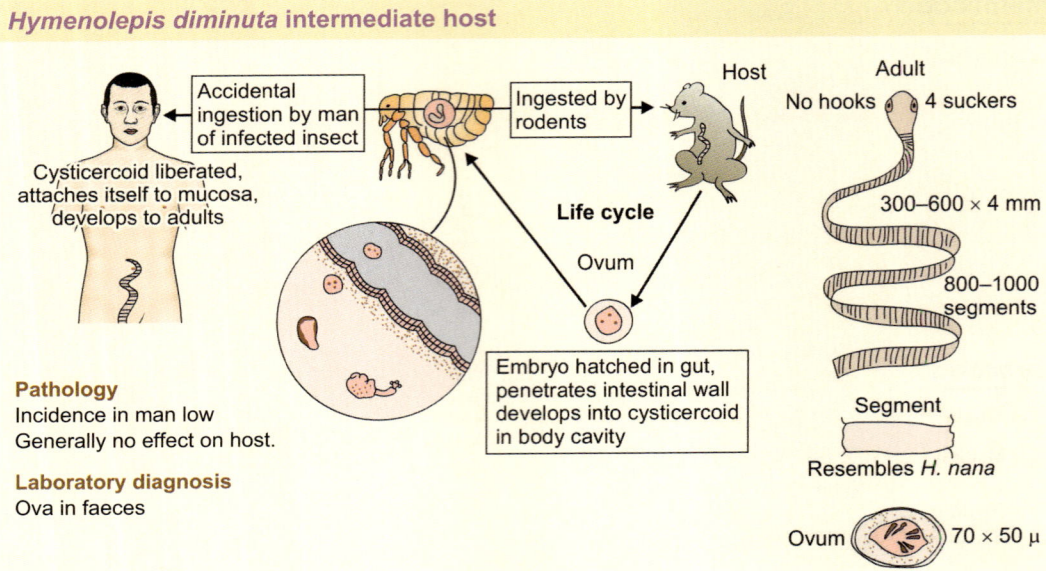

Pathology
Incidence in man low
Generally no effect on host.

Laboratory diagnosis
Ova in faeces

Resembles *H. nana*

OTHER CESTODES OF LESSER SIGNIFICANCE (CYCLOPHYLLIDEAN TAPEWORMS)

Larval stage only described in man, causing *Coenurus cerebralis*

Life cycle

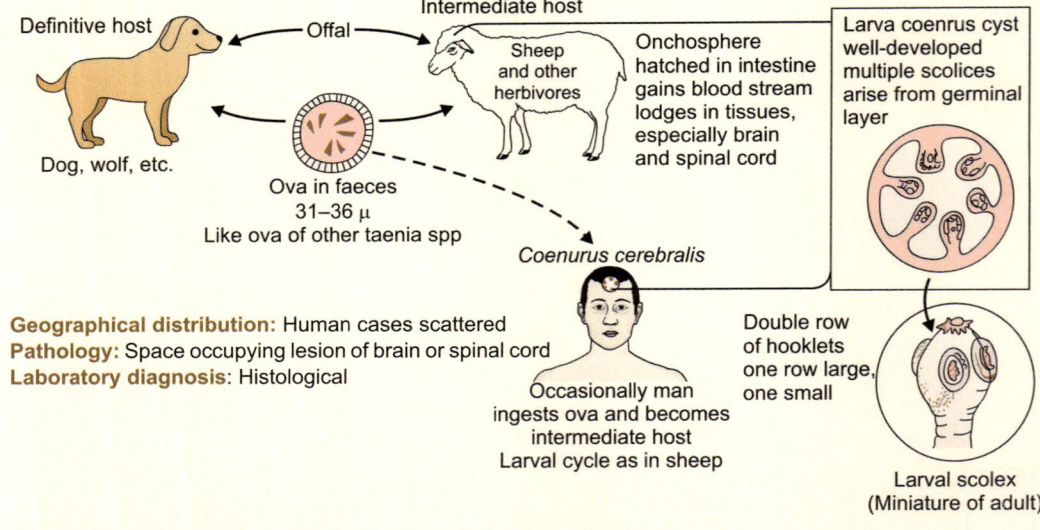

Geographical distribution: Human cases scattered
Pathology: Space occupying lesion of brain or spinal cord
Laboratory diagnosis: Histological

Related species recorded as causing Coenurus infection in man

Species	Definitive host	Intermediate host usually
Multiceps glomeratus	Unknown	Gerbille
M. senialis	Dogs, wolves, foxes	Rabbits and other rodents

Multiceps (or taenia) multiceps (the gid worm)

Intermicapsifer spp

Life cycle probably:

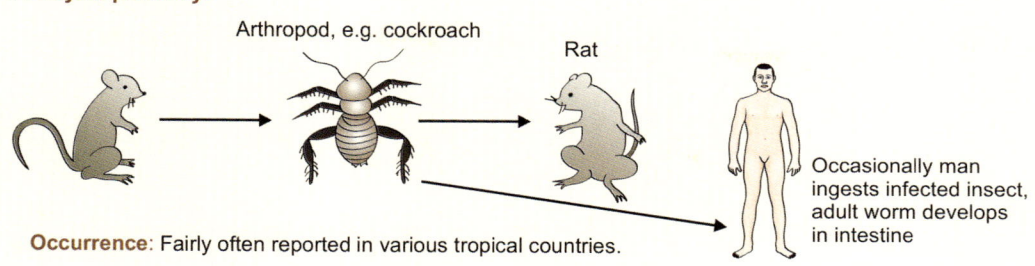

Arthropod, e.g. cockroach

Rat

Occasionally man ingests infected insect, adult worm develops in intestine

Occurrence: Fairly often reported in various tropical countries.

Bertiella studeri

Life cycle

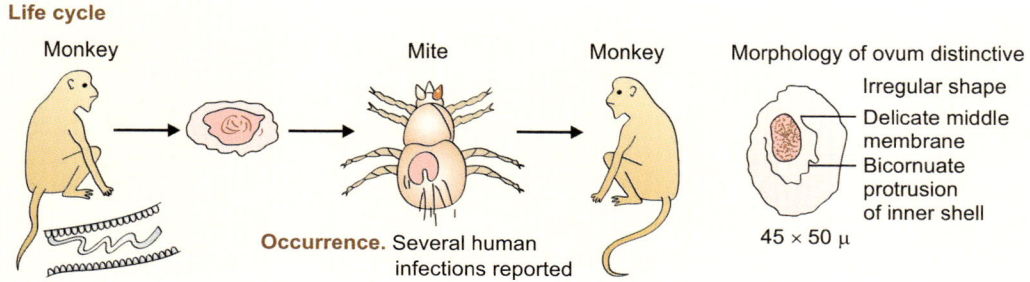

Monkey

Mite

Monkey

Morphology of ovum distinctive

Irregular shape

Delicate middle membrane

Bicornuate protrusion of inner shell

45 × 50 μ

Occurrence. Several human infections reported

Dipylidium caninum (The double-pored dog tapeworm)

Life cycle

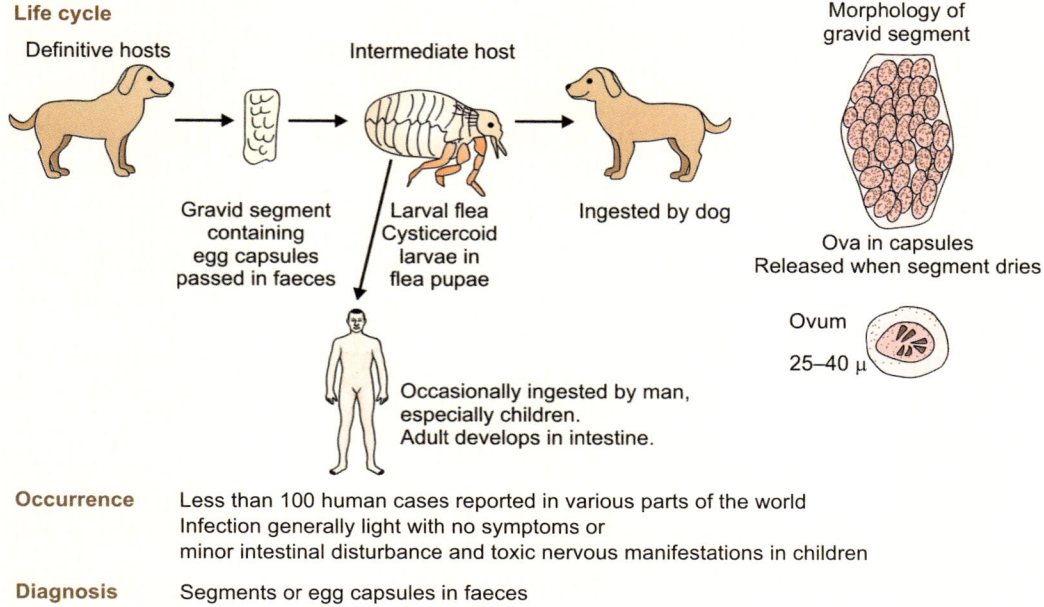

Definitive hosts

Intermediate host

Morphology of gravid segment

Gravid segment containing egg capsules passed in faeces

Larval flea Cysticercoid larvae in flea pupae

Ingested by dog

Ova in capsules Released when segment dries

Occasionally ingested by man, especially children. Adult develops in intestine.

Ovum

25–40 μ

Occurrence   Less than 100 human cases reported in various parts of the world
Infection generally light with no symptoms or
minor intestinal disturbance and toxic nervous manifestations in children

Diagnosis   Segments or egg capsules in faeces

Raillietine madagascarensis and other spp.

Life cycle: Not studied   **Occurrence:** Occasionally adults found in man

Phylum Platyhelminthes
Class Trematoda

Trematoda means pierced with holes. Species that affect mankind are of the type that need two separate hosts to complete their life cycle.

General Features of Digenetic Trematodes

A. Are leaf-shaped flattened unsegmented worms called flukes.

B. Size is variable from a mm to several cm.

C. Attachment organs are two strong muscular cup-shaped depressions, called suckers. One sucker surrounds the mouth and is called the *oral sucker* and the other, on the ventral surface of the body, is called the *ventral sucker* or the *acetabulum.*

D. Sexes are by and large not separate, i.e. each individual worm is a hermaphrodite (monecious) excepting the Schistosomes which have separate sexes and are unisexual.

E. They do not have any body cavity.

F. An incomplete alimentary canal is present. Anus is lacking. The oesophagus bifurcates in front of the ventral sucker into a pair of blind intestinal caeca or crura that may be simple (as in *C. sinesis)* or branched and compound (as in *Fasciola hepatica)* or may reunite to form a single caecum (as in Schistosomes).

G. Both, excretory and nervous systems are present. Excretory system consists of 'flame cells' and collecting tubules that open posteriorly into the excretory pore. The flame cell pattern provides the basis for identification of species.

H. A highly developed reproductive system exists in each individual and the genital organs lie between the two branches of the intestine.

I. Trematodes are oviparous and discharge eggs.

J. All eggs excepting those of Schistosomes are operculated and can develop only in water. In most cases they are immature when laid. Trematode eggs do not float on saturated solution of common salt.

General Morphology

A. *Hermaphroditic spp.* (All except genus Schistosoma)

General Morphology

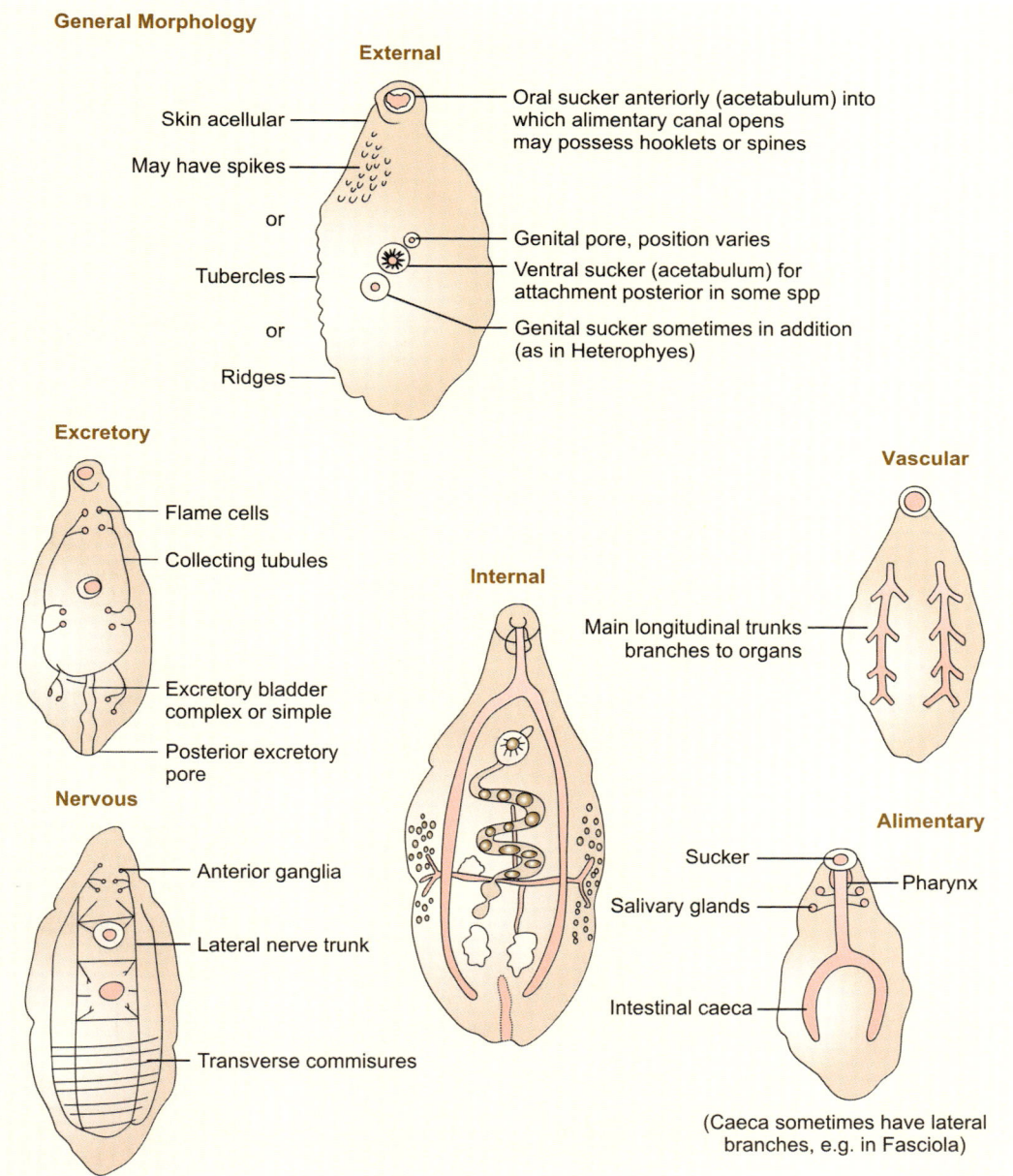

External

Skin acellular —

May have spikes —

or

Tubercles —

or

Ridges —

Oral sucker anteriorly (acetabulum) into which alimentary canal opens may possess hooklets or spines

Genital pore, position varies

Ventral sucker (acetabulum) for attachment posterior in some spp

Genital sucker sometimes in addition (as in Heterophyes)

Excretory

Flame cells

Collecting tubules

Excretory bladder complex or simple

Posterior excretory pore

Vascular

Main longitudinal trunks branches to organs

Internal

Nervous

Anterior ganglia

Lateral nerve trunk

Transverse commisures

Alimentary

Sucker —

Pharynx

Salivary glands —

Intestinal caeca —

(Caeca sometimes have lateral branches, e.g. in Fasciola)

Reproductive System

Male genital system: Consists of two testes (excepting Schistosomes) in the posterior part of the body, two vasa efferentia and one was deferens. Vas deferens is dilated into a seminal vesicle followed by a narrowing (the ejaculatory duct) before finally opening into the genital atrium. The distal part of the vas deferens is a muscular cirrus that serves as the copulatory organ. The prostate gland surrounds the narrowed portion of the vas deferens. The terminal vesicle, cirrus and the prostate gland are all enclosed in the cirrus sac.

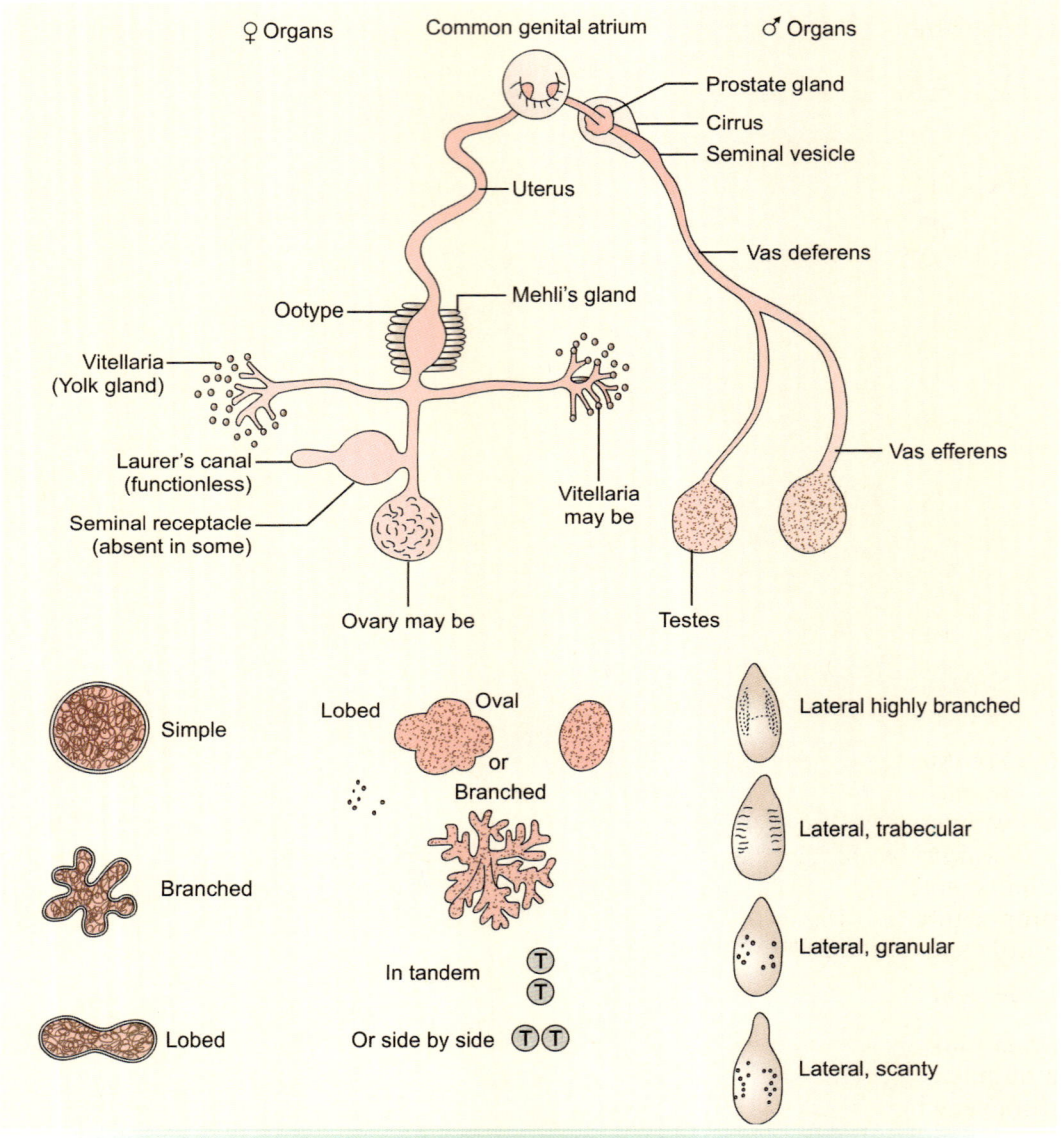

Fig. 9.1: Reproductive (schematic)

Female genital system: Consists of an ovary, its ducts, two vitellaria (yolk glands) and their ducts on either side, a vestigeal vagina (called Laurer's canal), seminal receptacle, uterus, ootype and Mehli's gland. *Ovary* lies in front of the testis. *Uterus* commences from ootype and after a tortuous course terminates in the genital atrium; the terminal part is called metraterm which, in the absence of the opening of Laurer's canal, acts as a vagina. Ootype is the fertilisation chamber. It lies between uterus and oviduct;

while, oviduct, in turn is joined by the common vitelline duct and the seminal recep-tacle. The two *vitelline ducts* from either side join to form the common vitelline duct that opens into the ootype. *Laurer's canal* is the vestigeal vagina and it may or may not open on the dorsal surface; if an opening is present it serves as vagina, permitting entrance of sperms and assisting in cross-fertilisation. *Mehli's gland* surrounds the ootype while the *genital atrium* opens on the ventral surface near the acetabulum.

Life Cycle of Trematodes in General

(Hermaphroditic Species)

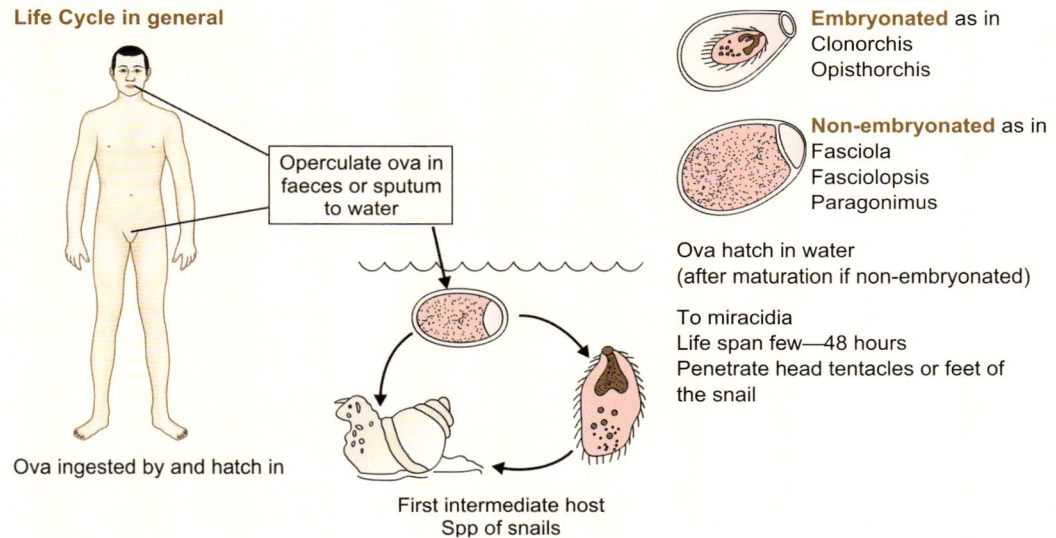

Life Cycle in general

Operculate ova in faeces or sputum to water

Ova ingested by and hatch in

First intermediate host
Spp of snails

Embryonated as in Clonorchis Opisthorchis

Non-embryonated as in Fasciola Fasciolopsis Paragonimus

Ova hatch in water (after maturation if non-embryonated)

To miracidia Life span few—48 hours Penetrate head tentacles or feet of the snail

Definitive host is generally man.

Intermediate host is usually a water snail or mollusc for larval development. A *second intermediate host* (fish or crab) is required for encystment in some trematodes.

The *eggs* discharged from the definitive host gain access to water. A free-swimming ciliated embryo—*the miracidium*—is hatched out. Miracidium then gains access to its proper intermediate host (snail or mollusc) and localises either in the liver or the lymph spaces for further development.

Development in Snail of Larvae

Miracidium gets transformed into a sac-like structure labelled as sporocyst. It contains a number of germ cells. Asexual multiplication does not occur here (except in schis-tosomes where a *second generation sporocyst* is formed).

↓

Sporocyst changes into a redia. A redia has an oral sucker, a pharynx, a sac-like intestine and a birth-pore through which the next generation escapes. Within the redia a fresh crop of germ cells is produced, which develop either into daughter rediae (*second generation rediae*) or into the next stage, the *cercariae*. *Asexual multiplication occurs at this phase in all trematodes* (in schistosomes, however, redia formation stage is missing).

↓

Cercaria represents the final development stage of larvae and is the stage infective to man. Cercaria has suckers and an intestine like that of the adult worm. It moves around assisted by the tail it possesses.

↓

The cercariae, when mature, escape from the snail into the water and may stay free in water or encyst (metacercaria or adolesceria) either in water-plants or in another intermediate host, a fresh-water fish or a crab.

So a single micracidium produces a large number of cercariae. Man is infected by drinking contaminated water or by ingesting encysted cercariae in the water-plant, fish or crab. Free cercariae can in a few cases penetrate through the skin too. After entering the definitive host, these young worms reach final sites of localisation to grow to adulthood, become sexually mature and the cycle is then repeated.

Modes of Infection

A. By ingestion of encysted cercariae through:
   (i) Vegetables—*F. hepatica, F. buski, W. watssni.*
   (ii) Flesh of crab or cray fish—*P. westermani.*
   (iii) Fish—*C. sinensis, H. heterophyes, M. yokogawai.*

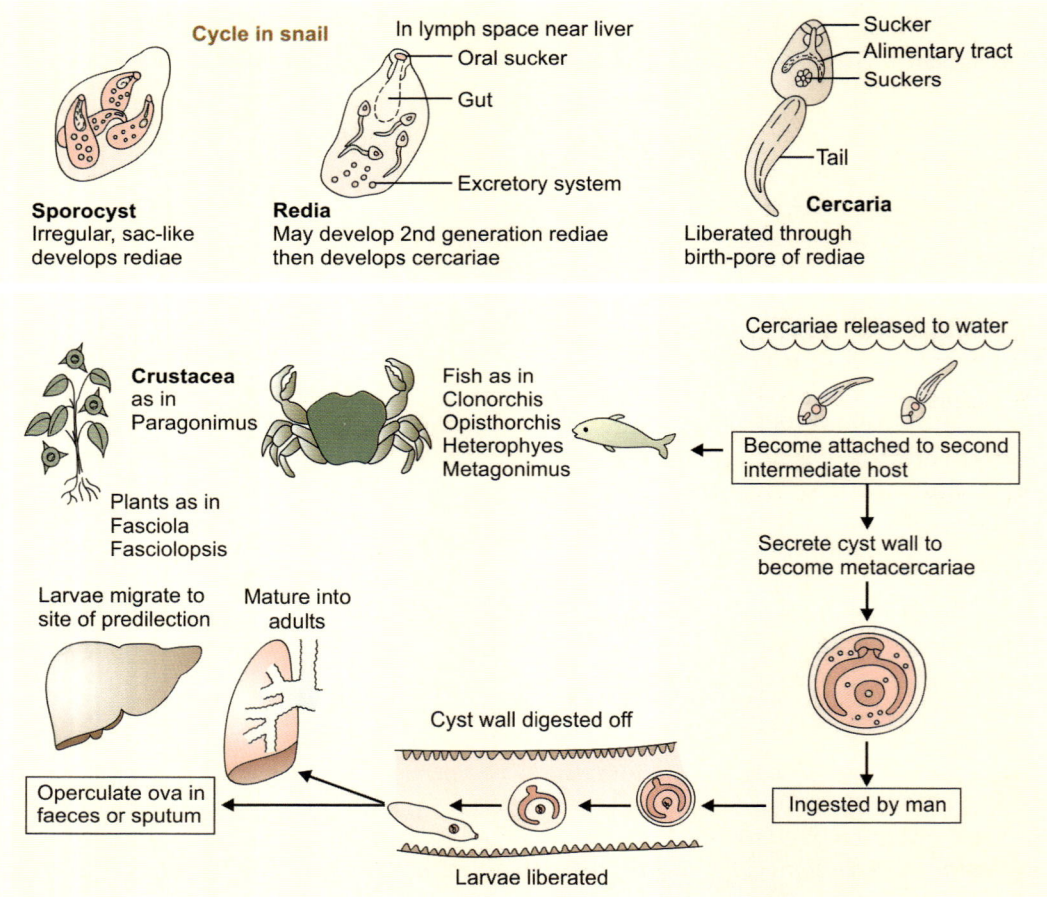

B. Skin penetration by cercariae as in *S. haematobium, S. japonicum* and *S. mansoni.*

Historical Aspects Related to Schistosomiasis

Ruffer in 1910 discovered schistosome eggs in the renal pelvis of a mummy dating back to 1250–1000 BC.

- 1847 Fuji described Katyama disease (caused by *S. japonicum)* in Japan.
- 1851 Bilharz (disease is also known as Bilharziasis) discovered the adult worm of *S. haematobium* from the mesenteric vein of a fellow Egyptian; he also described lateral-spined eggs.
- 1903 Manson described lateral-spined eggs in faeces of a patient who did not suffer from haematuria.
- 1904 Katsurada observed *S. japonicum* eggs in human faeces.
- 1904 Fujinami recovered an adult female of *S. japonicum* in the portal vein of a man at autopsy.
- 1907 Sambon specified that the lateral-spined eggs belonged to species *S. mansoni.*
- 1913 Miysiri and Suzuki (in the following year) explained the life cycle of *S. japonicum.*
- 1915 Leiper explained the life cycle of *S. haematobium* in Egypt. Also specified *S. mansoni* as belonging to a different species.
- 1918 McDonagh prescribed tartar emetic for treating vesical schistosomiasis.

Classification of Trematodes

According to habitat of the trematodes/flukes

Intestine : Ileum—*F. buski, H. heterophyes, M. yokogawai, W. watsoni;* Colon—*G. hominis.*
Liver : *C. sinensis, O. felineus, F. hepatica.*
Lung : *P. westermani.*
Blood : In vesical venous plexus—*S. haematobium.*
      : In rectal venous plexus—*S. mansoni, S. japonicum.*

Systematic Classification

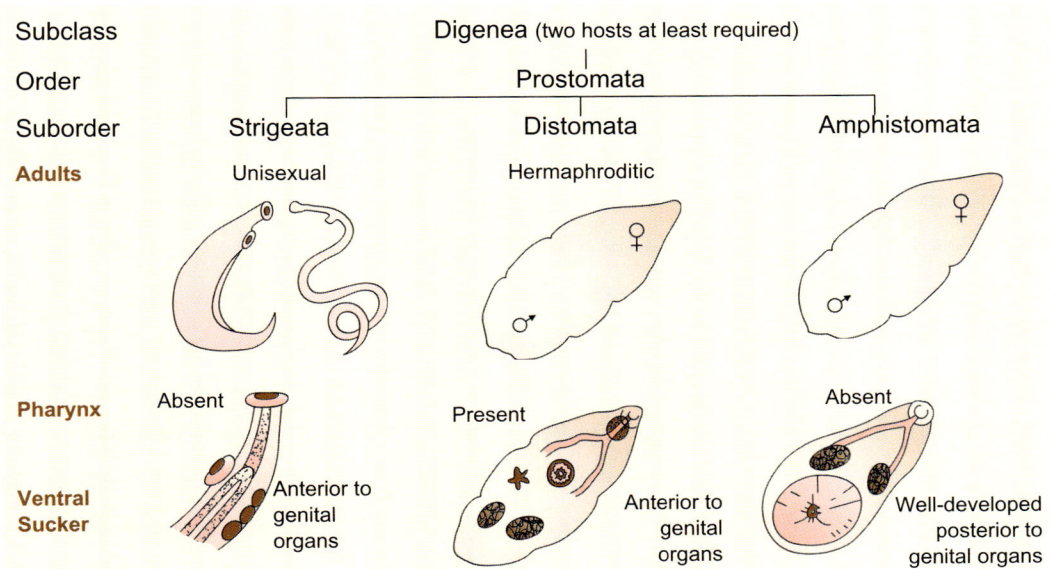

Subclass	Digenea (two hosts at least required)		
Order		Prostomata	
Suborder	Strigeata	Distomata	Amphistomata
Adults	Unisexual	Hermaphroditic	
Pharynx	Absent	Present	Absent
Ventral Sucker	Anterior to genital organs	Anterior to genital organs	Well-developed posterior to genital organs

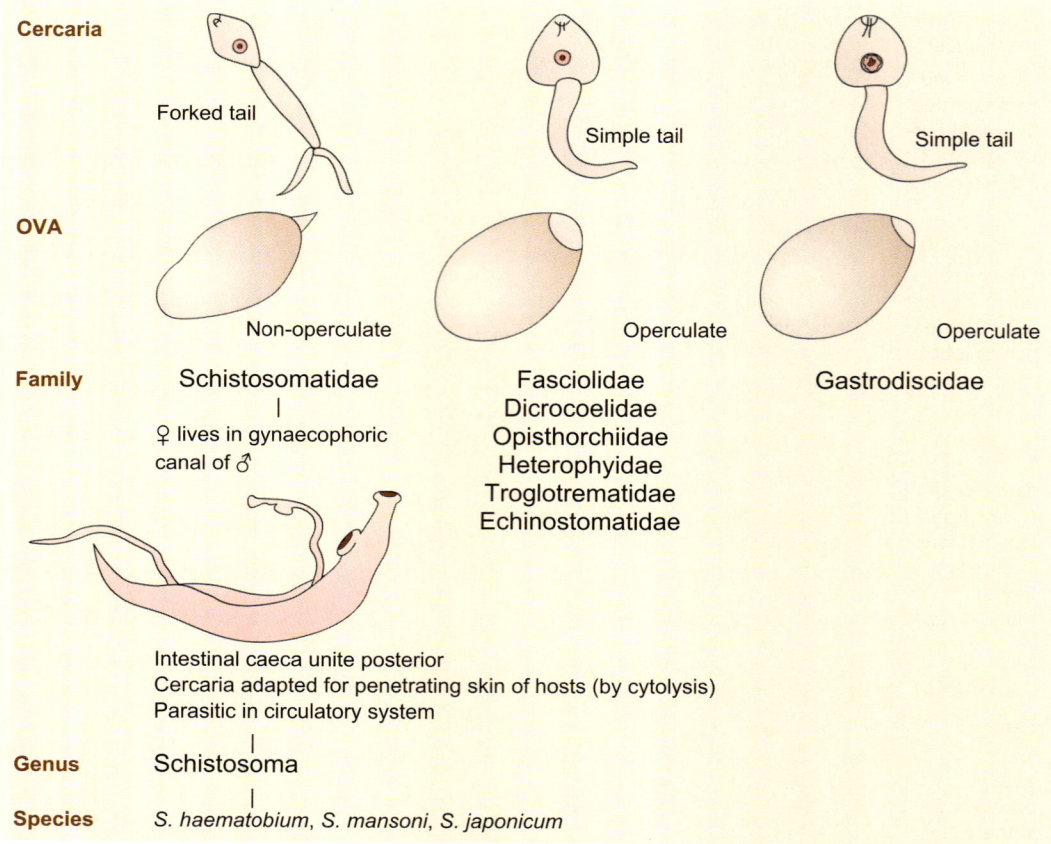

Cercaria

Forked tail

Simple tail

Simple tail

OVA

Non-operculate

Operculate

Operculate

Family

Schistosomatidae

Fasciolidae
Dicrocoelidae
Opisthorchiidae
Heterophyidae
Troglotrematidae
Echinostomatidae

Gastrodiscidae

♀ lives in gynaecophoric canal of ♂

Intestinal caeca unite posterior
Cercaria adapted for penetrating skin of hosts (by cytolysis)
Parasitic in circulatory system

Genus   Schistosoma

Species   *S. haematobium, S. mansoni, S. japonicum*

Suborder Family	Distomata Genital formula	Cercariae Encyst on	Site of Parasitisation	Genus	Species
Fasciolidae Ovary greatly branched anterior to Testes in tandem greatly branched	O T T	Vegetation	Bile ducts Intestine	Fascioia Fasciolopsis	F. hepatica F. gigantica F. buski
Dicrocoeliidae Testes side by side slightly lobed Ovary round Uterus posterior to genitalia	TT O	Ant	Bile ducts Pancreatic ducts	Dicrocoelium	D. dentriticum
Opisthorchiidae Ovary branched or lobed anterior to Testes in tandem branched or lobed	O T T	Freshwater fish	Bile ducts Pancreatic ducts	Clonorchis Opisthorchis	C. sinenisis O. feineus

Heterophyidae (very small) Ovary round anterior to testes side by side around Genital sucker may be present	O TT	Freshwater fish	Intestinal tract	Heterophyes	H. heterophyes
				Metagonimus	M. yokogowai
Troglotrematidae Ovary deeply lobed anterior to testes side by side deeply lobed	O T T	Freshwater crustacea	Lungs and other tissues	Paragonimus	P. westermani
Echinostomatidae Collar of spines Ovary round or lobed anterior to Testes in tandem round or lobed	O T T	Freshwater molluscs	Intestinal tract	Echinostoma	various spp.
Suborder **Amphistomata** Family **Gastrodiscidae** Testes obliquely placed, lobed, anterior to ovary lobed	Large ventral sucker posteriorly	T T O	Not known	Intestinal tract	Gastro-discoides / Watsonius	G. hominis / W. watsoni

SCHISTOSOMATOIDEA

(Superfamily)

General Features of Schistosomes

A. Schistosomes have separate sexes (are diecious).
B. Males are shorter and stouter than females. Lateral margins of males are ventrally folded to form a gynaecophoric canal in which the females are received.
C. Suckers are armed with delicate spines.
D. There is no muscular pharynx.
E. Intestinal caeca reunite behind the ventral sucker to form a single canal the length of which varies with different species.
F. In males the number of testes varies from 4 to 8.
G. No Laurer's canal exists in the females.
H. Eggs are non-operculated and are laid fully embryonated (contain a single embryo-miracidium).
I. Cercariae have bifid tails, do not encyst and penetrate through the skin of the host.
J. Adult worms reside in the lumen of the portal vein and its radicles.

General morphology

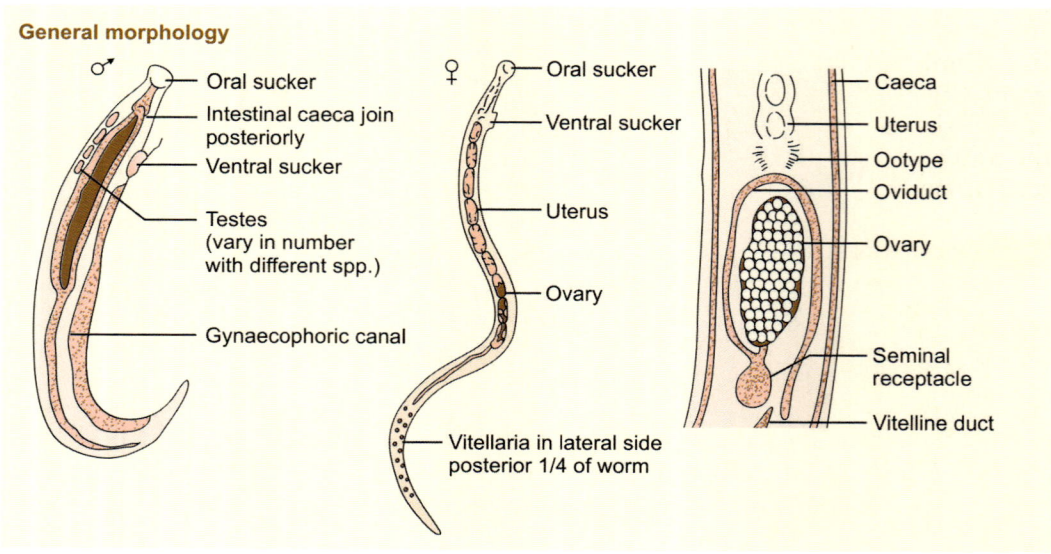

♂
- Oral sucker
- Intestinal caeca join posteriorly
- Ventral sucker
- Testes (vary in number with different spp.)
- Gynaecophoric canal

♀
- Oral sucker
- Ventral sucker
- Uterus
- Ovary
- Vitellaria in lateral side posterior 1/4 of worm

- Caeca
- Uterus
- Ootype
- Oviduct
- Ovary
- Seminal receptacle
- Vitelline duct

Life cycle in general

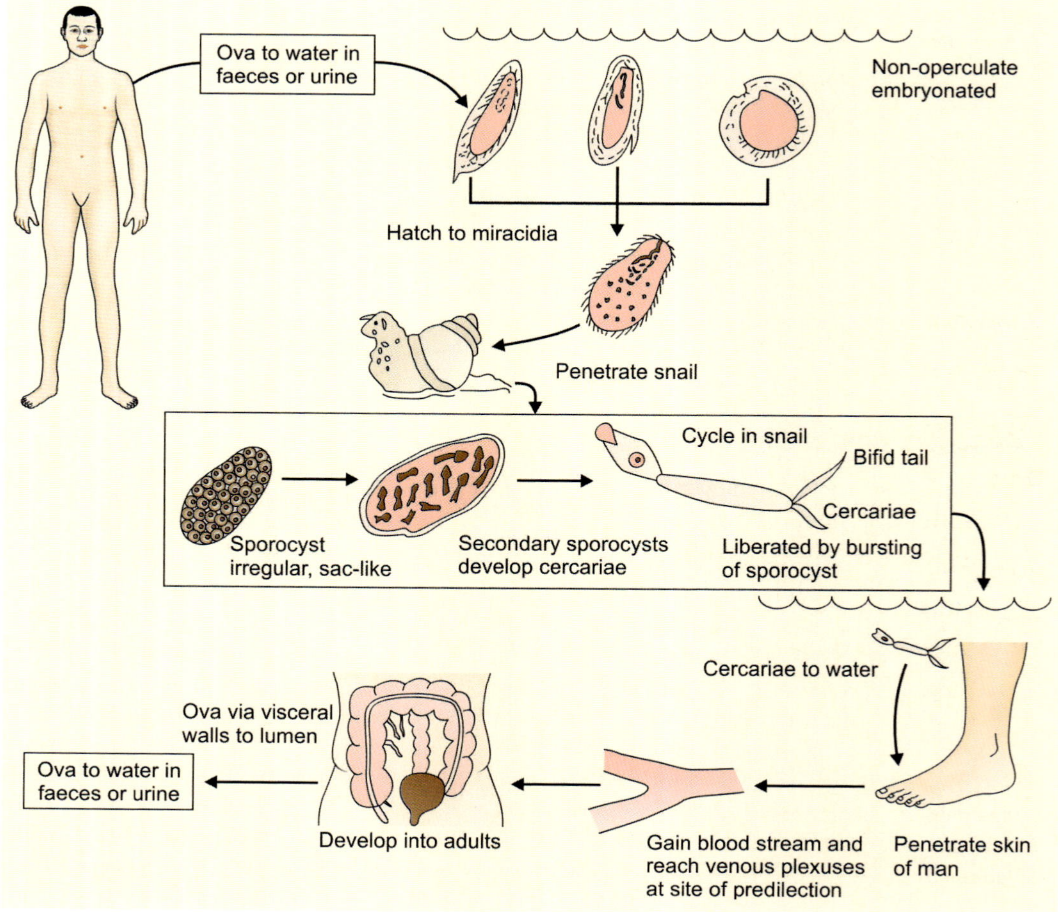

Ova to water in faeces or urine

Non-operculate embryonated

Hatch to miracidia

Penetrate snail

Cycle in snail

Bifid tail

Cercariae

Sporocyst irregular, sac-like

Secondary sporocysts develop cercariae

Liberated by bursting of sporocyst

Cercariae to water

Ova via visceral walls to lumen

Ova to water in faeces or urine

Develop into adults

Gain blood stream and reach venous plexuses at site of predilection

Penetrate skin of man

Immunity in Schistosomiasis

In endemic regions schistosomiasis is predominantly a disease of the young and the immunity develops gradually taking several years. As the age increases, the number of eggs discharged becomes less with reduction in severity of symptoms. However, the adult worms established within the host cannot be killed but the young schistosomulae are destroyed. The adult worms that provoke immunity are themselves

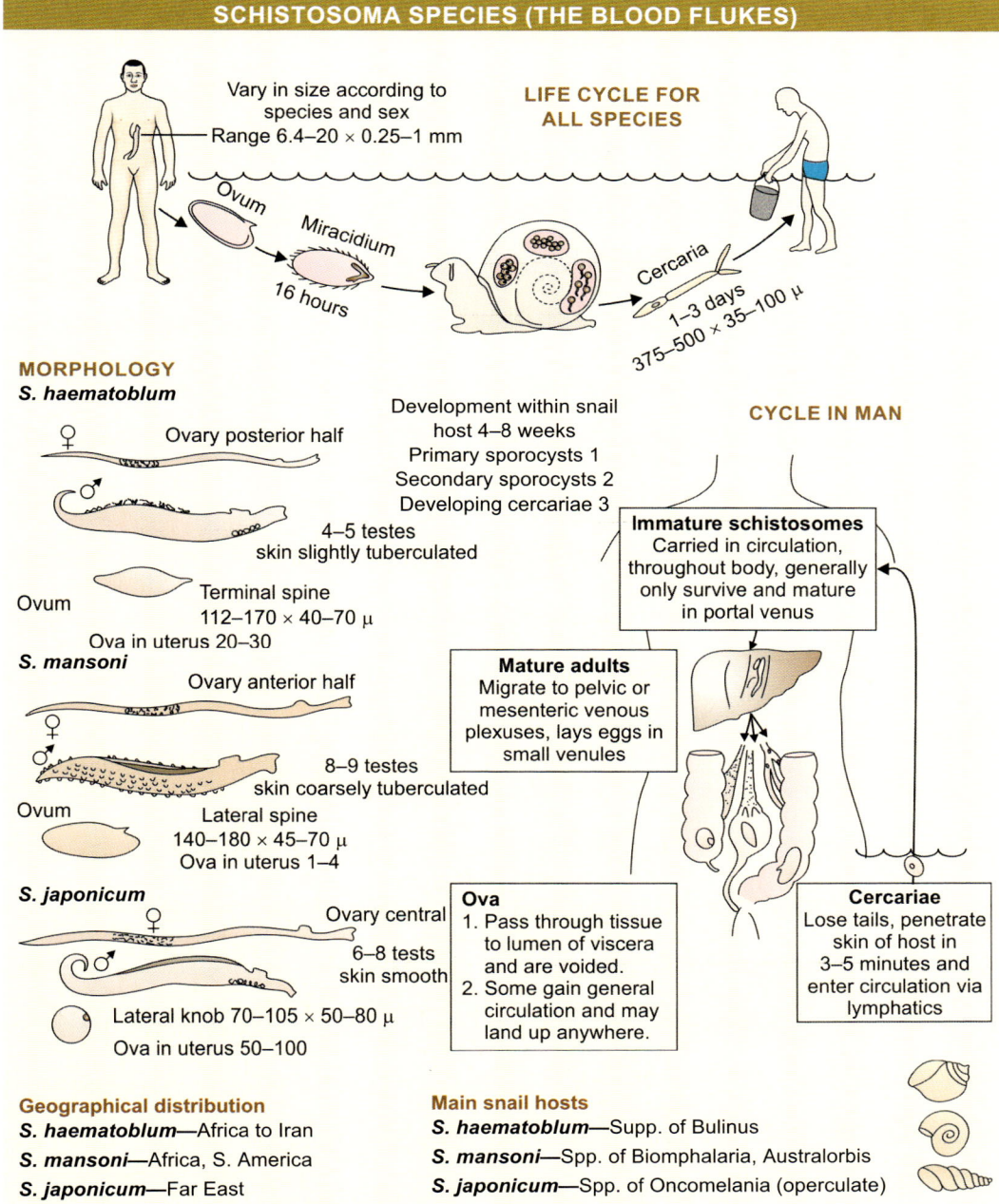

SCHISTOSOMA SPECIES (THE BLOOD FLUKES)

Vary in size according to species and sex
Range 6.4–20 × 0.25–1 mm

LIFE CYCLE FOR ALL SPECIES

Ovum
Miracidium
16 hours
Cercaria
1–3 days
375–500 × 35–100 μ

MORPHOLOGY
S. haematoblum

Ovary posterior half
♀
♂
4–5 testes
skin slightly tuberculated

Ovum
Terminal spine
112–170 × 40–70 μ
Ova in uterus 20–30

S. mansoni
Ovary anterior half
♀
♂
8–9 testes
skin coarsely tuberculated

Ovum
Lateral spine
140–180 × 45–70 μ
Ova in uterus 1–4

S. japonicum
♀
Ovary central
♂
6–8 tests
skin smooth

Lateral knob 70–105 × 50–80 μ
Ova in uterus 50–100

Development within snail
host 4–8 weeks
Primary sporocysts 1
Secondary sporocysts 2
Developing cercariae 3

CYCLE IN MAN

Immature schistosomes
Carried in circulation, throughout body, generally only survive and mature in portal venus

Mature adults
Migrate to pelvic or mesenteric venous plexuses, lays eggs in small venules

Ova
1. Pass through tissue to lumen of viscera and are voided.
2. Some gain general circulation and may land up anywhere.

Cercariae
Lose tails, penetrate skin of host in 3–5 minutes and enter circulation via lymphatics

Geographical distribution
S. haematoblum—Africa to Iran
S. mansoni—Africa, S. America
S. japonicum—Far East

Main snail hosts
S. haematoblum—Supp. of Bulinus
S. mansoni—Spp. of Biomphalaria, Australorbis
S. japonicum—Spp. of Oncomelania (operculate)

not affected because the worms also incorporate host's material into their covering tissues which are not attacked by host's antibodies (called concomitant immunity). A heterologous immunity develops in schistosomiasis and infection with zoonotic (animal) schistosomes acts as a natural zooprophylaxis in human infection.

DIFFERENTIATING FEATURES OF SCHISTOSOME SPECIES			
Feature	Schistosoma haematobium	Schistosoma mansoni	Schistosoma japonicum
Male			
Size	1–1.5 cm × 1 mm	1 cm × 1 mm	1.2–2 cm × 0.5 mm
Cuticle	Finely tuberculated	Coarsely tuberculated	Not tuberculated
Testes	4–5, in aggregates	8–9, arranged in a zigzag fashion	6–8 in a single row
Female			
Size	2 cm × 0.25 mm	1.4 cm × 0.25 mm	2.6 cm × 0.3 mm
Ovary	Behind the middle of the body	Anterior to middle of the body	In the middle portion
Uterus contains	20–30 eggs	1–3 eggs (often only one)	50 or more eggs
Reunited intestine	Long, reunion occurs at roughly the middle of the body	Longest of all three species, reunion occurs in the anterior half	Shortest, Reunion occurs in the posterior fourth of the body.
Egg			
Size	112–170 × 40–70 μ	140–180 × 45–70 μ	70–105 × 50–80 μ
Spine position	Terminal spine	Lateral spine	Have a lateral knob (not spine)
Cercariae (Cephalic glands)			
Oxyphilic	2 pairs	2 pairs	5 pairs
Basophilic	3 pairs	4 pairs	None
Intermediate snail host	Spp. of Bulinus	Spp. of Biomphalaria and Australorbis	Spp. of Oncomeiania
Definitive host	Man	Man	Man and domestic animals
Geographical distribution	Africa to Iran	Africa and South America	Far East
Habitat	Vesical, prostatic or uterine venous plexus	Mesenteric plexus of sigmoidorectal area (inferior mesenteric vein and its radicles)	Mesenteric plexus of ileocaecal region (superior mesenteric vein) and its radicles

Schistosoma haematobium

(Vesical Blood Fluke)

Geographical distribution: Prevalent in Africa and Middle East.

Habitat: Adult worms reside in the pelvic venous plexus—the vesical, prostatic and uterine plexus of veins.

Morphology: By and large, the three species are morphologically identical. The differentiating features are given in the table presented earlier. Life span of schistosomes is 20 to 30 years.

Egg laying and expulsion mechanism

Ova are laid in the venules of the vesical plexus. Female while being held in the gynaecophoric canal of the male, extends its anterior end far into the smallest venules and lays the eggs longitudinally one at a time. After laying an egg, the worm withdraws a short distance and lays another one, thus creating a row. When a venule gets filled with eggs pointing backwards; the two worms in copula move to an adjacent venule. Spines assist in holding the eggs in place and once the worms move out the vasoconstriction also helps. Eggs, later through the vessels reach to the mucosa of the urinary bladder and subsequently reach the cavity to be the finally passed out with the later part of the stream of the urine.

Life cycle

Definite host: Man.

Intermediate host: Freshwater snails.
Throughout Africa—*Bulinus truncatus*
Morocco and Portugal—*Planorbarius metidjensis*
India—*Ferrisia tennis*

The micturated embryonated—eggs reach water to develop into miracidia that move about freely in search of their intermediate host—the freshwater snail. Once located, they penetrate into the soft tissues of the snail to be later lodged into its liver. It loses its cilia and other organs and undergoes developmental changes in 4 to 8 weeks. Miracidium is transformed into a tubular sporocyst which multiplies and forms a second generation of sporocysts. Weeks later, the daughter sporocysts give rise to the final larval forms, the fork-tailed cercariae that are infective to man. The cercariae break off from the sporocyst and escape from the snail into water. On coming in contact with human skin, it penetrates. Once in the subcutaneous region, they shed off their tail (known as Schistosomulae at this stage) and reach a peripheral venule. After crossing the right heart, they reach the pulmonary capillaries. After a few days, the larvae pass through the pulmonary capillaries to reach the left heart and then into the systemic circulation. Most are shunted in the abdominal aorta to gain access into the mesenteric artery. Next, they pass through the capillary bed in the intestine and enter portal circulation (takes 5 days to reach liver). In the intrahepatic portion of the portal blood stream the larvae grow into adults (3 weeks time is required). Once sexually differentiated and matured, they get out of liver against the blood current, migrate through the inferior mesenteric vein to reach rectal venous plexus, pelvic veins, to ultimately reach the vesical plexus of veins. Period required from skin penetration to reach vesical plexus is from 1 to 3 months. Copulation occurs, eggs are released and the whole cycle is repeated.

(*No rediae are produced in schistosomes and asexual multiplication occurs only in the sporocyst stage*).

Pathology

Cercariae, on coming in contact with human skin stick to it by means of their ventral suckers (acetabula) and as skin surface dries they penetrate. Then rest of the life cycle in the human host ensues.

The terminal spined eggs of *S. haematobium* may erode blood vessels causing haemorrhage. These eggs behave like foreign protein and evoke round cell infiltration and connective tissue hyperplasia, leading to formation of a 'pseudotubercle' around each egg (also known as egg granuloma). Initially the granulomas show infiltration by eosinophils, foreign body type of giant cells, monocytes and lymphocytes but later they exhibit only a whorl of fibro-collagenous tissue surrounding a central degenerated region containing the egg which may be calcified. The host reaction to the soluble substances secreted by the egg evoke an immunological reaction and the sensitisation can be transferred by lymphoid cells and inhibited by immunosuppressants.

Clinical features: Infection caused by *S. haematobium* is also referred to as Schistosomiasis haematobia or urinary schistosomiasis or bilharziasis or endemic haematuria. Disease process takes the undermentioned course.

   (i) By the cercariae at skin—cause dermatitis, especially pronounced by cercariae of non-human schistosomes.

  (ii) The toxic metabolites liberated during the growth of schistosomulae in the hepatic portal blood may cause anaphylactic reaction, fever, urticarial rashes, eosinophilia and hepatosplenomegaly. Symptoms appear between fourth and fifth weeks of infection. It is commonly encountered with *S. japonicum* and rarely with *S. haematobium*.

 (iii) **During egg laying period:** The symptoms occur within 3 to 9 months of infection. There is painless terminal haematuria (haematuria seen in the later part of the stream). To begin with their is granulomatous reaction to be followed later by irreversible fibrosis and calcification. Vesical schistosomiasis is also associated with carcinoma of urinary bladder.

 (iv) **Ectopic lesions:** If the eggs and worms escape into pelvic veins, they may be carried to the lungs where the eggs excite an initial granulomatous reaction followed by fibrosis, pulmonary endarteritis, pulmonary hypertension culminating in chronic cor-pulmonale. Eggs and adult worms if carried from portacaval system to other distant parts cause lesions there—in the brain a space occupying lesion is seen (more common with *S. japonicum*), in the spinal cord transverse myelitis like syndrome (common in *S. mansoni* and *S. haematobium* infection).

Diagnosis: Eggs can be demonstrated in the centrifuged deposit of urine and the vesical mucosa biopsy. The excised piece of tissue is cut into two pieces. One piece is processed by histopathological examination and the other piece is compressed between two slides in order to squeeze the egg out and it is examined microscopically under the low power objective.

Miscellaneous investigations:
- Peripheral blood—eosinophilia
- Aldehyde test—positive because of raised globulins.
- Complement fixation test—patient's serum reacts with cercarial antigen obtained from infected snail's liver.
- Intradermal skin test—the cercarial antigen causes an allergic reaction (called Fairley's test).

Other useful immunological tests are:
- Precipitin formation around schistosome eggs [circumoval protein or (OP) test of Oliver-Gonzalez].
- Miracidial immobilisation test
- Development of pericercarial membranes around Schistosoma cercariae. (The immunological tests are group but not species specific).
- Fluorescent antibody technique (FAT) has been used for early detection of schisto-somiasis, using both cercariae and miracidia as antigens.

Treatment: Specific drugs are nitrothiazole compound niridazole (Ambilhar), nilodin, hycanthone, trivalent antimony compounds, e.g. tartar emetic, foucidin, anthiomaline and antimony dimercaptosuccinate.

Prophylaxis: Measures include:
 (i) Disease eradication in man.
 (ii) Preventing water from getting polluted by human excreta.
 (iii) Elimination of snail vector in endemic regions.
 (iv) Avoid swimming, bathing or washing in infected water.

Schistosoma mansoni

(Manson's blood fluke)

Geographic distribution: South America and parts of Africa.

Habitat: Adult worms reside in the mesenteric veins of sigmoidorectal area; also in branches of the portal vein in liver.

Morphology: See the table and figures given earlier.

Life cycle: Similar to that of *S. haematobium*.

Definitive host: Man.

Intermediate host: Freshwater snails.
    (*Biomphalaria alexandrina* in Africa and *Australorbis glabratus* in South America)
    Life cycle is from man to snail through water and from snail to man also through water. The schistosomulae are carried to liver where they grow to adulthood. Later they migrate against the blood stream into the inferior mesenteric vein to reach the capillaries of the sigmoidorectal region where the eggs are laid. Finally they escape through faeces.

Pathology: Disease is labelled *Schistosomiasis mansoni* or intestinal bilharziasis or schis-tosomal dysentery. The visceral type is called visceral schistosomiasis or Egyptian splenomegaly. The localising symptom is chiefly intestinal, causing dysenteric attack. *Ectopic lesions* include hepatomegaly, periportal fibrosis, portal hypertension (inducing splenomegaly and haematemesis), cor-pulmonale and myelitis.

Diagnosis: Demonstration of eggs of *S.mansoni* in:
— microscopic examination of faeces.
— rectal tissue biopsy and crush preparation as for *S. haematobium* vesical biopsy.
— other investigations same as for *S. haematobium*.

Visceral Schistosomiasis: Digest the biopsy taken with potash solution (lung or liver biopsy) and later examine for eggs.

Treatment and prophylaxis: As for *S. haematobium*.

Schistosoma japonicum

(Oriental blood fluke)

Geographic distribution: Far East. Found in China, Japan, Phillipines, Celebes and Shan States of Myanmar (Burma).

Habitat: Adult worms reside in the following locations:
- (i) Intrahepatic portion of portal venous system,
- (ii) Mesenteric veins draining the ileo-caecal region,
- (iii) Rectal or haemorrhoidal plexus of veins.

Morphology: See the table and figures given earlier.

Definitive host	: Domestic animals (cat, dog, pig and cattle)
	: Man (field mice serve as infection reservoirs)
Intermediate host	: Freshwater snail (Genus: Oncomelania).

The schistosomulae are carried to liver and grow to adulthood in the intrahepatic portion of the portal venous system. Later they migrate against the blood stream to superior mesenteric vein and then on to the capillaries in the last part of the ileum, caecum and ascending colon. Finally, the eggs escape through faeces.

Pathology: Disease is called *Schistosomiasis japonica* or intestinal and hepatic schistosomiasis of the Orient or as Katayama disease. The lesions produced are severer than *S. mansoni* (as greater number of eggs are produced). Localising symptom is dysenteric attacks. Liver is involved more frequently.

Liver: Periportal cirrhosis. It is a granulomatous fibrosis pylephlebitis with terminal scarring development around the eggs which are lodged in the smallest portal venules. No liver nodules are seen but there is neovascularisation to a considerable extent giving the portal field an angiomatoid appearance. Kupffer cells may show haematin pigment (the pigment is regurgitated by the adult worm after digesting blood in its alimentary tract, because the intestine terminates blindly).

Schistosomal hepatic fibrosis: Conglomeration of many egg-granulomas leads to confluent progressive fibrosis. These are prominent along the portal ramifications. *S. mansoni* and *S. japonicum* eggs can produce diffuse hepatic fibrosis, however, hepatic functions stay unaltered on account of compensatory increase in hepatic artery blood flow.

Splenomegaly and oesophageal varices result from pre-sinusoidal portal hypertension. In brain one may find space-occupying lesions while lung involvement may cause cor-pulmonale.

Diagnosis, Treatment and Prophylaxis: As for *S. haematobium.*

Pathology of Schistosomiasis

1. *Penetration of skin by cercariae:*
   - (a) Pathogenic spp.: Only slight local reaction (petechiae).
   - (b) Non-human spp.: Cause cercarial dermatitis (swimmer's itch)
     Papules—macules—vesicles—intense itching.

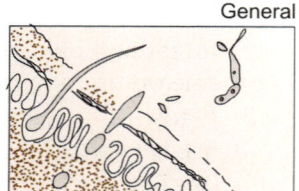

General

2. *Migration of immature worms:* General toxic and allergic symptoms (eosinophilia up to 50%).

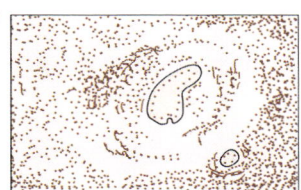

3. *Damage by eggs in tissue* (result depends on parasite load) Inflammatory reaction with: Epithelial, giant
                                  plasma, eosinophil cells
                                  fibroblasts
   Subsequent fibrosis and calcification.
4. *Sequelae of such damage*: Local—ectopic.

Urinary schistosomiasis (mainly due to *S. haematobium*)
   1. Initial toxic and allergic symptoms not marked.
   2. **(a) Bladder and ureters typically involved with:**
        Hyperaemia—papules—papillomata—ulceration.
        Hypertrophy of bladder, later contraction.
        Cystitis and calculus formation.
        Development of fistulae. Ova in urine.
      (b) Genitalia and renal pelvis sometimes affected,
        intestine occasionally.
   3. Ectopic lesions less severe than in other spp.

Particular

Intestinal schistosomiasis (*S. mansoni*)
   1. Initial toxic and allergic symptoms marked.
   2. (a) Large intestine and rectum typically involved with:
        Papules—abscesses—ulcers—papillomata—
        fistulae—ova in faeces.
      (b) Bladder sometimes involved, pathology as for
        urinary type.
   3. Ectopic lesions:
      (a) Liver frequently involved (eggs via portal vein)
        with
        Inflammatory⎤   ⎡Portal hypertension
        reaction   ⎟ leading to   ⎟Splenomegaly
                    ⎟ cirrhosis   ⎟
        Fibrosis   ⎦ with   ⎣Ascites
      (b) Elsewhere (brain, etc.)

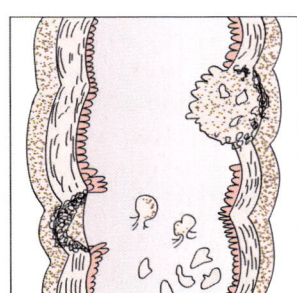

Oriental Schistosomiasis (*S. japonicum*):
   1. Initial toxic and allergic symptoms marked.
   2. Intestinal lesions like mansoni infection, small intestine often involved.
   3. Ectopic lesions:
      (a) Liver frequently affected as in mansoni.
      (b) Brain, etc. more frequent.

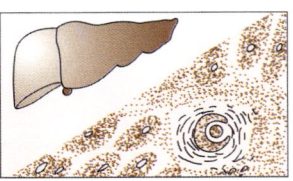

DISTOMATA (Suborder)

FASCIOLIDAE (Family)

Adults reside in the intestine and biliary passages of herbivorous animals and man. Eggs, when laid, are large, operculated and immature, each containing an unsegmented ovum. Miracidium develops within the eggs in water and has cross (x) shaped eye spots. Intermediate hosts are fresh-water molluscs where the miracidium passes through the stages of sporocyst and two or more generations of rediae. Cercariae encyst on vegetation and in fish which are the sources of infection to the definitive host. Two genera infect man:
— *Fasciola hepatica.*
— *Fasciola buski.*

Fasciola hepatica

(Sheep liver fluke or common liver fluke)

Historical: Jehan de Brie first described it in 1379, Linnaeus described further details in 1758.

Geographic distribution: Cosmopolitan.

Habitat: Basically a parasite of herbivorous animals (sheep, goat and cattle), living in the biliary passages of the liver. It is occasionally found in man.

Morphology: *Adult worm* is a large leaf-shaped fluke, measuring 30 × 13 mm, brown to pale grey in colour. Have two suckers, oral sucker is smaller. The anterior end bearing the oral sucker forms a conical projection. Posterior portion is broadly pointed. Acetabulum is situated in a line with the two shoulders formed by the broadening of the conical projection posteriorly. Both the intestinal caeca have a number of lateral branches. Genital system follows the same general pattern identical to that of other trematodes.

Life span of an adult worm in sheep is about 5 years, while in man it is from 9 to 13 years.

Eggs: Eggs are large, operculated, ovoid and brownish yellow in colour (being bile stained). They measure 130–150 × 63–90 μ. They contain a large unsegmented ovum in a mass of yolk cells. They are excreted with the bile into the duodenum to be later passed out with the faeces. They do not float on saturated solution of common salt. They can develop further only in water.

Life cycle: *F. hepatica* needs two hosts to complete its life cycle.

Definitive hosts: Sheep, goat, cattle and man. Adult worm stays in the biliary passages. Sheep is the reservoir host.

Intermediate host: Snails of genus Lymnaea or Succinea. Larval development takes place in the snail. Egg matures in water and in 2 to 3 weeks miracidium is developed which finds its way in a suitable intermediate host. Inside the mollusc's lymph spaces it passes through a stage of sporocyst, two generations of rediae and finally evolve into cercariae (this cycle in the intermediate host takes 1 to 2 months). Cercariae, at maturity, escape from the snail into the water to encyst in blades of grass or

Morphology

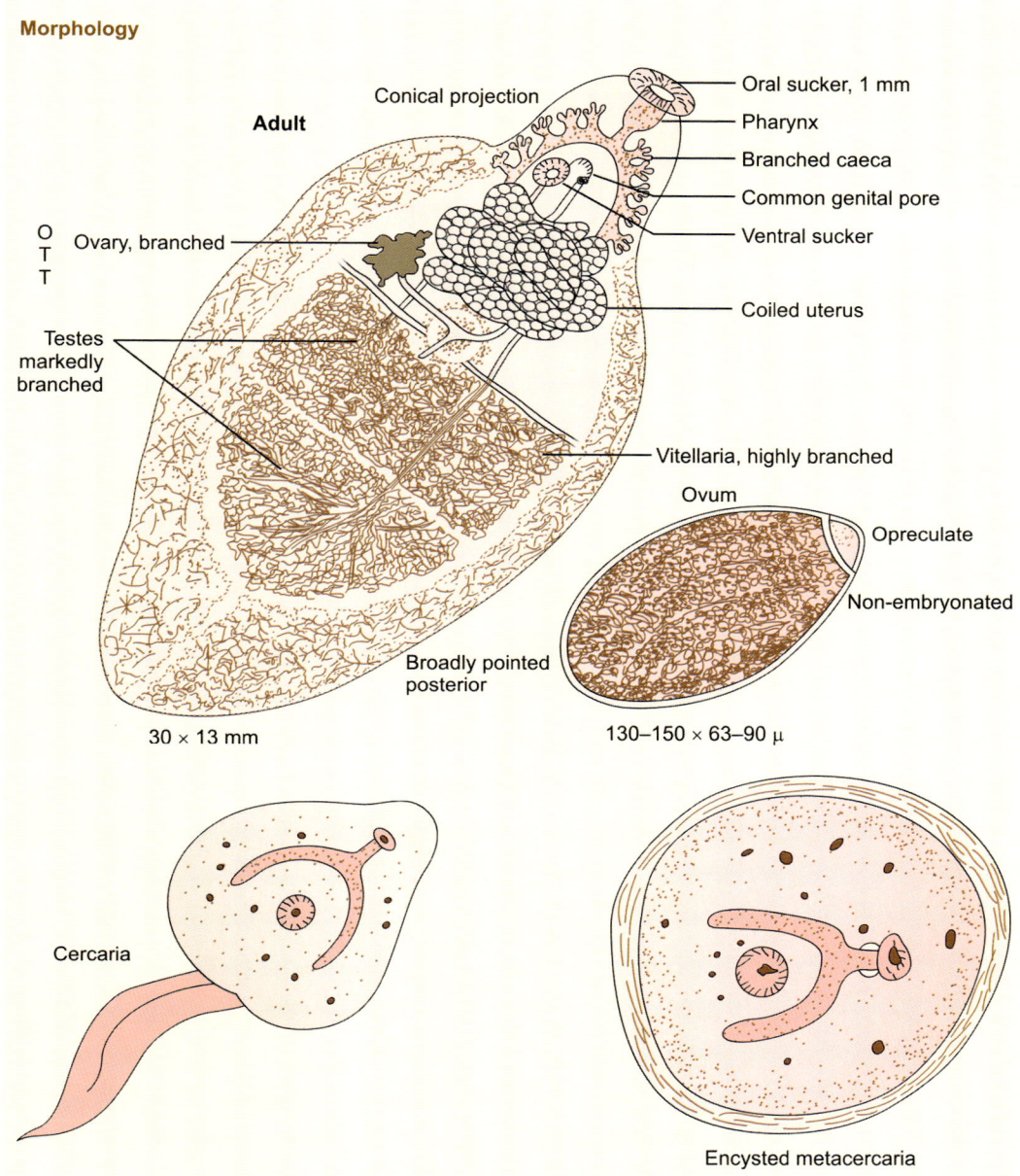

Adult

Conical projection

Oral sucker, 1 mm

Pharynx

Branched caeca

Common genital pore

Ventral sucker

O
T
T

Ovary, branched

Coiled uterus

Testes
markedly
branched

Vitellaria, highly branched

Ovum

Operculate

Non-embryonated

Broadly pointed
posterior

30 × 13 mm

130–150 × 63–90 μ

Cercaria

Encysted metacercaria

Fig. 9.2: *Fasciola hepatica*

water-cress. These encysted cercariae are swallowed along with the grass by herbivorous animals and occasionally by man. Once in the duodenum, the cercariae excyst, migrate through the intestinal wall into the peritoneal cavity, penetrate the hepatic capsule (Glisson's capsule), go past the parenchyma to ultimately settle in the biliary passages (this migratory phase takes about 30 days) and there they grow to adulthood and sexual maturity. The eggs are liberated with faeces through the bile in 3 to 4 months after infection. The cycle is then repeated.

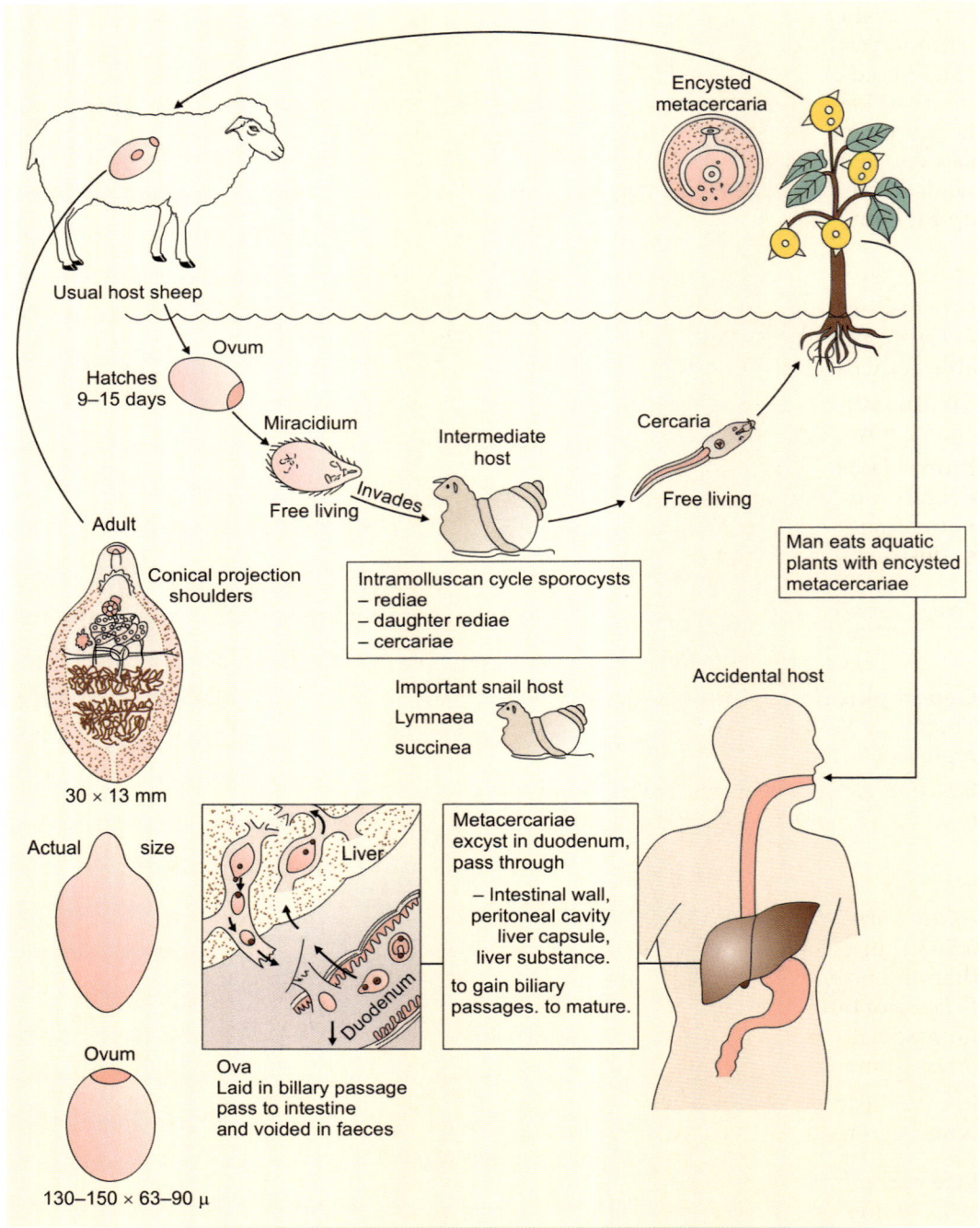

Fig. 9.3: Life cycle

Pathology

Symptoms of fascioliasis include biliary colic, vomiting, persistent diarrhoea, painful hepatomegaly and peripheral eosinophilia. Fascioliasis is most common in sheep and cattle-raising nations. Pharyngeal infection *(Halzoum)* was earlier attributed to local irritation caused by adults (present in raw flesh of sacrificial goats), however, now it is considered to be due to ingestion of nymphs of *Linguatula serrata.* In animals it causes *liver rot.* While passing through liver, extensive hepatic damage is caused which in heavy infections terminate into portal cirrhosis. Present in the biliary passage they can cause obstructive jaundice. They cause cystic dilatation of the bile ducts, the walls of which become massively thickened because of associated fibrosis. The lining epithelium of the biliary passages may proliferate and produce adenomas.

Diagnosis

Is based on demonstration of eggs in stool or bile obtained by duodenal intubation. *F. hepatica* eggs are identical to those of *F. buski.* Immunological investigations available are CFT and skin test.

Treatment: Emetine injection has been found to be useful. Bithionol is the drug of choice now.

Prophylaxis: Measures include:
- eradication of disease in animals,
- treatment of infected animals, and
- destruction of molluscan hosts.

Fasciolopsis buski

(Large intestinal fluke)

Geographical distribution: Basically an Asiatic trematode. Reported from China, Thailand, Malaysia, West Bengal, North-Eastern states of India and other oriental regions.

Habitat: Adult worm resides in the small intestine of pig and man. Pig serves as the reservoir of infection for man.

Morphology

Adult worm: The largest trematode parasitising man. Measures 2–7 × 0.5–2 cm and 0.5–3 mm thick. It is elongated and oval-shaped with the anterior end narrower than the posterior end. A large acetabulum lies close to the oral sucker. It resembles *F. hepatica* but it does not possess any cephalic cone and the two intestinal caeca have no associated lateral branches. Genital system follows the usual general pattern of other trematodes.

Life span is not more than 6 months. Eggs are identical to those of *F. hepatica.* Each worm can lay up to 25000 eggs a day.

Life cycle: It needs two hosts:
    Definitive host: Man and pig.
    Intermediate host: Aquatic snails of Genus Segmentina and Hippeutis.
    Life cycle is similar to that of *F. hepatica.*
    Cercariae after exiting the snail, encyst on freshwater plants. On being swallowed by the definitive host, the metacercariae excyst in the duodenum and the young worms so liberated attach to the intestinal wall, developing into adult worms in about 3 months time. The eggs released by sexually mature worms repeat the whole cycle.

Morphology

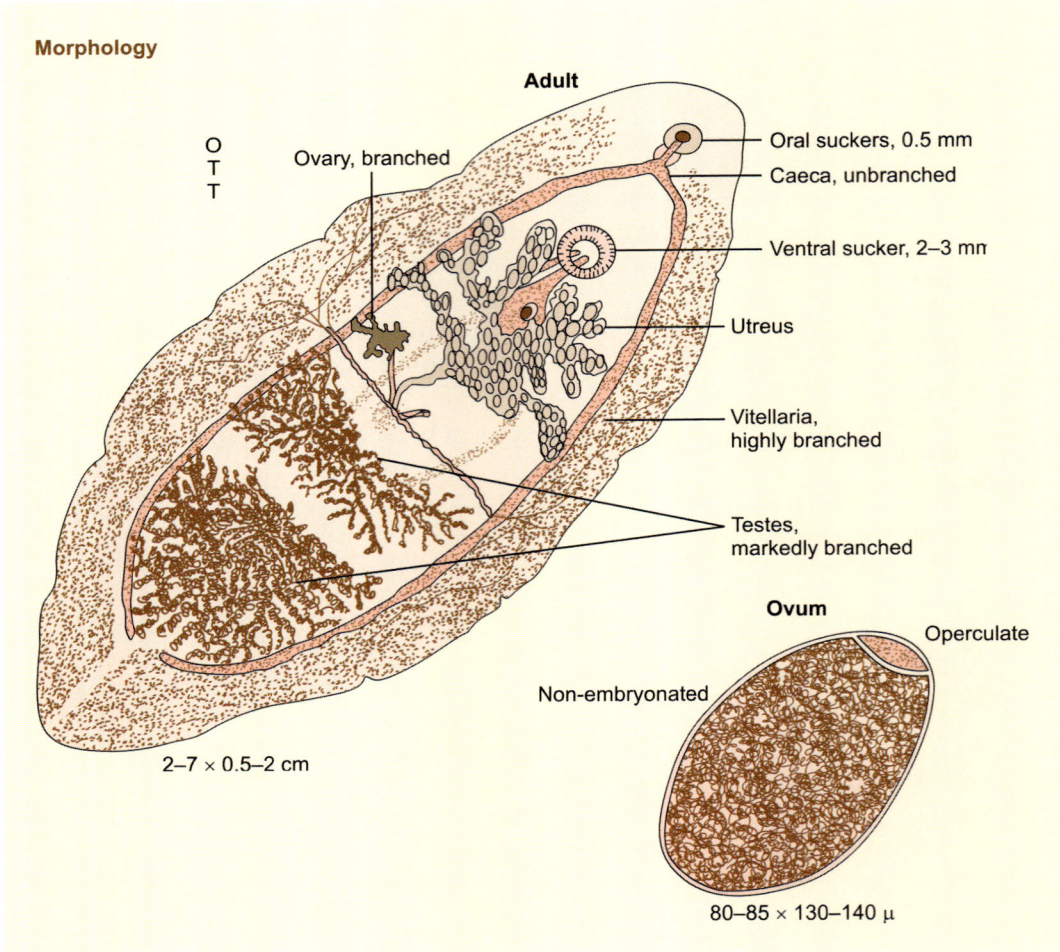

Adult

O
T
T

Ovary, branched

Oral suckers, 0.5 mm

Caeca, unbranched

Ventral sucker, 2–3 mm

Utreus

Vitellaria,
highly branched

Testes,
markedly branched

2–7 × 0.5–2 cm

Ovum

Operculate

Non-embryonated

80–85 × 130–140 µ

Pathology: Fasciolopsiasis (with *F. buski*) causes asthenia, mild anaemia and chronic diarrhoea. Absorption of toxic by-products of the worm can also cause oedema and peripheral eosinophilia.

Diagnosis: Is established by eliciting a history of residence in an endemic zone and by demonstration of eggs in stool on microscopic examination. Adult worms may be recovered by a purgative or anthelmintic drug.

Treatment: Specific drug of choice is tetrachlorethylene.

Prophylaxis: Measures include:
• Sterilisation of night-soil before being used as a fertiliser.
• Destruction of molluscan hosts by copper sulphate solution (1:50,000).
• Avoidance of consumption of raw vegetables or immersion of these vegetables in boiling water for a few minutes before being eaten.

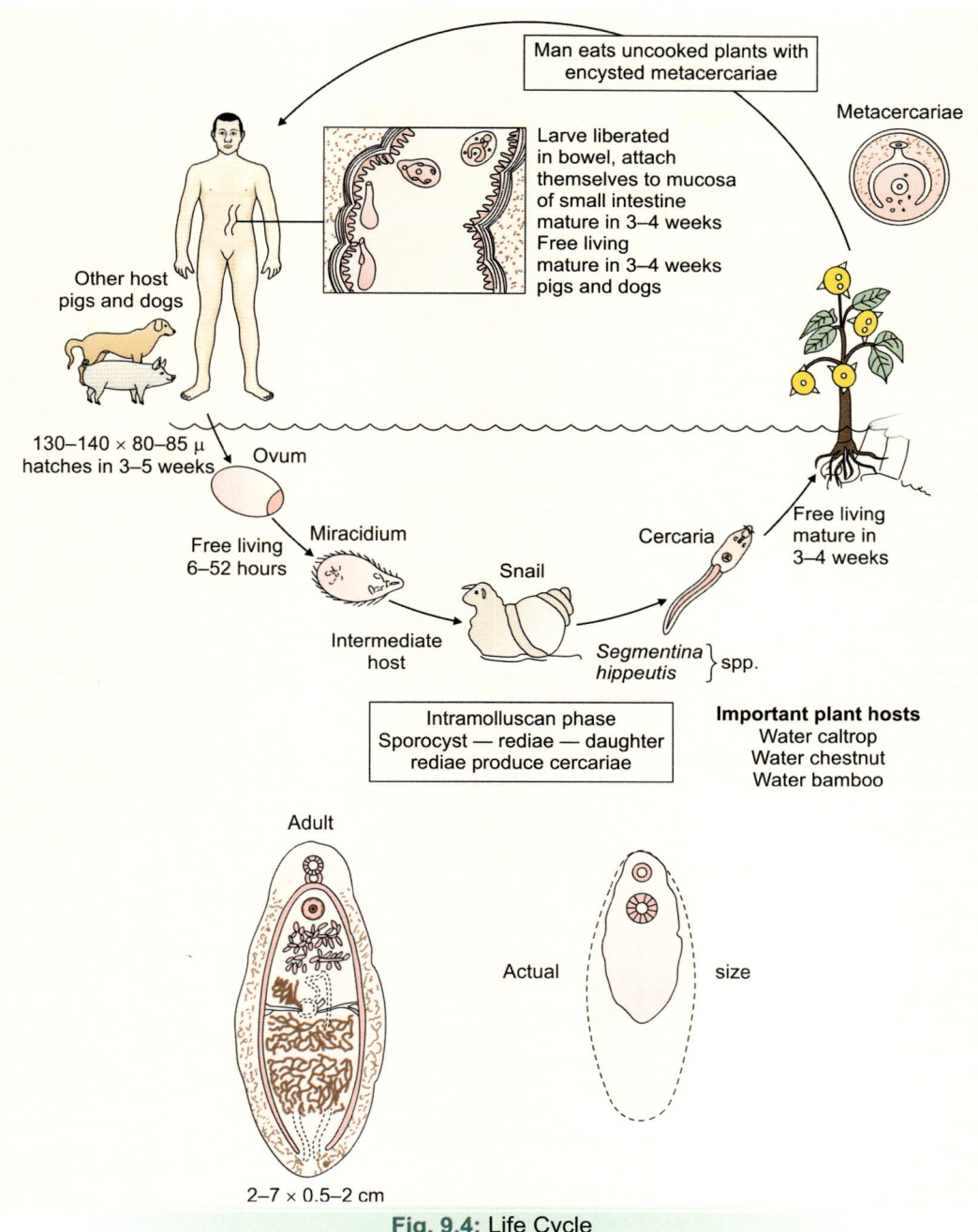

Fig. 9.4: Life Cycle

Fasciola gigantica

(The giant liver fluke)

Similar to *F. hepatica* somewhat larger eggs. 160–190 × 70–90 μ.

Occurrence: In herbivores in Africa and Far East. Occasionally described in man.

DICROCOELIIDAE (FAMILY)

Dicrocoelium dentriticum

(The lancet fluke)

Morphology

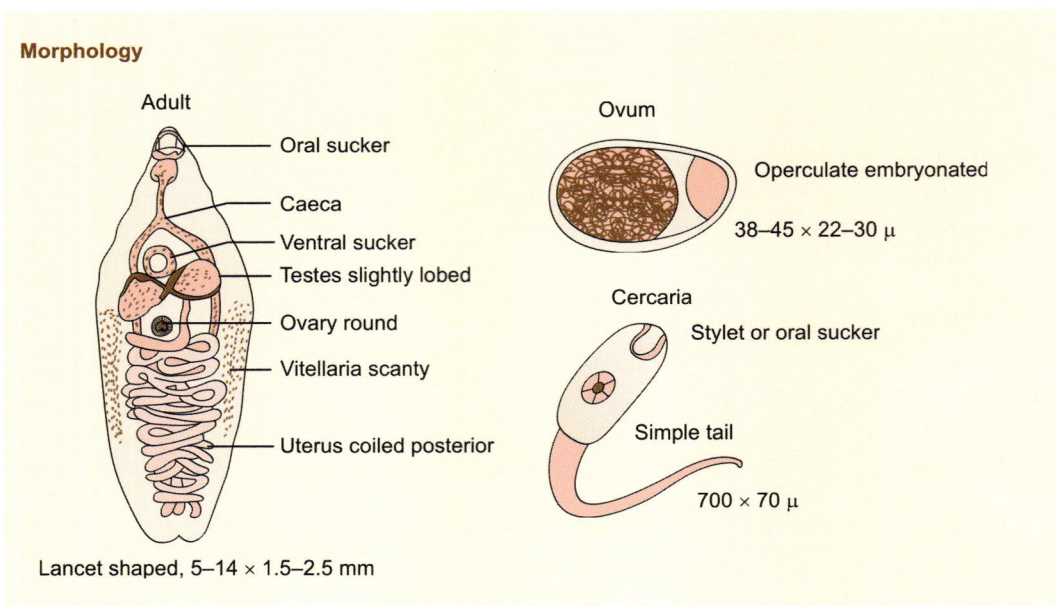

Adult
- Oral sucker
- Caeca
- Ventral sucker
- Testes slightly lobed
- Ovary round
- Vitellaria scanty
- Uterus coiled posterior

Lancet shaped, 5–14 × 1.5–2.5 mm

Ovum
- Operculate embryonated
- 38–45 × 22–30 μ

Cercaria
- Stylet or oral sucker
- Simple tail
- 700 × 70 μ

Life cycle

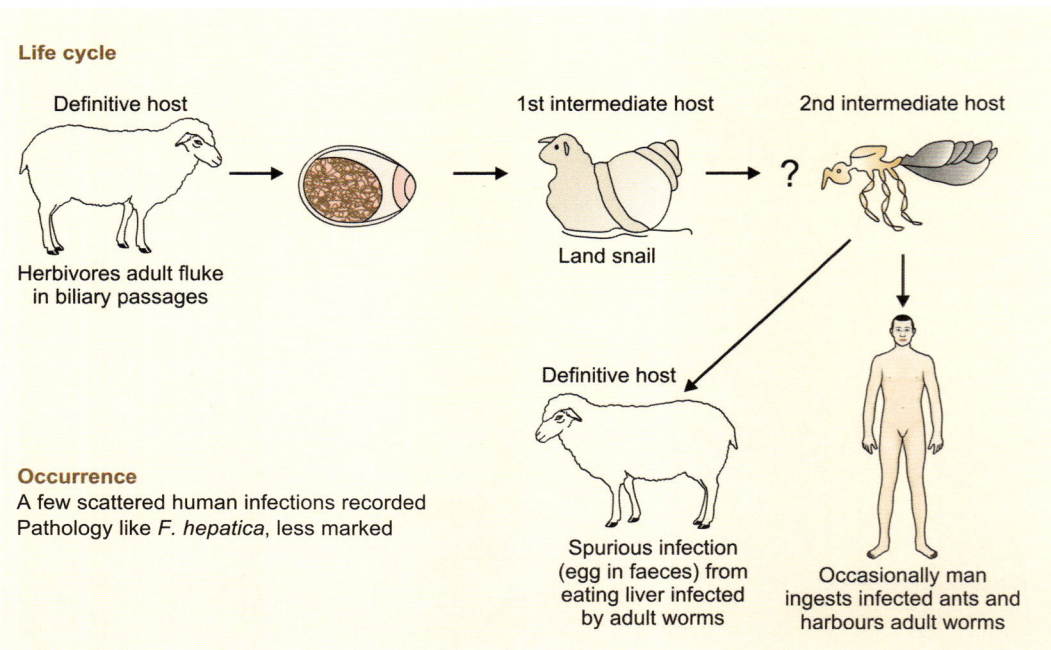

Definitive host — Herbivores adult fluke in biliary passages

1st intermediate host — Land snail

2nd intermediate host — ?

Definitive host — Spurious infection (egg in faeces) from eating liver infected by adult worms

Occasionally man ingests infected ants and harbours adult worms

Occurrence
A few scattered human infections recorded
Pathology like *F. hepatica*, less marked

OPISTHORCHIIDAE (FAMILY)

These are flat, transparent, medium-sized worms living in the biliary passages of fish-eating animals. Eggs are very small, thick-shelled, operculated and at the time of being laid contain a fully developed miracidium that does not hatch in water but only after being ingested by an appropriate mollusc host belonging to Genus Bythinia.

Clonorchis sinensis

(Chinese or Oriental liver fluke)

Historical: First detected by McConnell in 1875 and detailed study later made by Faust and Khaw in 1927.

Geographic distribution: Far East, endemic regions are Korea, Japan, Southern China, Vietnam and Cambodia.

Morphology

Adult worm: Is narrow, oblong and flattened with a somewhat pointed anterior end. It measures 10–20 × 3–4 mm. Oral sucker is slightly larger than the ventral sucker, the latter located at the junction of the anterior and the middle-third of the body. Blind intestinal caeca are simple and extend to the caudal region. Reproductive organs are similar to those of other trematodes. The two testes are large, extensively branched and lie in the posterior third of the body, one behind the other.

Life span of an adult worm is from 2 to 3 decades.

Eggs: Are yellowish brown in colour (bile-stained), flask-shaped and operculated. Possess a terminal hook-like spine. Measure 29 × 16 μ. When laid, contains a ciliated embryo (miracidium). Hatch only within the mollusc host. Do not float on saturated common salt solution. Infective only to snails.

Morphology

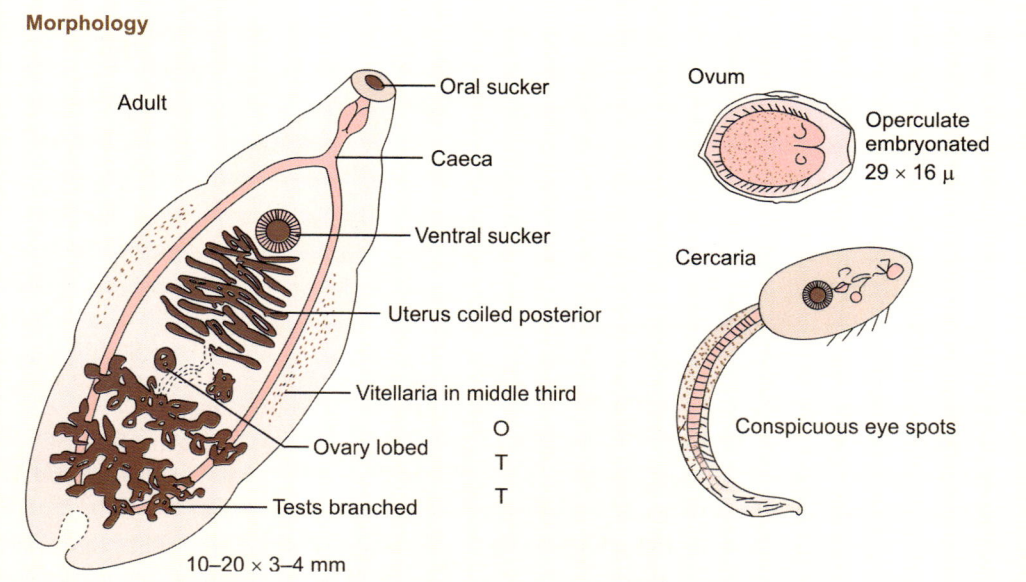

Adult — Oral sucker, Caeca, Ventral sucker, Uterus coiled posterior, Vitellaria in middle third, Ovary lobed, Tests branched, 10–20 × 3–4 mm, O T T

Ovum — Operculate embryonated 29 × 16 μ

Cercaria — Conspicuous eye spots

Life cycle: *C. sinensis* needs 3 hosts to complete its life cycle.

Definitive hosts: Man, cat, pig, dog. Adult worms in biliary tract of the liver.

Intermediate host first: Snails of genera Bulimus, Parafossarulus and Alocinma.

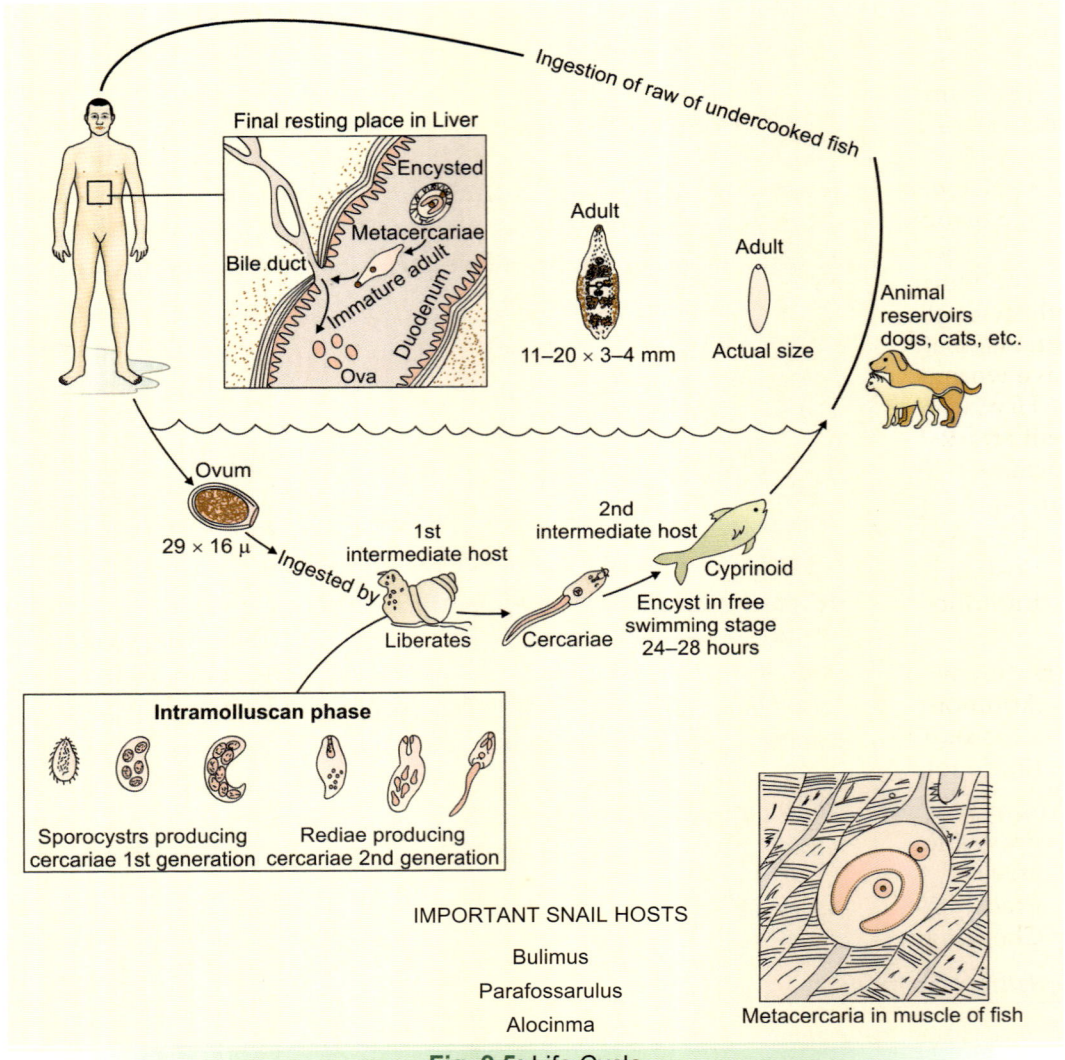

Fig. 9.5: Life Cycle

Intermediate host second: Cyprinoid fish.

Miracidia containing eggs are passed with the faeces of definitive hosts and on reaching water, they are ingested by an appropriate mollusc host. Miracidia that hatch in the mid-gut of the snail, penetrate the intestinal wall to reach the vascular spaces where it passes through the stages of sporocyst—redia—cercaria, this development takes up to 21 days. The cercariae escape from snail into water, to attack fish of the family cyprinidae. Cercariae get rid of their tails and encyst in the scale or the flesh of the above mentioned fish. These encysted metacercariae when eaten by the definitive host, excyst in the duodenum. Next, they attach themselves to the mucosa in the region of the common bile duct, pass through the ampulla of Vater and migrate to the distal biliary passages of the liver where they settle down to attain maturity in about 30 days.

Pathology: Man gets infected after eating raw, ill-cooked, dried, salted or pickled freshwater fish, harboring the encysted metacercariae. Disease caused is labelled clonorchiasis.

The immature worm while traversing upwards along the bile duct assisted by its suckers, often causes damage to the bile duct epithelium. It causes:

- Epithelial proliferation—adenoma.
- Neovascularisation in the peribiliary plexus.
- Surrounding inflammatory reaction, sometimes secondary infection.
- Association between clonorchiasis and cirrhosis of liver is debatable.

The worm thrives on protein and glucose of blood and on mucous secreted by biliary duct epithelial cells. Adult worms cannot reach gall bladder unless the cystic duct is dilated. If it happens to reach gall bladder, it quickly dies in its environment. Live worms have, however, been recovered from the pancreatic duct.

Heavy infections are characterised by chronic diarrhoea, hepatomegaly and recurrent attacks of jaundice. Other complications include cholangitis, intrahepatic calculi formation, cholangiocarcinoma.

Diagnosis: Based on —
- Demonstration of eggs in faeces or aspirated bile.
- Eosinophilia in peripheral blood.
- Immunodiagnosis: CFT and haemagglutination test.
               Intradermal test (immediate type of hypersensitivity reaction).

Treatment
- Antimony compounds (sodium antimonyl tartarate, tartar emetic and fouadin)
- Chloroquin.
- Bithionol.

Prophylaxis: Measures include —
- Prevention of water contamination with human night-soil and faeces of reservoir hosts.
- Eradication of snail hosts.
- Checking the habit of eating raw fish.

Opisthorchis felineus

(The cat liver fluke)

Morphology

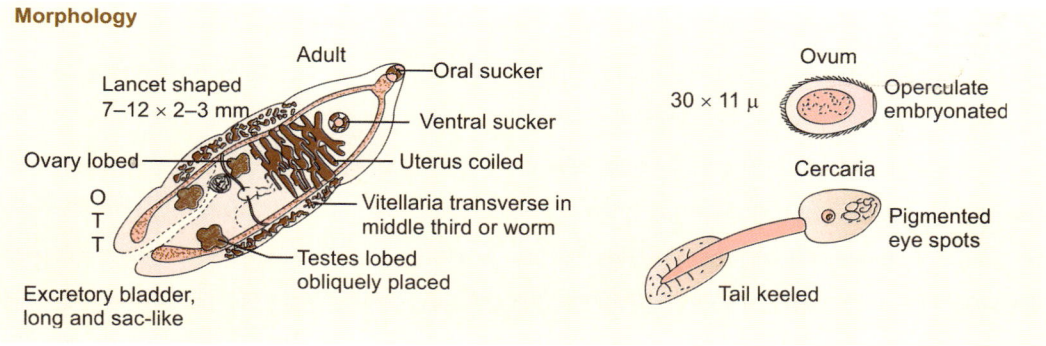

Adult
Lancet shaped
7–12 × 2–3 mm
Oral sucker
Ventral sucker
Uterus coiled
Ovary lobed
O T T
Vitellaria transverse in middle third or worm
Testes lobed obliquely placed
Excretory bladder, long and sac-like

Ovum
30 × 11 μ
Operculate embryonated

Cercaria
Pigmented eye spots
Tail keeled

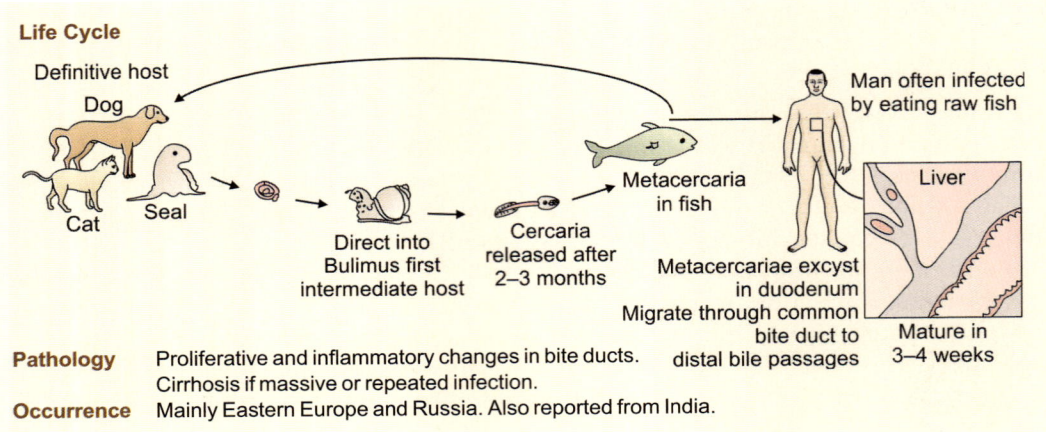

Life Cycle

Definitive host

Dog

Cat   Seal

Direct into
Bulimus first
intermediate host

Cercaria
released after
2–3 months

Metacercaria
in fish

Man often infected
by eating raw fish

Liver

Metacercariae excyst
in duodenum
Migrate through common
bite duct to
distal bile passages

Mature in
3–4 weeks

Pathology   Proliferative and inflammatory changes in bite ducts.
Cirrhosis if massive or repeated infection.

Occurrence   Mainly Eastern Europe and Russia. Also reported from India.

HETEROPHYIDAE (family)

These are small egg-shaped flukes which are normally parasites in the intestinal tract
of fish-eating animals.

Heterophytes heterophytes

Morphology

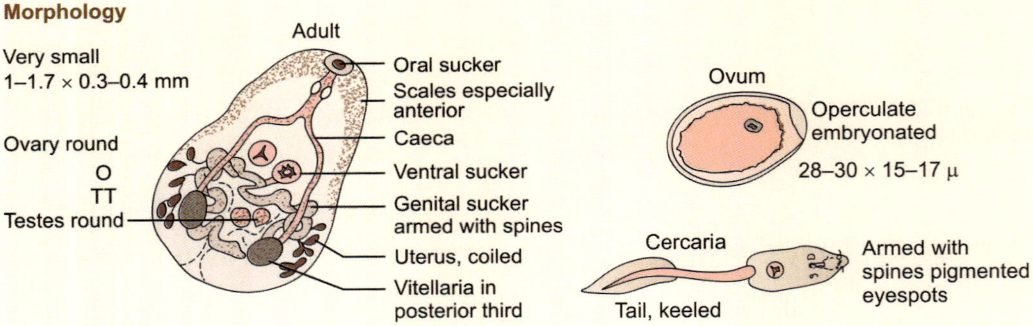

Adult

Very small
1–1.7 × 0.3–0.4 mm

Ovary round

O
TT

Testes round

Oral sucker
Scales especially
anterior
Caeca
Ventral sucker
Genital sucker
armed with spines
Uterus, coiled
Vitellaria in
posterior third

Ovum

Operculate
embryonated

28–30 × 15–17 µ

Cercaria

Tail, keeled

Armed with
spines pigmented
eyespots

Life cycle

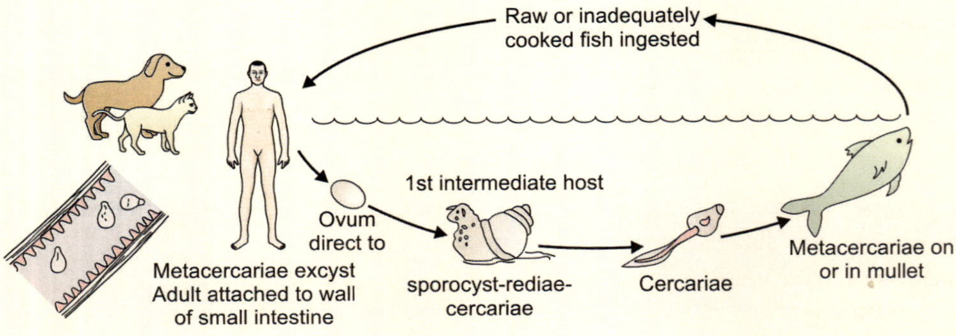

Raw or inadequately
cooked fish ingested

1st intermediate host

Ovum
direct to

Metacercariae excyst
Adult attached to wall
of small intestine

sporocyst-rediae-
cercariae

Cercariae

Metacercariae on
or in mullet

Pathology mild inflammatory reaction   Ectopic ova reported in heart and brain

Occurrence Nile delta: Far East   **Treatment:** Tetrachloroethylene and piperazine derivatives.

Metagonimus yokogawai

Morphology

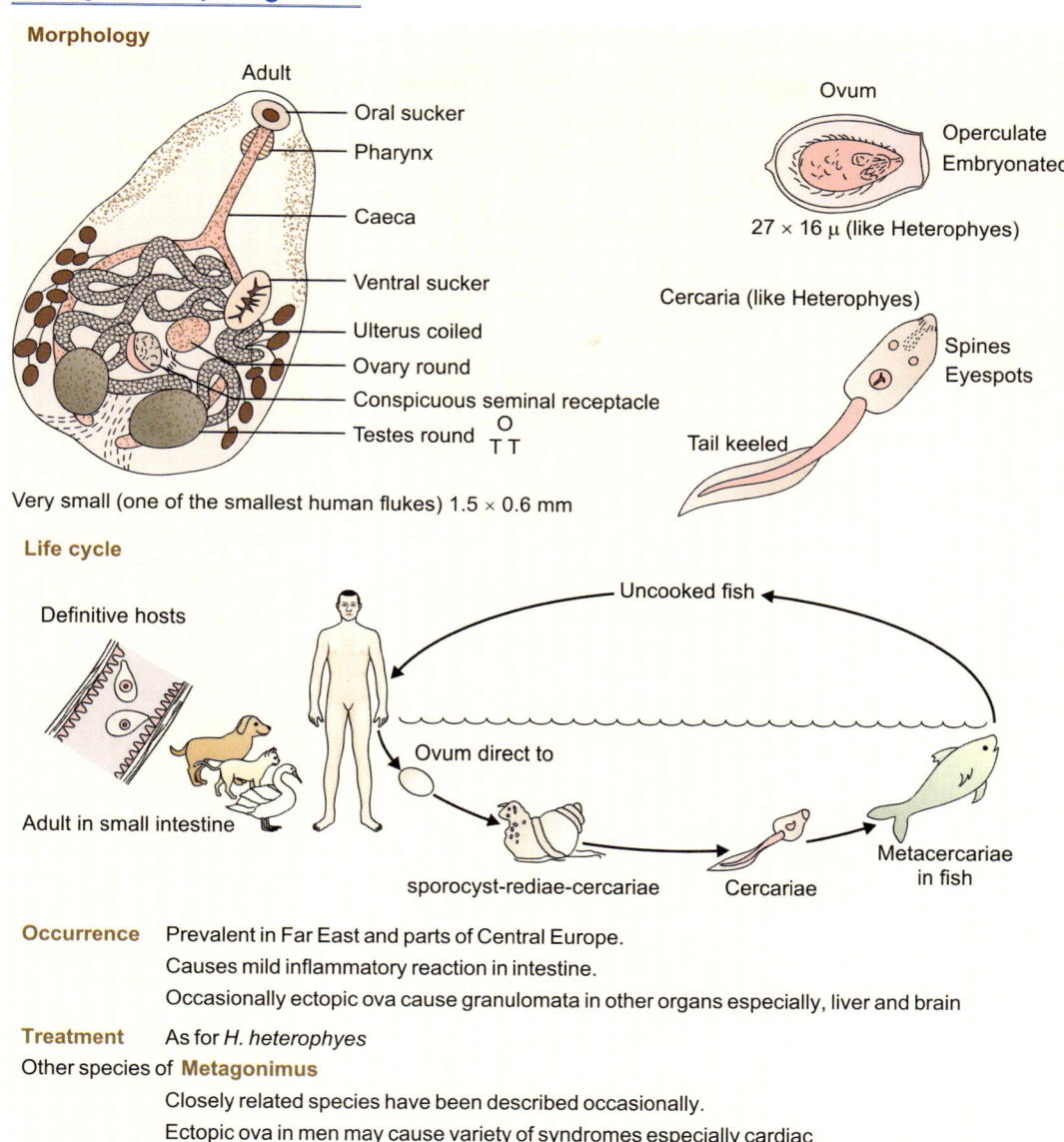

Adult
- Oral sucker
- Pharynx
- Caeca
- Ventral sucker
- Ulterus coiled
- Ovary round
- Conspicuous seminal receptacle
- Testes round O / T T

Very small (one of the smallest human flukes) 1.5 × 0.6 mm

Ovum
Operculate
Embryonated
27 × 16 μ (like Heterophyes)

Cercaria (like Heterophyes)
Spines
Eyespots
Tail keeled

Life cycle

Definitive hosts

Adult in small intestine

Uncooked fish

Ovum direct to

sporocyst-rediae-cercariae   Cercariae

Metacercariae in fish

Occurrence Prevalent in Far East and parts of Central Europe.
Causes mild inflammatory reaction in intestine.
Occasionally ectopic ova cause granulomata in other organs especially, liver and brain

Treatment As for *H. heterophyes*

Other species of **Metagonimus**

Closely related species have been described occasionally.
Ectopic ova in men may cause variety of syndromes especially cardiac like beriberi and cerebral haemorrhage.

TRIGLOTREMATIDAE (FAMILY)

The adults of this family are parasitic in carnivores and reside in the lungs. The worm possesses integumentary spines and an excretory vesicle that is tubular and Y-shaped. Genital pore lies behind the acetabulum and the cirrus sac is lacking. Vitellaria are well-developed and occupy whole of the lateral fields. Miracidia do not possess eye spots. Larval development is accomplished in two intermediate hosts, the first a snail and the second, a crustacean. Cercariae have knob-like tails and oral stylets.

Paragonimus westermani

(Oriental lung fluke)

Historical: First described by Kerbert in 1878 and later by Braun in 1899.

Geographic distribution: Far East (Korea, Japan, China, India—West Bengal, North Eastern States and South India). Also reported from Nepal, South America and occasionally Africa.

Habitat: Adult worms reside in the respiratory tract of man.

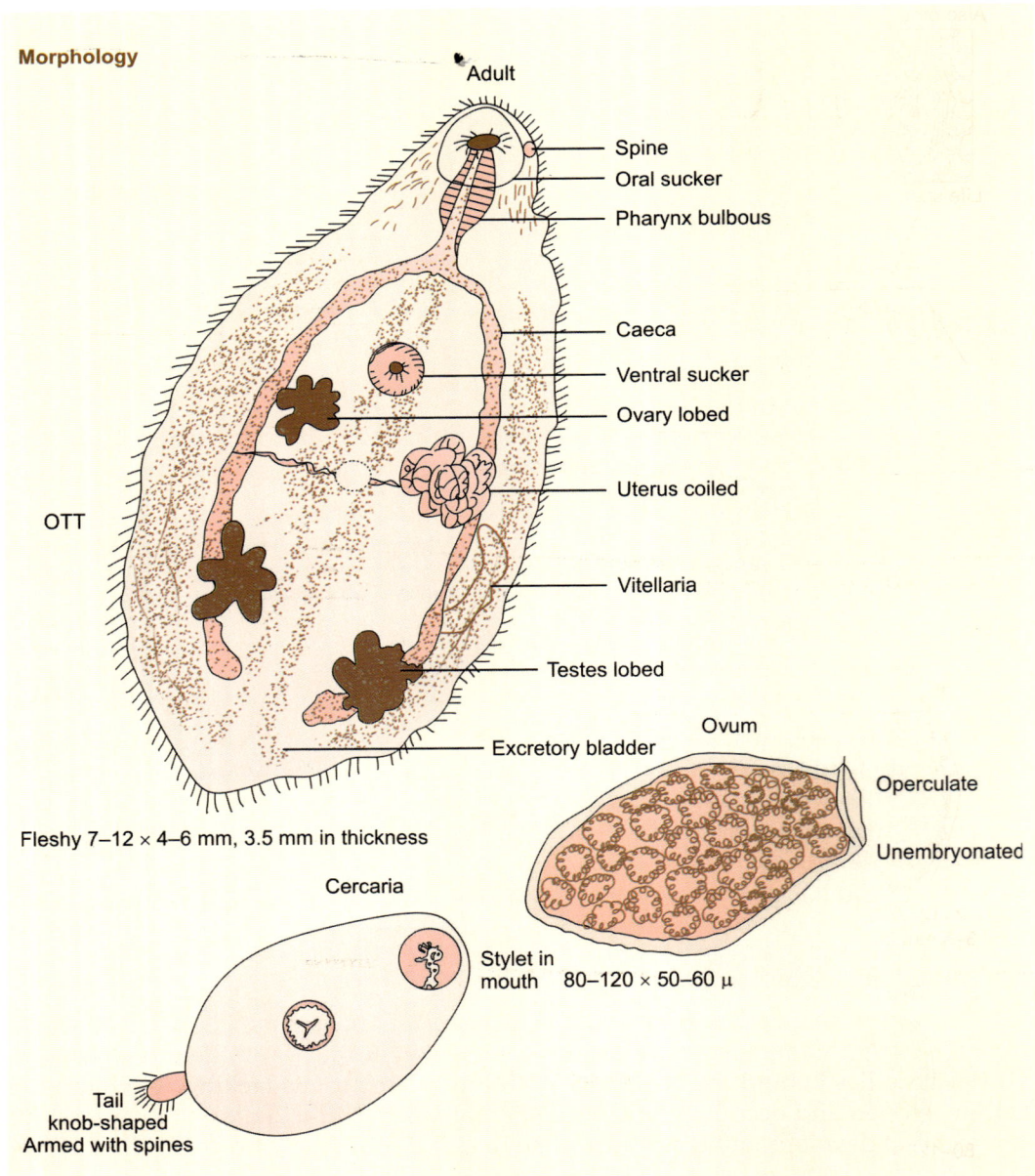

Morphology

Adult

- Spine
- Oral sucker
- Pharynx bulbous
- Caeca
- Ventral sucker
- Ovary lobed
- Uterus coiled
- Vitellaria
- Testes lobed
- Excretory bladder

OTT

Fleshy 7–12 × 4–6 mm, 3.5 mm in thickness

Ovum

Operculate

Unembryonated

80–120 × 50–60 µ

Cercaria

Stylet in mouth

Tail
knob-shaped
Armed with spines

Morphology

Adult worm is thick, fleshy and egg-shaped. The anterior end is slightly broader than the posterior end. It measures 7–12 x 4–6 mm and 3.5 mm in thickness. Ventral sucker is almost at the middle of the body. The excretory vesicle is large extending from anterior region to the posterior extremity and thereby dividing the body into two equal halves. The two blind intestinal caeca are urbranched and extend till the caudal region. Reproductive organs are identical to those of other trematodes.

Life Cycle

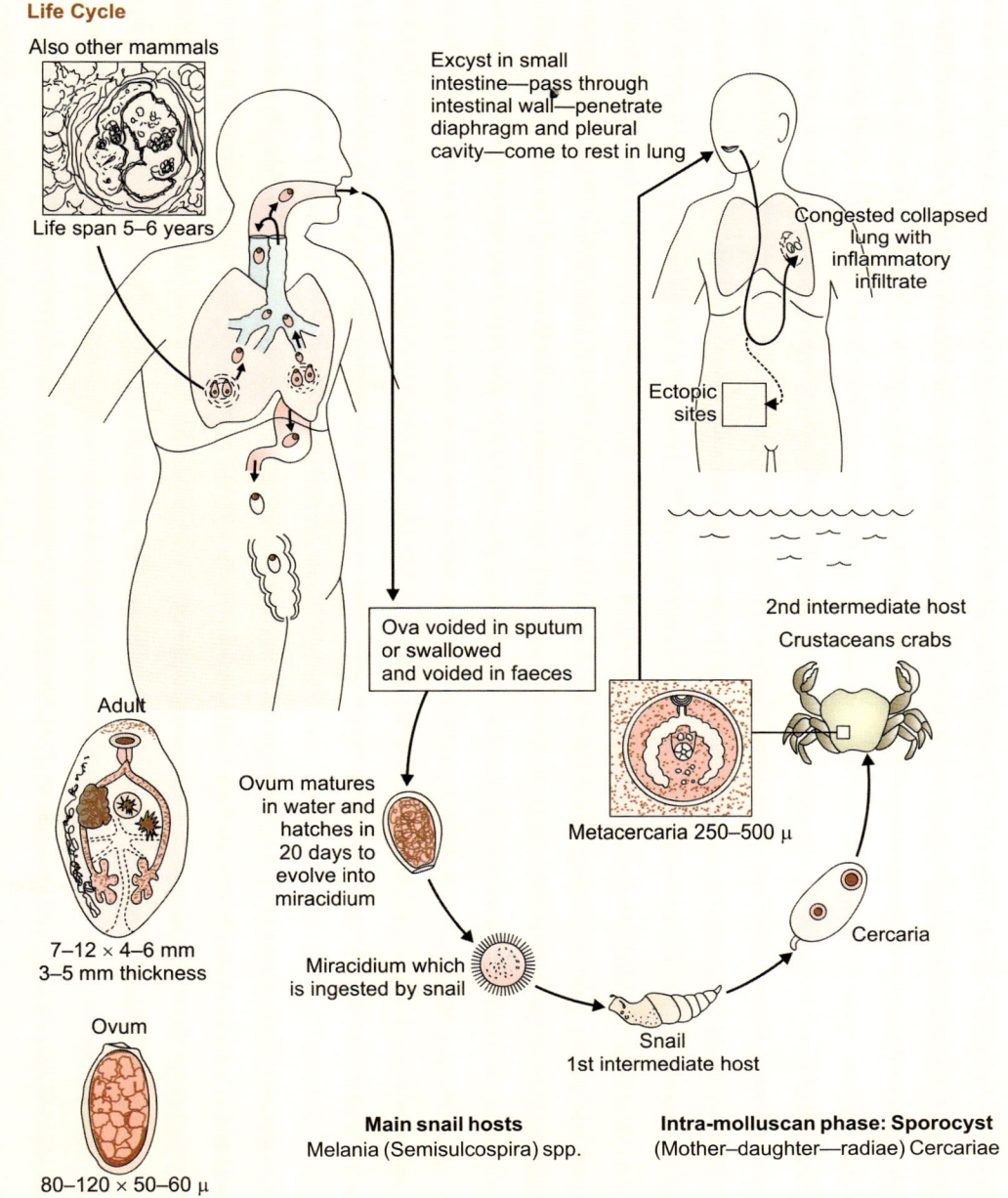

Also other mammals

Life span 5–6 years

Excyst in small intestine—pass through intestinal wall—penetrate diaphragm and pleural cavity—come to rest in lung

Congested collapsed lung with inflammatory infiltrate

Ectopic sites

2nd intermediate host

Crustaceans crabs

Adult

7–12 × 4–6 mm
3–5 mm thickness

Ovum

80–120 × 50–60 μ

Ova voided in sputum or swallowed and voided in faeces

Ovum matures in water and hatches in 20 days to evolve into miracidium

Metacercaria 250–500 μ

Cercaria

Miracidium which is ingested by snail

Snail
1st intermediate host

Main snail hosts
Melania (Semisulcospira) spp.

Intra-molluscan phase: Sporocyst
(Mother—daughter—radiae) Cercariae

Life span of an adult worm is about 6–7 years.

Eggs: Are golden brown in colour, oval in shape and possess a flattened opercula. Measure 80–120 × 50–60 μ. They contain an unsegmented ovum enclosed within yolk cells.

Life cycle: It needs three hosts to complete its life cycle.

Definitive host: Man and domestic animals. Common hosts in Asia are tiger and leopard. Feline hosts serve as reservoirs of infection.

First intermediate host: Freshwater snail of the Genus Melania.

Second intermediate host: Freshwater crayfish or crab.

Adult worms reside in the respiratory tract of the definitive hosts. Eggs are usually expectorated with the sputum, some are passed out with the faeces. On reaching water, in 2–7 weeks' time, a ciliated miracidium is released which then searches for its snail host of genus Melania. In the snail it gets rid of its tail and passes through the stages of sporocyst and two generations of rediae being finally transformed into cercariae (this cycle takes 10 to 12 days). Mature cercariae find their way into water to enter their second intermediate host, a freshwater crab or crayfish. In the crustacean host they encyst in the viscera, muscles and gills.

On ingestion of the raw flesh of an infected crayfish or crab by man or other definitive hosts, the cyst-wall is dissolved by the gastric secretions and the adolescariae are released in the duodenum. These young worms then penetrate the intestinal wall to later enter the abdominal cavity. Subsequently they migrate upwards, pierce the diaphragm and the two pleural layers (parietal and visceral pleural layers) to gain entrance into the lungs where they settle to become sexually mature (this migratory phase takes two weeks). Eggs are then discharged into a bronchiole to be expectorated out with sputum. The cycle is then repeated.

Pathology: Disease entity is designated paragonimiasis. The adult worm causes worm cysts and burrows by their mechanical actions. Eggs evoke a foreign body granulomatous reaction which may soften in the centre to form cavities, the wall of which is composed of fibrous granulation tissue (one finds epithelioid cells, lymphocytes, plasma cells, giant cells, eosinophils and fibroblasts).

Clinical features: Subdivided into pulmonary and extrapulmonary paragonimiasis.

Pulmonary paragonimiasis causes chronic cough with recurrent attacks of haemoptysis (clinically simulating pulmonary tuberculosis or bronchiectasis).

Extrapulmonary paragonimiasis: Liver, intestine, peritoneum or other organs may be involved. Therefore, the symptoms vary according to the organ involved. Abdominal involvement causes abdominal pain, diarrhoea and hepatomegaly. Cerebral involvement may induce epileptic seizures. Generalised paragonimiasis causes fever, generalised lymphadenitis and skin ulcers.

Diagnosis: Established by demonstration of eggs in the sputum. Sometimes the eggs may be found in stool examination too.

Immunological tests: Intradermal injection of a saline extract of *P. westermani* produces an immediate type of hypersensitivity reaction. CFT has also been used.

A chest skiagram may show abnormal shadows (nodular, cystic or infiltrative) in the middle or lower lung fields identical to those seen in pulmonary tuberculosis. Shadows of tunnels and burrows mimic bronchiectasis.

Treatment

Emetine and chloroquine have been used earlier but were not found to be very effective.

Bithionol has given encouraging results.

Prophylaxis: Measures include—
- Making sputum and faeces disinfective.
- Eradication of mollusc host.
- Avoidance of eating raw, ill-cooked or fleshy salted crabs and crayfish.

ECHINOSTOMATIDAE (family)

Echinostoma Species

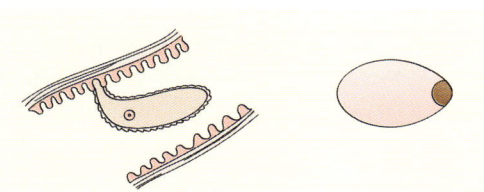

Intestinal flukes found in indigenous populations particularly in the Far East as common or occasional infections.

Relatively unimportant, but ova may be passed in faeces and require identification, mainly based on size.

GASTRODISCIDAE (FAMILY)

Gastrodiscoides hominis

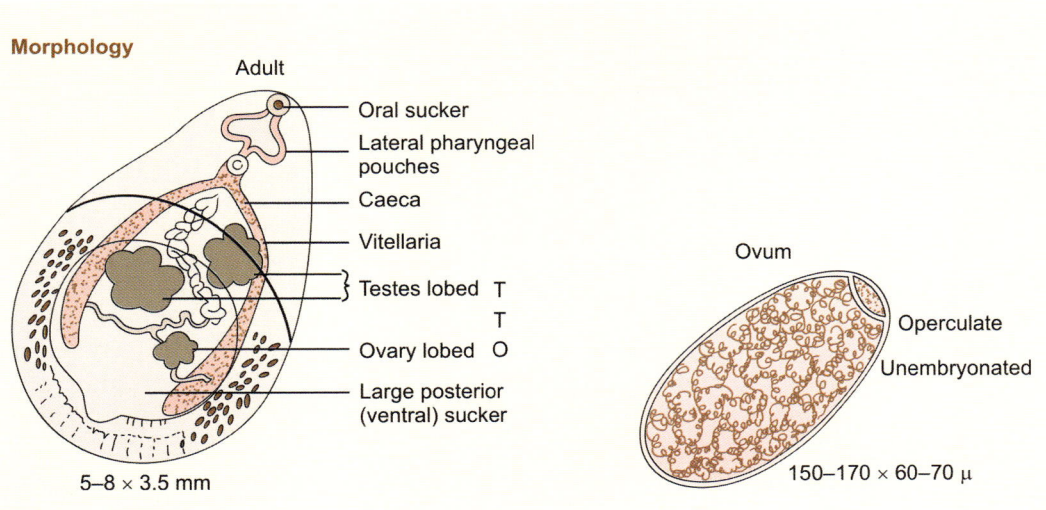

Morphology

Adult
- Oral sucker
- Lateral pharyngeal pouches
- Caeca
- Vitellaria
- Testes lobed T
                T
- Ovary lobed O
- Large posterior (ventral) sucker

5–8 × 3.5 mm

Ovum
- Operculate
- Unembryonated

150–170 × 60–70 µ

Life Cycle

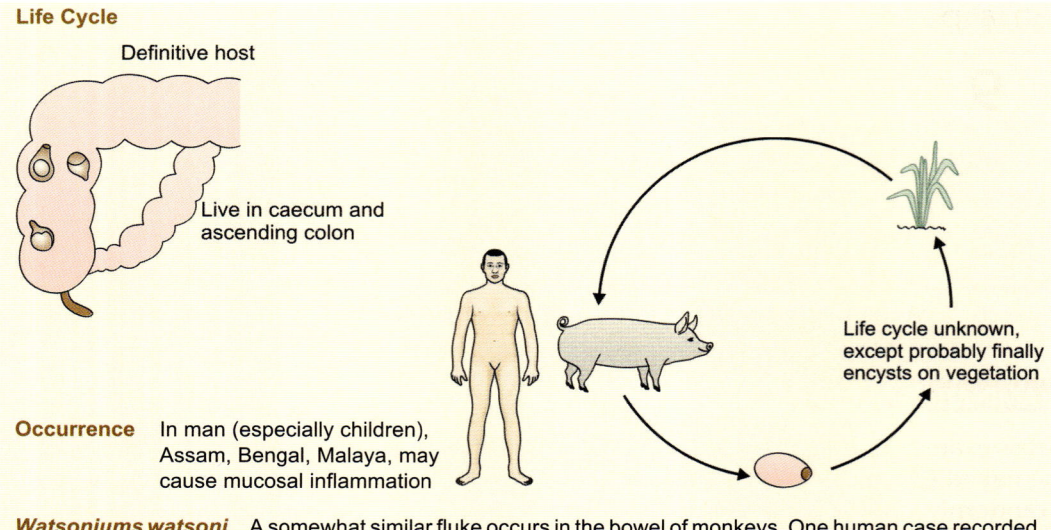

Definitive host

Live in caecum and ascending colon

Life cycle unknown, except probably finally encysts on vegetation

Occurrence   In man (especially children), Assam, Bengal, Malaya, may cause mucosal inflammation

Watsoniums watsoni   A somewhat similar fluke occurs in the bowel of monkeys. One human case recorded.

Practical Parasitology

EXAMINATION OF STOOL FOR PARASITES DIAGNOSING PROTOZOAL INFECTIONS

Gross examination of stool is a must for all samples, though, no protozoa are visible to the naked eye. Select stool sample from mucoid or bloody part if present, otherwise, a randomly selected part may be used for microscopic study.

For showing trophozoites an unstained preparation is examined, for seeing nuclear characters clearly stained preparation is useful and for examining cysts an iodine-stained preparation is used (this also helps in defining the nuclear characters). So, both stained and unstained preparations should be examined for all the samples.

On a slide put a drop of normal saline on one side and a drop of iodine solution on the other. Take stool sample on an applicator stick and dilute faeces, both in normal saline and iodine solution. Having done this put a coverslip on saline and also on iodine side and examine microscopically using both low power (10x) and high power (40x) objectives. If parasite movement is to be observed the microscope stage should be warm (to 37°C). In no case should the slides be allowed to dry. No oily preparation or barium or bismuth salts be given to the patient a day or two before the examination.

E. histolytica—Microscopic Examination

Stool should be fresh and passed into a clear and dry container. Urinary admixture should not be there. If necessary, a rubber catheter (inserted through the anus into the rectum) or a proctoscope or a sigmoidoscope may be used for procuring the stool sample.

Saline and iodine preparations must be studied.

UNSTAINED PREPARATION

Useful for demonstrating motile forms of E. histolytica often seen in symptomatic amoebasis. Pick mucoid portion of the stool and mix it in the normal saline drop. The resulting mixture should be neither too thick nor too thin. It should allow a newspaper to be read through. Put a coverslip, take the condenser to a lower level and partially shut the iris diaphragm to obtain a clear view. Besides trophozoites cysts can also be examined in unstained preparation. If the examination needs a longer period, seal the edges of the coverslip with vaseline. Examine the entire field and later discard the slide in a vessel containing 5% lysol.

STAINED PREPARATION

Useful for detecting cysts and dead trophozoites for defining nuclear characters. Iodine preparation is sufficient, however, if a permanent preparation is wanted, the film is first fixed and then stained with iron-haematoxylin.

When direct examination yields a negative result and the stool is formed, concentration method may become mandatory to detect cystic forms (trophozoites are destroyed by employing this technique). Method of Faust et al (ZnSO$_4$ floatation technique) is good.

STAINING METHODS

Iodine Solution

Lugol's iodine solution should be diluted 5 times before use. This stain should be prepared fresh every fortnight.

Constituents of Lugol's iodine solution

Iodine crystals (powdered)	5 gm
Potassium iodide	10 gm
Distilled water	100 ml

Staining for permanent preparation

Make uniform smears on a clean glass slide.

Fixative: Schaudinn's fluid.

Saturated solution of mercuric chloride in distilled water	200 ml
95% or absolute alcohol	100 ml
Glacial acetic acid	15 ml

Keep in this fluid for 5–10 minutes. Later, wash the smear in 50% alcohol and iodised 70% alcohol from 10 to 30 minutes.

Stain: Heidenhain's haematoxylin, employs 2 solutions:

(i) Haematoxylin crystals — 1 gm
　　Alcohol 90% — 10 ml
　　Distilled water — 90 ml
　　(This is the staining solution)
　　(Ripen this mixture for 10 days in sun, use when it turns brown).

(ii) Iron alum — 2 gm
　　Distilled water — 50 ml
　　(This is the mordant).

Place the slide in distilled water for 10 minutes after fixation. Next place it in the mordant for 6 hours. Wash with distilled water. Place in the staining solution for at least 6 hours (or overnight). The smear now becomes dark black in colour.

Differentiation: Dilute mordant with three parts of water, place the slide in this solution, black colour gradually comes off. Wash slide in distilled water, examine under the microscope from time to time, till the nuclear structure is distinctly visible.

Dehydration: Wash in distilled water or running tap water. Pass the slide through ascending series of alcohol (70, 80 and 90% and then to absolute alcohol), keep the slide in each solution for 5 minutes. Clear the smear with xylene, and mount and examine.

For Helminthic Infections

Always examine the stool grossly. One may observe adult worms of *Enterobius vermicularis, Trichuris trichiura, Ascaris lumbricoides, Ancylostoma duodenale* and the different intestinal flukes or parts of the adult tapeworms (segments) may be seen. A still better way is to dilute the stool sample with water and pour it on a sieve (with 30 meshes to an inch). The faecal matter would be washed away while the worms would be visible against the mesh background. The worms may be passed out with the stool spontaneously or after giving a purgative or following the administration of an anthelmintic.

Eggs are usually present in stool samples of infected individuals. If necessary stool samples of 3 consecutive days should be examined. Always note the shape, size, colour and markings on the egg surface, look for yolk granules, ovum or a differentiated embryo. Operculum, booklets, etc, should also be noted. Helminthic egg examination needs no staining.

Direct smear

Low power examination of a direct smear would usually reveal the eggs or larvae when present in large numbers. Sometimes stool washing is necessary.

Concentration techniques: Floatation or sedimentation techniques are employed. The same methods may also be used for protozoal cysts.

Floatation method

Faeces are dissolved in solution of a higher density than that of the eggs. On doing so the eggs float on the fluid surface. All helminthic eggs float except unfertilised eggs of *A. lumbricoides,* eggs of *T. solium* and *T. saginata,* eggs of all intestinal flukes. Strongyloides larvae also do not float on salt solution.

Simple floatation method

One needs:
1. A glass or metal container (15–20 ml capacity), having a flat-bottom, vertical edges and diameter not in excess of an inch and a half.
2. Glass slides 3" × 2" (and not 3" × 1").
3. Saturated salt solution of specific gravity 1.200. Prepared by letting an excess of common salt to boil in a basin until a scum forms on the surface. When cooled it is stored in glass bottles, leaving an excess of undissolved salt at the bottom.
4. A sheet of glass on which the container is to be kept.

Method: To one ml of faeces add a few drops of the salt solution in the container. Stir with a glass rod to make an even emulsion. Add more salt solution now to nearly fill the container. Keep stirring continuously. At this moment, any coarse matter that comes to the surface should be removed (eggs take 20 to 30 minutes to reach the surface). Now place the container on a level surface. Next fill the container drop by drop until a convex meniscus is formed. Now carefully place the 3" × 2" slide atop the container so that its centre is in contact with the fluid. Now let this stand for 20 to

30 minutes, quickly lift the slide, gently turn it over and examine microscopically. A coverslip need not be used but the surface of the film is to be focussed with 2/3rd in objective, for the detection of the eggs.

Direct centrifugal floatation or DCF method

One needs:
1. Special bucket (for containing the centrifuge tube) with flat bottom and ground-off top, having special carriers with guards to keep the coverslip from slipping out of position.
2. Special coverslip 19 x 19 mm x 0.5 mm thickness.
3. Lane's centrifugal machine.

Method: Mix 1 to 2 grammes of faeces with water in a Clayton Lane's centrifuge tube. Centrifuge the faecal emulsion at 1000 rpm for 2 minutes. Pour off the supernatant, add saturated solution of common salt (specific gravity 1.200) to fill 3/4 of the tube. Shake the mixture vigorously. Fill the tube till the brim and put the thick coverslip on top. Centrifuge at 1000 rpm for 2 minutes. Lift off the coverslip and examine like a hanging-drop preparation.

Zinc sulphate centrifugal floatation: To 10 ml of lukeworm distilled water add a gram of stool and prepare a fine faecal suspension. Remove the coarse particles by straining through a wire mesh (40 meshes to an inch). Collect the filtrate into a Wassermann tube and centrifuge for 1 minute at 2500 rpm. Pour off the supernatant, add distilled water to the sediment. Shake well, centrifuge and repeat the process 2 or 3 times till the supernatant is clear. Finally, to the sediment add 3 to 4 ml of 33% zinc sulphate solution having a specific gravity 1.800. Stir the sediment and add further zinc sulphate solution to fill to the top and centrifuge at 2500 rpm for at least one minute. The surface film is then removed by a platinum wire loop of 5 mm diameter, on a clean glass slide, put on a coverslip and examine microscopically.

For protozoal cysts add a drop of iodine before putting the coverslip on.

Sedimentation Method

Fluid of density less than that of the eggs is used, so eggs settle at the bottom or sediment.

Simple sedimentation: Adequate amount of faeces is thoroughly shaken with 10–20 times its volume of tap water, let settle in cone-shaped flask (urine container) for an hour or two. Discard supernatant. Repeat the process till supernatat becomes clear. Finally, examine the sediment for eggs. This process is not suitable for protozoal cysts.

Formol-ether concentration: Emulsify a gram of faeces in 7 ml of 10% formol-saline and keep for 10 minutes. Strain through a wire mesh (40 meshes to an inch) and collect the filtrate in a centrifuge tube. Add 3 ml ether and shake the mixture vigorously for one minute. Centrifuge at 2000 rpm for 2 minutes and then let it settle. Loosen the debris with a stick, decant the supernatant, remove the fatty debris too, leave only 1 to 2 drops at the bottom. Shake this deposit and pour on a glass slide, place a coverslip and examine microscopically. No structural distortion occurs and takes only 5 minutes to complete the whole process.

Counting of eggs: Done to estimate the worm load. Roughly it is taken that each female worm produces 100 eggs per gram of faeces per day. In hermaphrodite species, as in Clonorchis and Fasciolopsis the total number of worms is calculated on this basis. In nematodes, considering that the sexes are equally divided, 50 eggs per gram of faeces represent one worm.

Method: Mix 4 grams of faeces with 56 ml of N/10 NaOH in a thick glass tube, mix thoroughly to make a uniform suspension. Done better by adding a few glass beads and closing the mouth with a rubber stopper and then shaking the tube vigorously. Place 0.15 ml of this emulsion on a large slide 3" × 2" size, coverslip it (size 22 × 40 mm) and count all the eggs in the coverslip field. Count the total number of eggs in two such preparations and multiply by 100 to get the number of eggs per gram of faeces. The average daily output of faeces being known the total egg-production. For calculating egg production in stools of loose consistency, multiply the count obtained by the relevant correction factor—correction factors for mush-formed, mushy stool, mushy diarrhoeic stool, frankly diarrhoeic and watery stool are 1.5, 2, 3, 4 and 5 respectively.

Kato's Cellophane-covered Thick Smear

Introduced by Kato and Miura in 1954, this method provides a semi-quantitative assessment. They used wettable strips 22 x 30 mm x 40–50 µ thickness soaked in glycerine-malachite green solution for 24 hours or more to clarify a measured amount of faeces (about 50 grams) spread in an even layer on a glass slide. The strips were placed over the faecal smear, permitted to dry at room temperature for an hour and then examined microscopically.

Faeces preservation: Treat up to 2 grams of faeces with about 10 ml of 10% formalin and keep in a closed container. Label the specimen properly. Use the emulsion as and when necessary.

Diagnosis of enterobiasis—anal swab: Anything that is conveniently available, e.g. scraping by curettes, spatula, glass slides, rods, etc. can be used.

NIH swab: NIH swab consists of one end of a glass rod (8–10 cm x 4 mm) covered with a piece of transparent cellophane (one square inch size) is held in place by a rubber band. This end of the rod is employed for swabbing the anal region. After swabbing, the cellophane end of the rod may be replaced in a test tube and the mouth closed. For examination—place a drop of saline on a slide and hold the cellophane end of the rod over it. Release the cellophane from the grip of the rubber band, now spread out and smoothen the cellophane in such a way so that the material adhering to the cellophane comes to lie in direct contact with the glass slide. Place a drop of saline over it and coverslip. The eggs, therefore, lie between the glass slide and the cellophane.

Scotch cellulose tape method: About 3–4" x 3/4" sized scotch cellulose tape with adhesive side out at the end of the blade of a wooden tongue depressor or a spatula is employed. The tape end is placed first on one side and then on the other side of the anal orifice. After swabbing, the tape is removed and placed with adhesive side down on a drop of toluene on a glass side and examined microscopically.

Faecal culture: Employed to diagnose different hookworm species and possibly Trichostrongylus or Ternidens in same regions.

Smear about half a gram of faeces on a strip of sterile filler-paper (15 x 1.5 cm) leaving clean spaces at both the ends which is put into sterile test tube along the side (with unsmeared surface in contact with the wall). The lower end of the paper should touch the column of sterile water (5–7 ml) already put in the tube. Plug the tube top with cotton. Incubate this at 24°–28°C for 7 to 10 days. The filariform larvae will be collected at the bottom of the tube which can be pipetted off to a microscope slide for observation and identification. To kill the larvae, the tube can be placed in 50°C water bath for 15 minutes or the larvae can be treated with iodine solution.

BLOOD EXAMINATION FOR PARASITES

Preparation of a thin blood film: A thin blood film is prepared by spreading a drop of blood evenly across a clean grease-free slide, using a smooth edged spreader. Let the film dry and label it.

Making thick smears: While thin smears are used for describing blood cells, the thick smears are helpful for detecting malarial parasites and microfilariae. A large drop of blood is taken on the centre of a slide and with the aid of a needle or a slide corner spread the drop over 1/2 an inch square area. When dry the thickness should be such that printed matter can be seen through it.

Thin and thick smears can be made on the same slide too.

Fixing of Blood Films

Before staining, the blood films need to be fixed with acetone free methyl alcohol for 30 to 60 seconds in order to prevent haemolysis when they come in contact with water while staining them with aqueous (water based) stains or when water has to be added subsequently. Alcohol denatures the proteins and hardens the cell contents. For Wright's stain and Leishman's stain no pre-fixation is required as these contain acetone free methyl alcohol but for Giemsa's stain pre-fixation is a must because the alcohol content is only 5% in the ready to use stain.

Staining of Blood Films

Blood cells have structures that are acidophilic and some basophilic structures, so they vary in their reaction (pH). The nuclei are basophilic and stain blue (also in the parasites too). The highly basophilic (acidic) basophil granules also stain blue. Haemoglobin (being basic) stains acidophilic or red.

Stains that are made up of combinations of acid and basic dyes are called Romanowsky stains and various modifications are available, e.g. Wright's, Leishman's, Giemsa's and Jenner's stains. Most use methylene blue as the basic stain, though, toludine blue is employed in some. Most use eosin as the acid stain, through Azure I and Azure II are also used.

The dried film can stay good for a couple of days in hot dry weather but gets bad if they are not fixed (in hot and humid climate that exists in India).

It is best to use neutral distilled water for diluting the stain. Stale distilled water becomes acidic after absorbing CO_2 from atomsphere. If the distilled water is alkaline the RBC's stain a dirty bluish green colour, the parts of WBC which should stain blue will be slightly purplish, the eosinophils appear bluish or greenish instead of pink and the granules of neutrophils are over-stained. If the water is acidic RBC's stain bright orange and nuclei of the white cells a very pale colour.

The ideal pH is 6.8 and in order to maintain this, buffered distilled water is used. Buffer water is a solution which tends to keep its original pH even on addition of small amount of alkali or acid.

Butter Solution used in the Laboratory

Solution No. I

NaOH (sodium hydroxide)	8 gm
Distilled water	1000 cc

Solution No. II

KH_2PO_4 (Potassium dihydrogen phosphate)	27.2 gm
Distilled water	1000 cc

Take 23.7 cc of solution I, add to it 50 cc of solution II. Add 20 cc of this solution to 1000 cc of distilled water. This has a pH of 6.8.

Stain Preparation and Staining

Wright's stain

Wright's stain (powder)	0.2 gm
Acetone-free methanol	100 cc.

Let this mature for a few days.
If the WBC granules do not stand out clearly try out a 0.25 or 0.3% solution.

Method: Cover the slide with stain for 1–2 minutes taking care that it does not dry on the slide. Now dilute this with equal amount of buffer water (If the stain is ripe a scum or film with a metallic sheen will form on the surface of the diluted stains on the slide). The diluted stain is allowed to act for 3–5 minutes and then flooded off with buffer or tap water. The stain should never be poured off or a precipitate of the stain will be deposited on the slide. Should this occur, it can sometimes be removed by flooding the slide with undiluted stain for 10–15 seconds and then washing it off again by flooding the slide once more with buffered water.

Leishman's stain

Powdered Leishman's stain	0.15 gm
Acetone free methanol	133 ml

Dissolve the stain completely (stain crystals should be well ground before), keep the stain in a glass stoppered bottle. Do not filter.

Method: Like that for Wright's stain but with double dilution of the buffer water. Pour few drops (about 8) on the slide. Wait for 2 minutes. Add double the amount (16 drops) of buffered water. Mix by rocking and not by blowing and wait for 7–10 minutes. The stain is flooded off with distilled water and this should be complete in 2–3 seconds. Longer washing will remove the stain. Stand in a rack to drain and air dry. A fan will expedite the process.

Giemsa's stain

Giemsa powder	0.3 gm
Glycerin	25 ml
Acetone-free methanol	25 ml

This makes stock solution and before use it has to be diluted by adding 1 ml of stain to 9 ml of buffered distilled water.

Method: Fix the blood film with methanol for a minute or two and dry. Pour on diluted stain and keep for 15 minutes or longer. Wash off with tap water or neutral distilled water and dry.

Staining of Thick Film

Thick films before staining or fixing need to be dehaemoglobinised.

Dehaemoglobinisation

(i) Place the film in distilled water for 5–10 minutes. When the film becomes white, take it out and let dry.

(ii) Prepare a solution of 2% glacial acetic acid and 2% crystalline tartaric acid in a ratio of 4 : 1. Flood the film with the above-mentioned mixture and when the blood film turns greyish-white in colour, drain off the fluid by tilting. Fix with methanol for 3–5 minutes. Wash the slide with buffer water to remove even the slightest trace of the acids used.

After dehaemoglobinisation, the films are used in the same way as for thin films for staining purposes. Other stains commonly used for thick films are:

1. Field's stain, and
2. Simeon's stain.

Field's Stain

Field's stain A

Methylene blue	0.8 gm
Azere 1	0.5 gm
Disodium hydrogen phosphate (anhydrous)	5.0 gm
Potassium dihydrogen phosphate (anhydrous)	6.25 gm
Distilled water	500 ml

Field's stain B

Eosin (yellow eosin, water soluble)	1.0 gm
Disodium hydrogen phosphate (onhydrous)	5.0 gm
Potassium dihydrogen phosphate (anhydrous)	6.25 gm
Distilled water	500 ml

Grind all solids well and dissolve in the said solvent, keep the stains for 4 hours for ripening and filter before use. Keep the stains in covered jars. The depth of the solution should be about 3 inches, the level should be maintained by adding more of the stain solution.

Method

Dip the film for one second in solution A.

Remove from solution A and immediately rinse by waving very gently in clean water for a few seconds, until the stain ceases to flow from the film and the glass of the slide is free from stain.

Dip for one second in solution B.

Rinse by waving gently by 2–3 seconds in clean water.

Place vertically in rack to drain and dry.

SIMEON'S MODIFICATION OF BOYE'S AND STERENEL'S METHOD

This stain can be used instead of Leishman's or Wright's stain when methanol is not available to prepare them.

Solution I

Eosin pure	1 gm
Distilled water	1000 ml

Solution II

(a) Methylene blue	1 gm dissolve completely
Distilled water	75 ml
(b) Potassium permanganate	1.5 gm dissolve completely
Distilled water	75 ml

1. Mix (a) and (b) in a flask. A massive percipate is formed.
2. Keep the flask in a water bath at boiling point for half an hour during which time the precipitate re-dissolves.
3. Filter. The stain is now ready for use, it needs no further dilution.

Method of staining thin films

1. Fix the smear by immersion into rectified spirit 1 minute.
2. Rinse with tap water: 4 seconds.
3. Immense into solution I: 10 seconds
4. Rinse with tap water: 4 seconds.
5. Immerse into solution II: 15 seconds.
6. Rinse with tap water: 4 seconds
7. Immerse again into solution I: 5 seconds.
8. Rinse with tap water: 4 seconds.
9. Allow to dry in an upright position.

Procedure for staining thick smears

1. Dehaemoglobinise by immersion in tap water, if necessary.
2. Immerse in Sterenel's blue (solution II): 6 seconds.
3. Wash in tap water.
4. Immerse in eosin solution (solution I): 12 seconds.
5. Wash in tap water, allow it to dry in air.

The stains are useful for screening purposes.

Mounting and Preservation of Films

Unstained films cannot be preserved well. Due to hardening of plasma they do not stain well after some time. Stained films if left unmounted tend to fade away rapidly. Canada Balsum should not be used as it decolourises the smear. Gurr's neutral mounting medium is quite satisfactory. Use only thin coverslips for mounting.

Examination of Blood for Malarial Parasite

Time for taking blood: Parasites are more easily detected in the film when the blood has been taken several hours after the peak has been reached. Schizogony of *P. vivax*,

P. malariae and *P. ovale* occurs in the peripheral blood, hence the parasites can be easily demonstrated both during the febrile and afebrile periods in these cases. The parasites in cases of *P. falciparum* infections, however, disappear from the peripheral blood during the afebrile period.

Always make both thin and thick smears either on the same slide or on different slides. First examine the thin stained smear. If positive, there is no need to see the thick smear. If thin smear is negative, thick smear should be examined. For species identification one should refer back to the thin smear. While examining the thin smear always pay greater attention to the smear margins and the tail. Examine at least 100 fields (it takes about 8–10 minutes). It is observed that in non-immune persons the clinical attack of malaria is associated with the presence of at least one parasite per 100 fields.

In thick films the only things visible are leucocytes and malarial parasites (red cells are destroyed during dehaemoglobinisation). Species identification is difficult on a thick smear. Thick films should never replace or become a substitute for thin films. Young trophozoites (ring forms) of all species appear as streaks of blue cytoplasm with detached nuclear dots. Various terms used to describe these forms are: *Comma*—cytoplasm forms a curved thread with red nucleus, *Swallow or gullswing*—dash of blue appears on either side of the red nucleus as two wings, *Exclamation marks*—where the red nucleus occurs below the blue line. Schizonts and gametocytes (crescent shaped) retain their normal appearance, although being smaller and less regular in outline; the pigments are seen more discretely. The nuclei of leucocytes stain a deep purple and are clearly defined; whereas cytoplasm always appears shredded. Platelets stain purple having a woolly texture and outline.

Examination of Blood for Microfilariae

Blood collection: Where micofilariae show nocturnal periodicity, the blood should be collected between 10 pm and 2 am where periodicity does not exist blood may be taken at any time, preferably in the morning.

Unstained preparation examination: Take a couple of drops of blood on a clean glass slide and place a coverslip on it. Seal the rim with vaseline so as to avoid drying. Leave it overnight. Examine next morning under low power objective, microfilaria, if present, may be seen wriggling about in the blood (microfilaria may stay alive in such a preparation for a day or two.)

Stained preparation study: Prepare a thick blood film and keep it covered. Dehaemoglobinise on the next morning, dry and fix in methanol and then stain with Leishman's, Giemsa or haematoxylin and eosin. Sometimes, microfilaria may be observed in a thin film.

H & E stain (Haematoxylin and Eosin stain): After fixing the thick dehaemoglobinised film, stain with Delafield's haematoxylin for 5 to 7 minutes. Wash the stain in running water for 7–10 minutes. Counterstain with diluted Giemsa or 5% aqueous eosin solution for 30 seconds. Do the final differentiation in running tap water.

Vital staining: Mix fresh blood or sediment of dehaemoglobinisation with methylene blue (1 in 5,000 in isotonic saline). The viable microfilariae of *L. loa, O. volvulus*, and *D. perstans* pick up the stain in 10 minutes, whereas those of *W. bancrofti* and *B. malayi* take longer time.

CONCENTRATION METHODS

Consist of taking 5–10 ml of blood and centrifuging it at 2000 rpm for 2–5 minutes. Decant the supernatant and examine them for microfilariae. Either the sediment can be made into a film, air dried, fixed and permanently stained; or else the whole sediment can be vitally stained. Various concentration methods employ different dehaemoglobinising agents—e.g. distilled water, 2% acetic acid, 2–5% formalin, 1–10% saponin.

For mass screening/survey: Two methods are often employed:
1. *Counting chamber technique* described by Denhan and associate in 1971, where a measured quantity of haemolysed blood is examined directly.
2. *Membrane filter concentration* method using millipore membrane or nucleopore filter, where the microfilariae liberated from measured quantity of heparinised blood are examined fresh, or after staining.

Hetrazan Provocative Test: A single 100 mg dose of Hetrazan (diethyclcarbamazine) induces appearance of nocturnally periodic Mf in the peripheral blood during daytime. Collect blood 30–45 minutes after giving Hetrazan and examine by concentration technique.

LABORATORY CULTIVATION

(Culture Methods)

Cultivation of *E. histolytica*

Media preparation (Modified Boeck and Drbohlav's method): Prepare tubes of inspissated horse blood serum by heating in a serum inspissator. To all the tubes add 3–5 ml of a solution of egg albumin so as to cover the solid part of the medium to a depth of 1 ml of the fluid. Preserve the medium in an incubator and take out just befor inoculation. Prior to inoculation add a little rice starch with a platinum loop. Ideal pH is 7.2 to 7.8. Intestinal bacteria that get inoculated along with are useful.

Egg albumin solution: Sterilise the surface of 4 eggs. Break open the shell with sterilised forceps, withdraw the white portion of the eggs by a 5 ml syringe and a thick 18 gauge needle. Dissolve the white of 4 eggs in one litre of sterile Ringer's solution.

Ringer's solution consists of 9 grams of solution chloride, 200 mg of potassium chloride, 200 mg of calcium chloride in 1000 ml of distilled water.

Rice starch is sterilised by heating it at 180° with dry heat for one hour.

Trophozoites as well as cysts can be used. Cultures are incubated at 37°C and subcultures made every 2–3 days. Inoculation is done with a 1 ml sterile capillary glass pipette. Use freshly passed stool only. Examine the cultures every 24 hours. Collect the material by 1 ml pipette from the sediment at the bottom of fluid cultures where amoebae abound if grown. Place a drop of fluid on a clean glass slide, coverslip and examine microscopically. If found negative, examine again after 48 hours, if this too does not reveal anything, a negative report can be signed out.
- Washing the faeces containing cysts is helpful as this removes an excystation inhibitory substance.
- Presence of some bacteria (heat-killed) and addition of a reducing substance (0.1 cystine hydrochloride or 0.3% thioglycollic acid neutralised) assists.

- Partial anaerobiasis also favours excystation.
- It is well understood that cultivation of bacteria-free excysted amoeba cannot be maintained unless a living bacterium or a flagellate (*T. cruzi*) is present in the culture medium.
- *Blastocystis hominis* usually present in every stool, grows readily and inhibits the growth of amoebae. To prevent this add a little rice starch or 1% dextrin.

Morphology in culture: Culture material reveals both excystation and encystation. Trophozoites are also observed. Cultures inoculated with cysts readily excyst. When trophozoites are inoculated, they multiply by binary fission rapidly.

Culture maintenance: Medium employed uses either an egg, an agar or serum slant covered with a fluid medium. By making subcultures every 48 hours, the strain can be maintained for up to 5 years. Attempts have also been made to obtain a culture free from bacteria. Pure cultures cannot, however, be maintained for over 2 generations.

SIGNIFICANCE OF CULTURE TECHNIQUE

Diagnosis: This method has increased the number of identifiable cases.

Morphological study of the parasite becomes easier.

May be used in research laboratories for assessing efficacy of amoebicidal drugs.

Methods can be employed to obtain amoebic antigen for subsequent use in specific immunological investigations.

Cultivation of Leishmaniae

N.N.N. medium, solid medium and semi-defined medium, etc. are available for laboratory cultivation of leishmania species.

N.N.N. medium (after discoverers Novy, Macneal and Nicolle): It consists of 2 parts of salt agar and 1 part of defibrinated rabbit's blood. Salt agar is prepared by dissolving 14 gm of agar and 6 gm of sodium chloride in 900 ml of distilled water. During cooling of liquid agar, add rabbit's blood. Let the tubes set in sloping stance. Rubber cap finally.

One can use blood/bone marrow/splenic pulp. The material to be cultured is inoculated in the water of condensation of the N.N.N. medium. Inoculate 4 such tubes. Incubate at 32°C for a period of 1 to 4 weeks. Examine the tubes for presence of promastigotes from tenth day onwards. The condensation of fluid is withdrawn by means of a capillary pipette or the material can be gently scraped from the surface of the medium and examined fresh. Flagellates, if present, can be seen moving in the field.

On the solid medium, the parasite grows as a thick, grayish white mucoid spreading lawn. No water of condensation is required. Usually the parasite grows within 2–3 days at 24°C which should then be subcultured. All strains cannot be grown on this medium.

Semi-defined liquid medium is an easily prepared inexpensive monophasic medium which supports continuous culture of Leishmania species.

Cultivation of Malarial Parasite

Hardly ever employed in routine diagnosis of malaria. RPMI 1640 medium can be used for *in-vitro* continuous culture technique. Readymade media are commercially available (Sigma, USA). Erythrocytes are inoculated in this medium at 38°C (medium is enriched with human serum, under 7% CO_2 and 1 to 15% oxygen atmosphere). The parasite material derived from owl monkeys (*Aotus trivirgatus*) is diluted more than 100 million times by addition of normal human RBC's (Group AB, Rh +) at 3 or 4 days intervals. The parasites continue to reproduce their normal asexual cycle of approximately 48 hours.

The method is useful
- For obtaining erythrocyte stages for the study of antigenic structure
- As a source of antigen for sero-epidemiological studies
- For assessing sensitivity/resistance to various drugs
- For studying immune-prophylactic activity

BIOPSY STUDIES

Splenic Puncture for Kala-azar Diagnosis

Quite useful though risky method. Positivity rates for splenic aspirate are 98%, for bone marrow 54–86% and for lymph nodes they are 64%. In acute visceral leshmaniasis, when the spleen is small and soft or impalpable, bone-marrow or lymph node aspiration is recommended.

Splenic puncture should not be done if patient's prothrombin time is more than 5 seconds longer than the control or if the platelet count is less than 40,000/cu.mm. Ensure that the needle does not stay within the spleen for more than a second and that the entry and exit axes of the aspirating needle are identical, to avoid tearing of the splenic capsule.

One requires

- Cotton swabs
- Microscope slides
- Needle, 21 gauge (32 × 0.8 mm). Should be sterile.
- Marker or pen for labelling.
- 5 ml disposable/sterile glass syringe
- Tubes for culture media.
- Tr. of iodine, alcohol, Tr benzoin Co or colloidin.

Method

Before starting, obtain patient's consent. Keep the material's tray ready. Palpate the spleen and outline its margins on the patient's abdomen with a pen. Ideally, the spleen should be palpable at least 3 cm below the costal margin on expiration. Use alcohol, Tr. iodine and again alcohol to sterilise the skin site to be punctured. With a 21 gauge needle attached to a 5 ml syringe, just penetrate the skin, midway between the edges of the spleen, 2–4 cm below the costal margin. Aim the needle cranially at 45° angle to the abdominal wall. Aspiration process—pull the plunger back to approximately 1 ml mark to create vaccum and with a quick in and out movement push the needle into the spleen to the full needle depth and then withdraw it completely, maintaining suction throughout.

After taking the needle out of the patient's body expel the contents of the syringe into the culture medium and on to glass studies. On slides make smears immediately.

Important: Record the patient's blood pressure every half an hour for 4 hours, then hourly for 6 hours. Patient must stay in bed for 12 hours. Seal the wound site with Tr. Benzoin Co.

LYMPH NODE PUNCTURE FOR KALA-AZAR AND AFRICAN TRYPANOSOMIASIS

Sterilise the skin over the node while holding it steady between the index finger and the thumb, insert a dry, sterilized hypodermic needle into the node. Lymph would come into the needle by capillary action. Withdraw the needle quickly and attach to a syringe. Expel the lymph fluid on to a glass slide, make smears, stain and examine microscopically. Cultures on NNN medium may also be made. This method is not useful in Indian Kala-azar. For demonstrating trypomastigote forms of *T. brucei*, the aspirated lymph can be examined fresh and unstained. This is a useful procedure for 'Gambian' sleeping sickness. Seal the wound site with Tr. Benzoin Co.

BONE MARROW ASPIRATION

Can be obtained from sternal puncture or iliac crest (anterior or posterior) puncture. Salah's or Klima's or Jamshedi's needles can be used. Take all sterile precautions and give local anaesthesia. Wait for 10–15 minutes. For sternal puncture site is mid-sternal region, a little away from the midline (patient lying on back supine), at the level of second or third intercostals space. Pierce the skin and subcutaneous tissues up to the periosteum, and marrow cavity is reached with a rotary motion. Loss of resistance implies that the marrow cavity has been reached. Take the stylet out and withdraw about 0.25 to 0.75 ml of marrow. Patient experiences a dragging pain when this is done. After bone marrow has been aspirated and needle withdrawn (with stylet reintroduced), seal the wound site with Tr. Benzoin Co.

Iliac crest puncture: The technique and procedure of aspiration are same as for sternal puncture.

For posterior iliac crest, the patient lies on one side with knees drawn up and back flexed as for lumbar puncture. The needle is inserted perpendicularly 1 cm below the posterior superior iliac spine.

For anterior iliac crest the patient lies on back and the needle is inserted into the iliac crest at a point behind the anterior superior iliac spine.

BONE MARROW BIOPSY

Bone marrow biopsy may be done with Nordin-Sacker trephine (more difficult and painful). Easier way out is using Jamshedi Swain needle to obtain biopsy from iliac crest. Bone marrow biopsy can be used for making marrow imprints as well as biopsy.

LIQUID BASED CYTOLOGY AS AN AID TO DIAGNOSE PARASITIC DISEASES/INFESTATION

For all FNAC brush cytologies, gynaecologic cytologies, all body fluids—like lymph/pleural fluid, peritoneal fluid/CSF, etc. where one expects parasites—we can now use LBC systems or THINPREP systems.

The sample is suspended in a presevative/separating fluid and after processing through an automated instrument it delivers a nice thin smear on a glass slide for eventual staining and visulisation through a microscope.

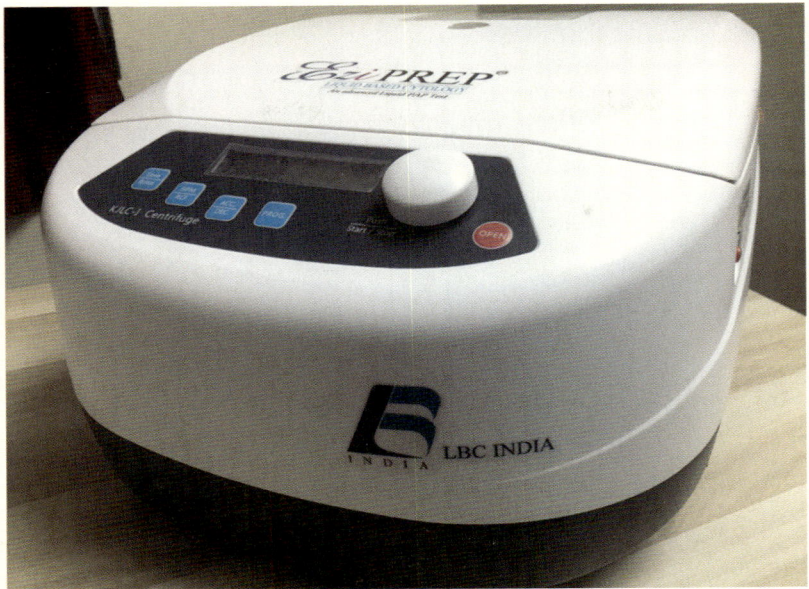

Fig. 9.1: LBC instrument (*Courtesy*: LBC INDIA)

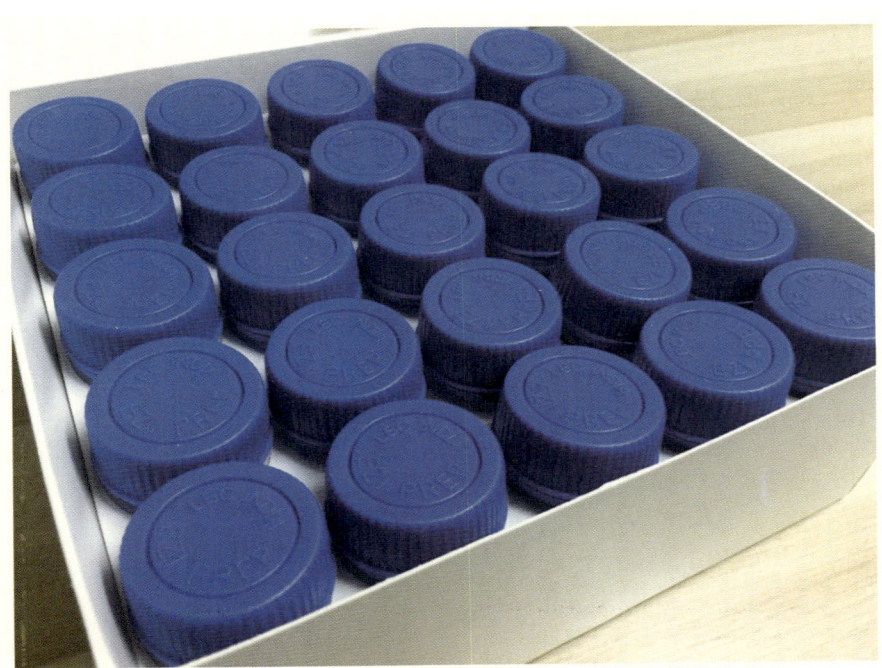

Fig. 9.2: Box of preservative liquid vials

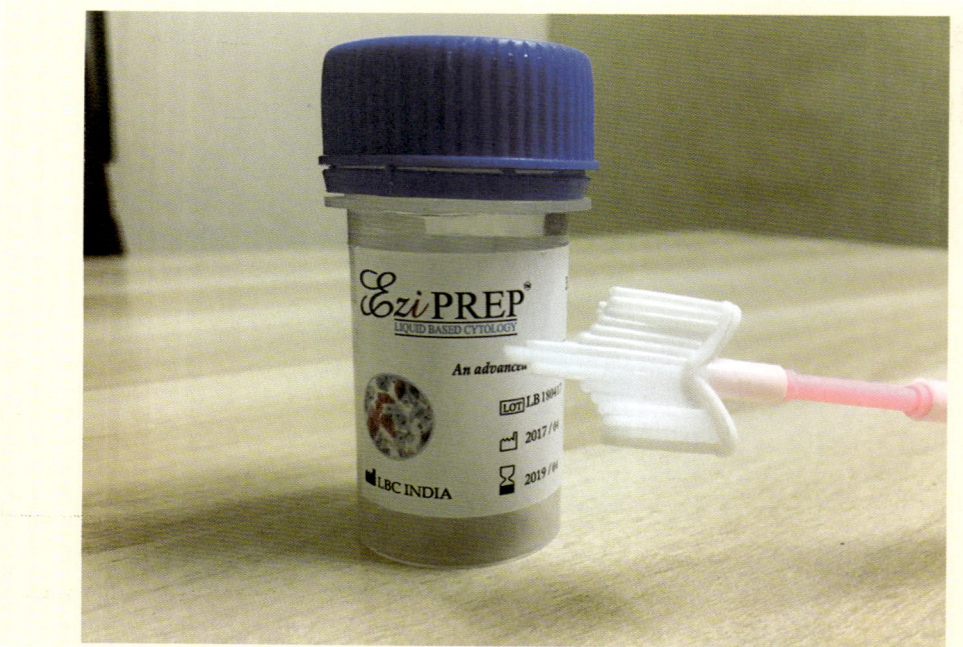

Fig. 9.3: Individual vial with the brush for taking a cervical cytology specimen

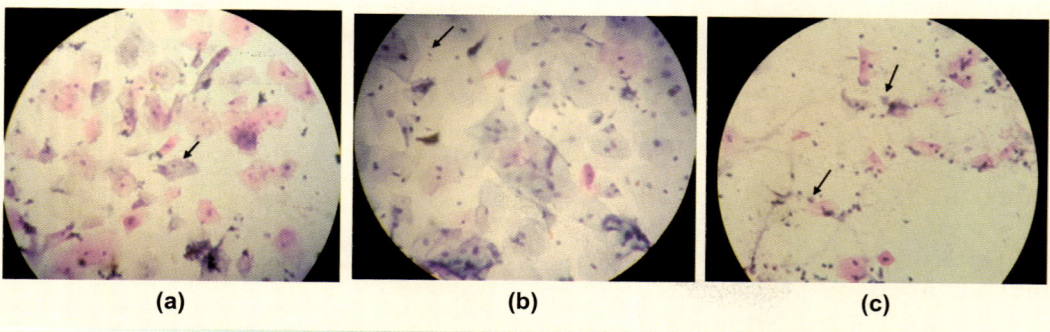

| (a) | (b) | (c) |

Fig. 9.4: (a) Bacterial vaginosis; (b) Clue cells (bacteria adherent to exfoliated squamous cells) and; (c) Arrows point to *Trichomonas trophozoites*

Discrete images after appropriate staining. The third image shows *Trichomonas trophozoites.*

The system can also be used for lymph and other body fluids in order to assess presence of Microfilariae, etc.

Immunodiagnostics in Parasitology

Parasitic infections are one of the world's major causes of human illness and suffering. Manifestations of disease range from the fevers of malaria to physical deformities, such as "river blindness" and elephantiasis, resulting from infections by certain parasites. Parasitic diseases lower the productivity of the human work force, and some of the apathy encountered in regions where these diseases are endemic may be directly traced to such infections. In the extreme, death results, either as a direct consequence of the parasitic infection or from viral, bacterial, nutritional or other diseases to which the body, weakened by the ravages of parasitic infections.

WHAT IS IMMUNODIAGNOSTICS?

One of the body's defences against parasites is its immunological system. On or in parasites and in their secretory or excretory products, are many proteins. Against some of these (antigens), the body is capable of generating other complex protein molecules (antibodies) that neutralize the antigens by binding to them. Techniques that measure these antibodies or antigens provide alternative tools for diagnosis. This method of diagnosis, which uses the immunological binding reaction between antibodies and antigens, is termed immunodiagnosis and the assays for measuring these antibodies or antigens, immunoassays.

In short, immunodiagnostics is a diagnostic methodology that uses an antigen–antibody reaction as their primary means of detection.

WHAT IS AN ANTIGEN?

Antigens may be proteins, nucleoproteins, lipoproteins, polysaccharides which are present on/in micro-organisms or parasite, in the environment or in the body.

The term antigen is used in two senses:
- To describe a molecule which generates antibody response and
- A molecule, which reacts specifically with antibodies.

Antigens which have both the above properties, i.e. the ability to generate antibodies and to react specifically with the antibody so produced are called complete antigens. Some antigens because of their low molecular weights cannot by themselves initiate an antibody response but they can however react with antibodies. These antigens are called Haptens. The hapten can react with the paratope on an antibody. Haptens can produce antibodies if they are attached to larger carrier molecule (normally proteins).

Haptens contain a single epitope. Antigens which can generate an immune response are called immunogens.

The defence mechanisms of the body mount an immune response only against antigens, which are 'foreign' or 'non-self', which is not a part of the host body. The immune systems must be able to discriminate between 'self' and 'non-self'; failure of the immune system to make this discrimination could lead to the synthesis of antibodies directed against components of its own body which could be detrimental. Such a condition leads to autoimmune disorders. Antigens possess a number of antigenic determinants. Antigenic determinants are small areas on the antigen, which possess a specific chemical structure and configuration, which determine the specificity of the antigen–antibody reaction.

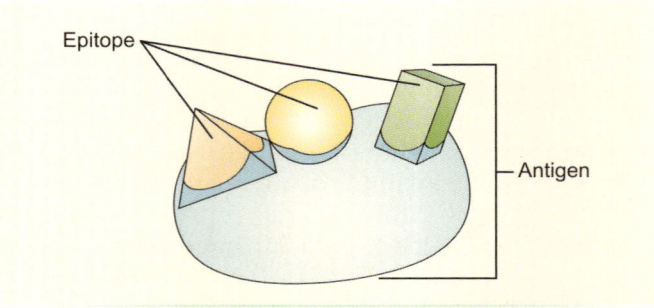

Fig. 10.1: Antigen structure (schematic)

Large antigens carry many different types of antigenic determinants. Antigenic determinants are also known as epitopes.

Antigens can be classified according to their source.

1. **Exogenous antigens:** Exogenous antigens are antigens that have entered the body from the outside, for example, by inhalation, ingestion or injection. The immune system's response to exogenous antigens is often subclinical.

2. **Endogenous antigens:** Endogenous antigens are generated within normal cells as a result of normal cell metabolism, or because of viral or intracellular bacterial infection.

3. **Autoantigens:** An autoantigen is usually a normal protein or protein complex (and sometimes DNA or RNA) that is recognized by the immune system of patients suffering from a specific autoimmune disease. Under normal conditions, these antigens should not be the target of the immune system, but in autoimmune diseases, their associated T cells are not deleted and instead attack.

4. **Neoantigens:** Neoantigens are those that are entirely absent from the normal human genome. As compared with nonmutated self-antigens, neoantigens are of relevance to tumour control, as the quality of the T cell pool that is available for these antigens is not affected by central T cell tolerance. Technology to systematically analyse T cell reactivity against neoantigens became available only recently.

5. **Viral antigens:** For virus-associated tumours, such as cervical cancer and a subset of head and neck cancers, epitopes derived from viral open reading frames contribute to the pool of neoantigens.

WHAT ARE ANTIBODIES?

All immunogens are antigens but all antigens may not be immunogens (e.g. haptens are antigens but they are not immunogens). Antibodies are plasma proteins produced in response to the introduction of foreign antigens. Antibodies react specifically with the antigen responsible for their production. The part of the antibody that binds to the antigen is called paratope.

Paratopes and epitopes have complementary structures, hence they react specifically with each other... Like a lock and key mechanism.

STRUCTURE OF ANTIBODIES

Antibodies belong to the group of proteins called gamma globulins and since they are involved with the immune system, they are also called immunoglobulins often abbreviated as Ig. All proteins are made of amino acid molecules linked by peptide bonds. Each antibody molecule consists of four types of polypeptide chains; two light (L) chains and two heavy (H) chains. The two identical heavy (H) polypeptide chains are held together by disulphide bonds. The light (L) polypeptide chains are attached to the heavy chains in the hinge region by disulphide bonds. Hinge region is the region where the molecule can bend or open and close.

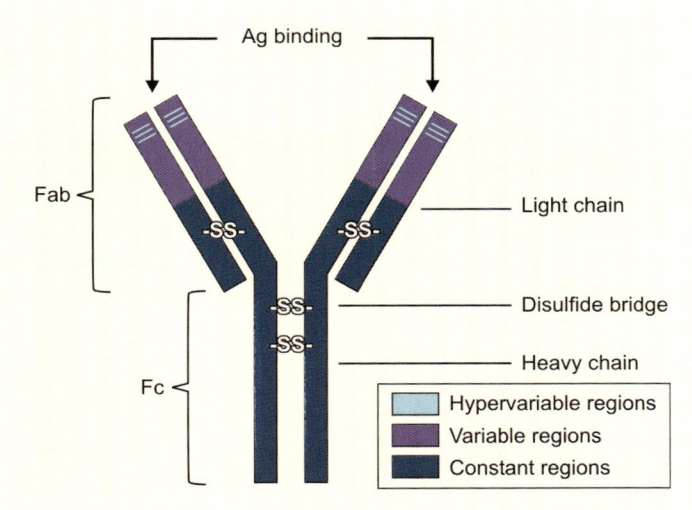

Fig. 10.2: Basic structure of antibody

The N terminal regions of the heavy and light chains have variable amino sequences, the remainder of the chains are constant in structure. The ability of an antibody to combine with an antigen depends only on these few variable amino sequences at the end of each chain. This portion of the antibody that combines antigen is called Fragment Antigen Binding (Fab). The remaining portion of the molecule is called the Fragment Crystallisable (Fc) because it can be crystallised. The Fc portion of the antibody reacts with the complement and is responsible for placental transport.

Types of Antibodies

1. **IgG:** IgG is the most abundant antibody isotype in the blood (plasma), accounting for 70–75% of human immunoglobulins (antibodies). IgG detoxifies harmful substances and is important in the recognition of antigen–antibody complexes by leukocytes and macrophages. IgG is transferred to the foetus through the placenta and protects the infant until its own immune system is functional.

2. **IgM:** IgM usually circulates in the blood, accounting for about 10% of human immunoglobulins. IgM has a pentameric structure in which five basic Y-shaped molecules are linked together. B cells produce IgM first in response to microbial infection/antigen invasion. Although IgM has a lower affinity for antigens than IgG, it has higher avidity for antigens because of its pentameric/hexametric structure. IgM, by binding to the cell surface receptor, also activates cell signalling pathways.

3. **IgA:** IgA is abundant in serum, nasal mucus, saliva, breast milk, and intestinal fluid, accounting for 10–15% of human immunoglobulins. IgA forms dimers (i.e. two IgA monomers joined together). IgA in breast milk protects the gastrointestinal tract of neonates from pathogens.

4. **IgE:** IgE is present in minute amounts, accounting for no more than 0.001% of human immunoglobulins. Its original role is to protect against parasites. In regions where parasitic infection is rare, IgE is primarily involved in allergy.

5. **IgD:** IgD accounts for less than 1% of human immunoglobulins. IgD may be involved in the induction of antibody production in B cells, but its exact function remains unknown.

Types of antibodies					
	IgM	IgG	IgA (Secretory component)	IgE	IgD
Heavy chain	μ (mu)	γ (gamma)	α (alpha)	ε (epsilon)	δ (delta)
MW (Da)	900 k	150 k	385 k	200 k	180 k
% of total antibody in serum	6%	80%	13%	0.002%	1%
Fixes complement	Yes	Yes	No	No	No
Function	Primary response, fixes complement. Manomer serves as B-cell receptor	Main blood antibody, neutralizes toxins, opsonization	Secreted into mucus, tears, saliva	Antibody of allergy and anti-parasitic activity	B cell receptor

ANTIGEN–ANTIBODY REACTIONS

By definition antigens and antibodies react with each other specifically and this is the basis for immune reactions both *in vivo* and *in vitro*. *In vivo* (inside the body), antigen–antibody reactions provide our body with the vital function of defence and *in vitro* (outside the body) these reactions help the physician in diagnosis.

The antibody's paratope interacts with the antigen's epitope. An antigen usually contains different epitopes along its surface arranged discontinuously, and dominant epitopes on a given antigen are called determinants.

Antibody and antigen interact by spatial complementarity (lock and key). The molecular forces involved in the Fab-epitope interaction are weak and non-specific, for example, electrostatic forces, hydrogen bonds, hydrophobic interactions, and van der Waals forces. This means binding between antibody and antigen is reversible, and the antibody's affinity towards an antigen is relative rather than absolute. Relatively weak binding also means it is possible for an antibody to cross-react with different antigens of different relative affinities.

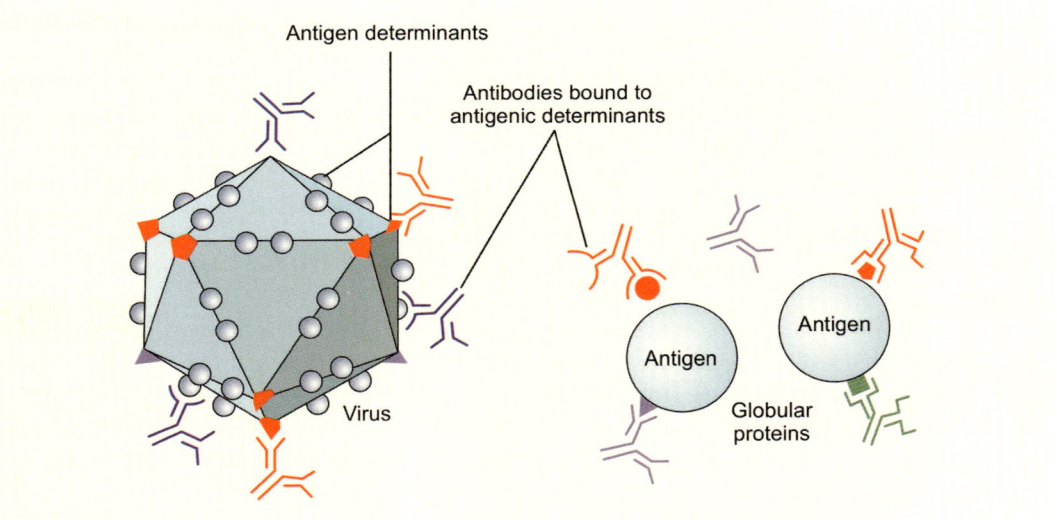

Fig. 10.3: Formation of antigen–antibody complex

Often, once an antibody and antigen bind, they become an immune complex, which functions as a unitary object and can act as an antigen in its own right, being countered by other antibodies. Similarly, haptens are small molecules that provoke no immune response by themselves, but once they bind to proteins, the resulting complex or hapten-carrier adduct is antigenic.

How do Antigen–Antibody Reactions Help in Diagnosis?

- Detection of either antigen or antibody helps in pinpointing the cause of the disease.
- Measurement of antigen/antibody helps in evaluating the extent of the disease, prognosis and the efficacy of treatment.

Tests based on immunological principles involve antigen and antibody and are termed immunoassays.

Tools for Diagnosis

Currently, the detection and diagnosis of parasite infections rely on several laboratory methods in addition to clinical symptoms, clinical history, travel history, and geographic location of patient.

The need for immunological tests is particularly great in assessing the effectiveness of treatment and in detecting infections in which a few parasites are available for microscopic examination. The available tests for antibody detection appear to be poor in this respect. However, measurement of antibodies has the advantage of providing indications of the immune response of the infected host.

Detection of parasitic antigens is a recent alternative to antibody detection, and several research groups developed assay systems. It now appears feasible to measure levels of antigens released by parasites in blood.

Types of Diagnostic Tests

1. **Microscopy:** For many years, microscopy has been the only tool available for the detection of parasites through inspection of blood smears, faeces, etc. However, sample preparation for direct observation is time-consuming, labour intensive, and proper diagnosis depends on qualified laboratory technicians. In the case of slide reading, a second independent reading is preferable, but not always required for accurate diagnosis. If need be, divided readings are resolved by a third reader. In endemic regions, where resources are limited, this proves to be difficult and misdiagnosis can significantly impact patient care. In reality, all major intestinal helminth infections are still solely dependent on microscopy for diagnosis. As for other parasite infections, many are confirmed by the use of microscopy in conjunction to other methods of diagnosis including serology-based assays and more recently molecular-based assays.

2. **Serology-based assays system:** In situations where biologic samples or tissue specimens are unavailable, serology alone is the gold standard for diagnosis. Although the ease of use and turnaround times for serologic assays are similar to microscopy, serology-based assays are more sensitive and specific. It becomes important for individuals whose blood smears do not permit identification of the parasite (e.g., differentiating between Babesia and Plasmodium) or for patients exhibiting low-parasitemia and/or who are asymptomatic (e.g. Chagasic patients). Classifying an infected asymptomatic patient as negative could lead to transmission of the parasite during blood transfusions.

   Serology based assays can be classified into the following types
   1. Rapid diagnostics tests
   2. Enzyme-linked immunosorbent assay (ELISA)
   3. Chemiluminescence immune assay (CLIA)

1. Rapid Detection Tests (RDTs)

Rapid diagnostic tests (RDTs) are a type of point-of-care diagnostic, meaning that these assays are intended to provide diagnostic results conveniently and immediately to the patient while still at the health facility, screening site, or other health care provider. Receiving diagnosis at the point of care reduces the need for multiple visits to receive diagnostic results, thus improving specificity of diagnosis and the chances the patient will receive treatment, reducing dependence on presumptive treatment, and reducing the risk that the patient will get sicker before a correct diagnosis is made. Rapid tests are used in a variety of point of care settings—from homes to primary care clinics or emergency rooms—and many require a little to no laboratory equipment or medical training.

There are two types of RDTS: 1. Flow-through RDT and 2. Lateral flow RDT

Lateral flow tests are the simplest type of RDT, requiring only very minimal familiarity with the test and no equipment to perform, since all of the reactants and detectors are included in the test strip. In a lateral flow test, the sample is placed into a sample well and migrates across the zone where the antigen or antibody is immobilized. The results are read after a certain amount of time has passed. Another type of RDT, a flow-through test, obtains results even faster than lateral flow tests, but requires an added wash and buffer step, which can limit its portability and stability.

Rapid diagnostics tests (RDTs) based on Immunochromatographic antigen detection have been implemented in many diagnostic laboratories as an adjunct to microscopy for the diagnosis of malaria. RDTs consist of capturing soluble proteins by complexing them with capture antibodies embedded on a nitrocellulose strip. A drop of blood sample is applied to the strip and eluted from the nitrocellulose strip by the addition of a few drops of buffer containing a labelled antibody. The antigen–antibody complex can then be visualized directly from the membrane.

In malaria—specific enzymes/antigen secreted by plasmodium parasites in host blood, these antigens are

1. Pf Specific HRP2 (Histidine Rich Protein-II)
2. Pv Specific pLDH (Plasmodium Lactate Dehydrogenase)
3. Pan Specific pLDH (secreted by all malaria causing parasites)

In malaria RDTs these specific antigens to be detected. There are number of RDTs which are available in the market for diagnosis of malaria. In this RDTs various parameters are included, some examples are given below for different parameters.

(a) Rapid test for P. falciparum malaria: Paracheck Pf

Test Principle: Paracheck Pf utilizes the principle of agglutination of antibodies/ antisera with respective antigen in immunochromatography format along with use of nano gold particles as agglutination revealing agent. As the test sample flows through

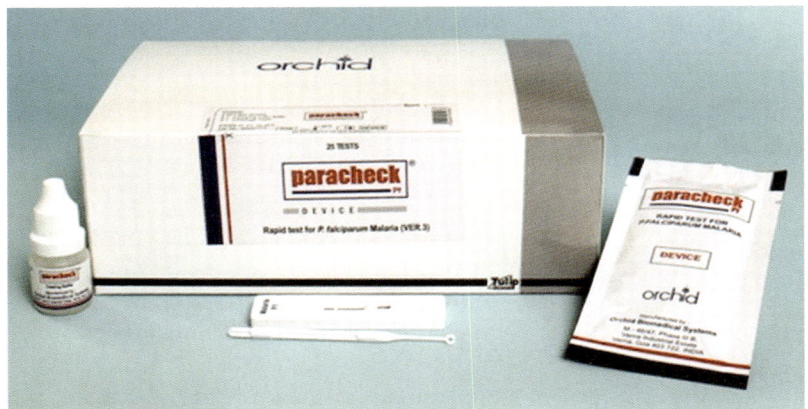

Fig. 10.4: Paracheck

the membrane assembly of the device after addition of the clearing buffer, the colored agglutinating sera for HRP-2-colloidal gold conjugate complexes the HRP-2 in the lysed sample. This complex moves further on the membrane to the test region where it is immobilised by the agglutinating sera for HRP-2 coated on the membrane leading to formation of a colored band which confirms a positive test result. Absence of this colored band in the test region indicates a negative test result.

Specimen use: Whole blood—5 µl

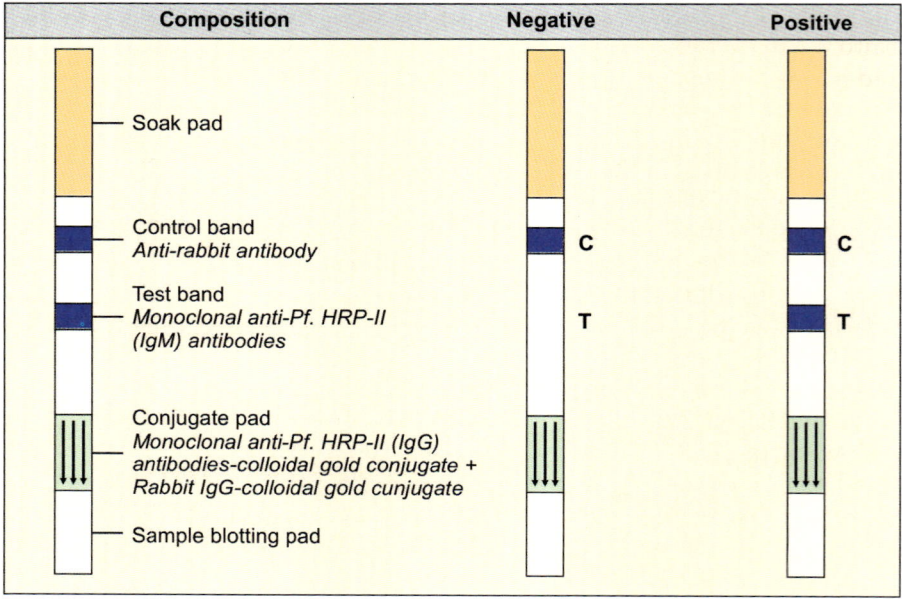

Fig. 10.5: Composition of Pf. HRP-II based assays

Interpretation

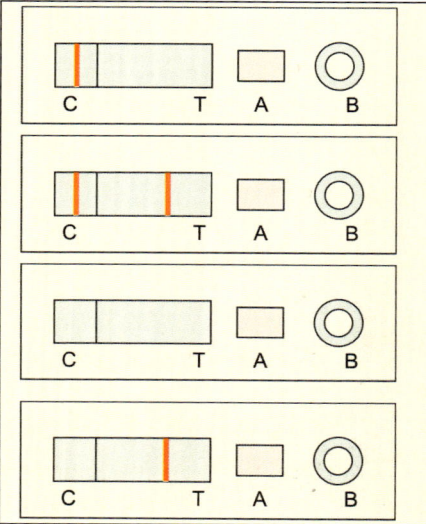

Negative for *P. falciparum* malaria: A colored band appears in control window 'C'.

Positive for *P. falciparum* malaria: In addition to the control band, a distinct colored band also appears in the test window 'T'.

Invalid: The test should be considered invalid if no colored band appears on the device. The test should also be considered invalid if a colored band appears only at the test window 'T' and not at the control window 'C'. In such cases, repeat the test with a new device, ensuring that the test procedure has been followed accurately.

(b) Rapid test for malaria (PAN), e.g. Parabank

Principle: Parabank utilizes the principle of agglutination of antibodies/antisera with respective antigen in immunochromatography format along with use of nano gold particles as agglutination revelling agent. As the test sample flows through the membrane assembly of the device after addition of the clearing buffer, the coloured agglutinating sera for Pan Malaria specific pLDH-colloidal gold conjugate complexes the protein in the lysed sample. This complex moves further on the test membrane to test region where it get immobilised by agglutinating sera for Pan malaria specific pLDH coated on the membrane leading to formation of pink-purple colour band which confirms positive test result. Absence of these colored band in the test region considered a negative test result.

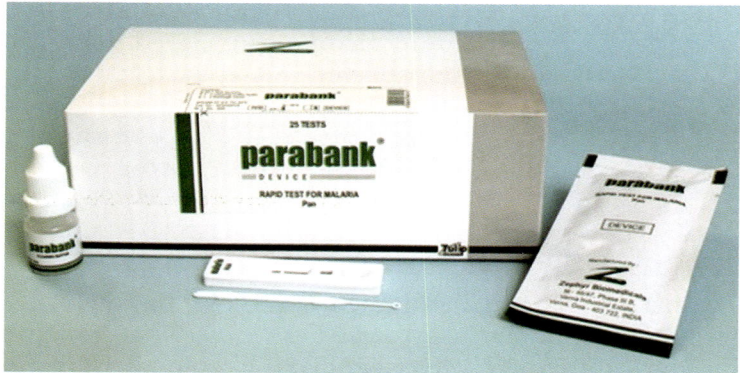

Fig. 10.6: Parabank

Specimen use: Whole blood—5 μl

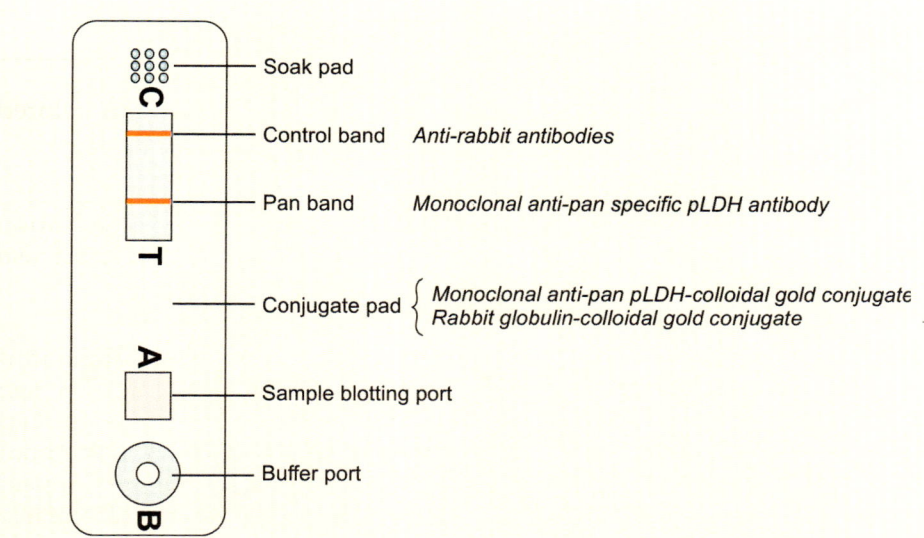

Fig. 10.7: Design and composition of parabank (device)

Interpretation

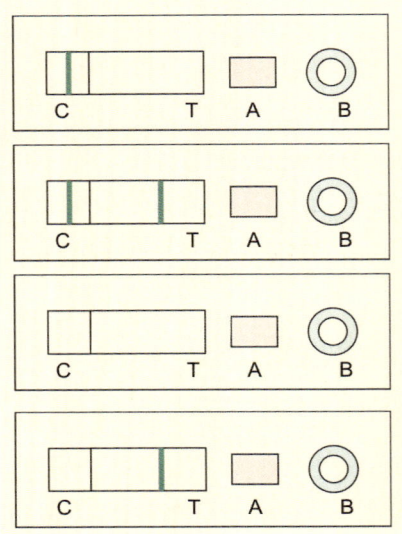

Negative for malaria: A colored band appears in control window 'C'.

Positive for malaria: In addition to the control band, a distinct colored band also appears in the test window 'T'.

Invalid: The test should be considered invalid if no colored band appears on the device. The test should also be considered invalid if a colored band appears only at the test window 'T' and not at the control window 'C'. In such cases, repeat the test with a new device, ensuring that the test procedure has been followed.

(c) Rapid test for malaria (PAN/Pf), e.g. Malascan Plus

A rapid test for malaria Pf and Pan which is a rapid, self-performing, qualitative, two-site sandwich immunoassay, utilising whole blood for the detection of *P. falciparum* specific histidine rich protein-2 (Pf. HRP-2) and Pan specific pLDH. The test may also be used for differentiation of *P. falciparum* and other malarial species in whole blood samples.

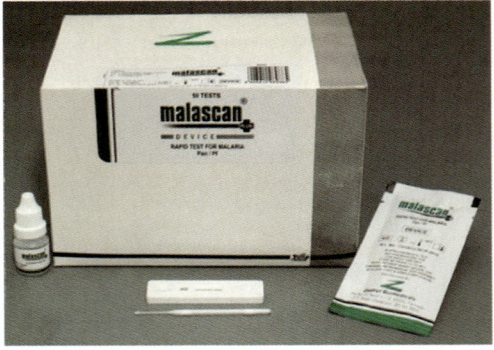

Fig. 10.8: Malascan

Test Principle: Utilizes the principle of immunochromatography. As the test sample flows through the membrane assembly of the device after addition of the clearing buffer, the colored monoclonal anti-Pf. HRP-2 (IgG) specific / monoclonal anti-Pan specific colloidal gold conjugate antibodies complexes the proteins in the lysed sample. This complex moves further on the membrane to the test region where it is immobilised by the monoclonal anti-Pf. HRP-2 (IgM) / monoclonal anti-Pan specific antibody coated on the membrane leading to formation of pink-purple colored band/s which confirms a positive test result. While both the bands will appear at the test region in falciparum positive samples, only one band will appear in non-falciparum malaria positive samples. Absence of this colored band/s in the test region indicates a negative test result.

Interpretation

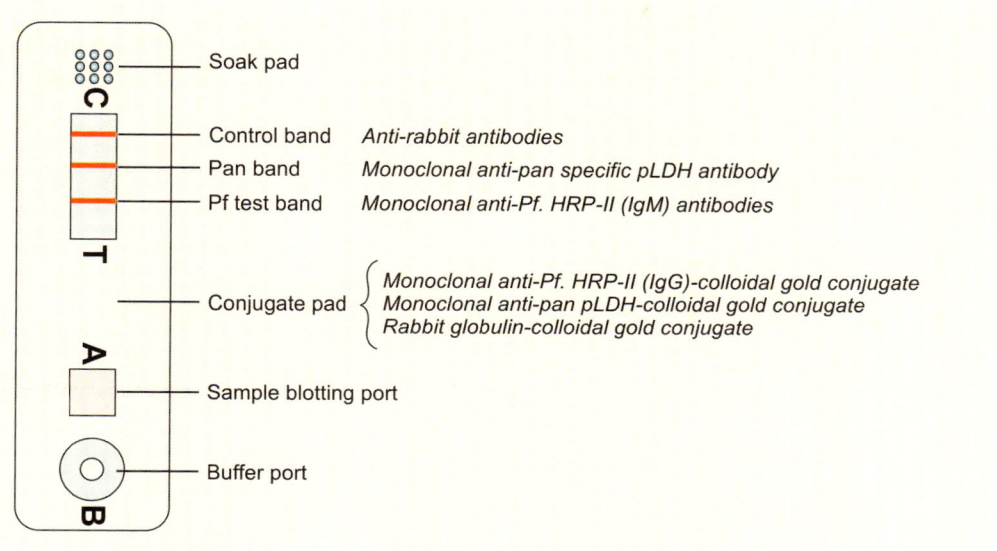

Fig. 10.9: : Design and composition of malascan plus (device)

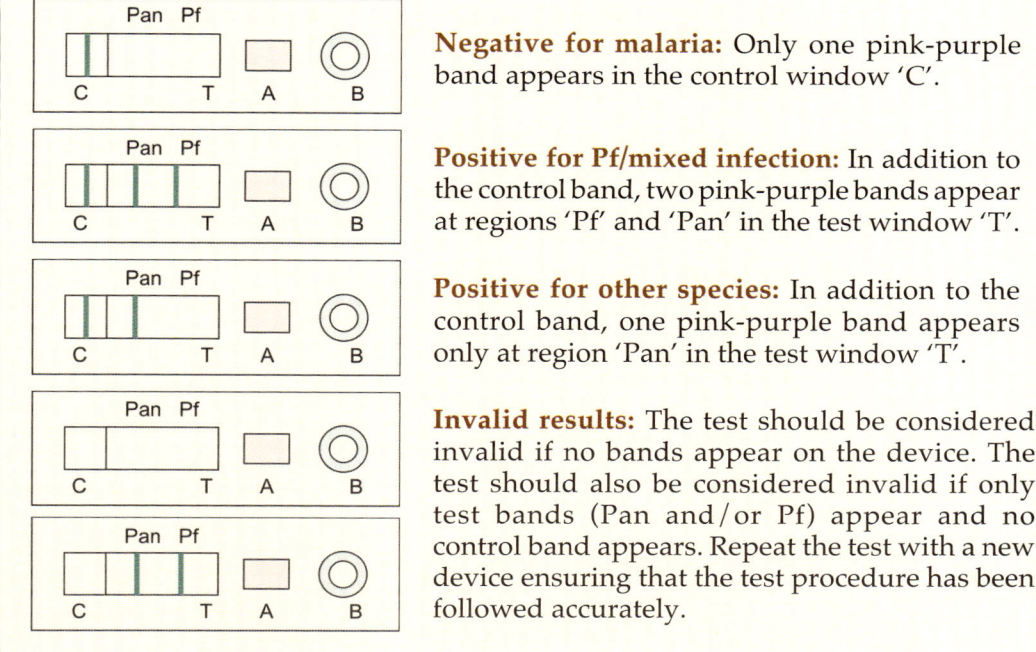

Negative for malaria: Only one pink-purple band appears in the control window 'C'.

Positive for Pf/mixed infection: In addition to the control band, two pink-purple bands appear at regions 'Pf' and 'Pan' in the test window 'T'.

Positive for other species: In addition to the control band, one pink-purple band appears only at region 'Pan' in the test window 'T'.

Invalid results: The test should be considered invalid if no bands appear on the device. The test should also be considered invalid if only test bands (Pan and/or Pf) appear and no control band appears. Repeat the test with a new device ensuring that the test procedure has been followed accurately.

(d) Rapid test for malaria Pv/Pf, e.g. FalciVax

Test Principle: Utilizes the principle of immunochromatography. As the test sample flows through the membrane assembly of the device after addition of the clearing buffer, the colored colloidal gold conjugates of monoclonal anti-Pf. HRP-2 (IgG) antibody and monoclonal anti-Pan specific pLDH antibody complexes the HRP-2/pLDH in the lysed sample. This complex moves further on the membrane to the test region where it is immobilized by the anti-vivax specific pLDH (monoclonal) antibody and/or the monoclonal anti-Pf. HRP-2 (IgM) antibody coated on the membrane leading to formation of pink-purple colored band/s which confirms a positive test result. A band will appear under Pf at the test region in falciparum positive samples, while a band will appear under Pv in vivax malaria positive samples. Appearance of band under Pf as well as Pv in the test region suggests a mixed infection. Absence of colored band/s in the test region indicates a negative test result.

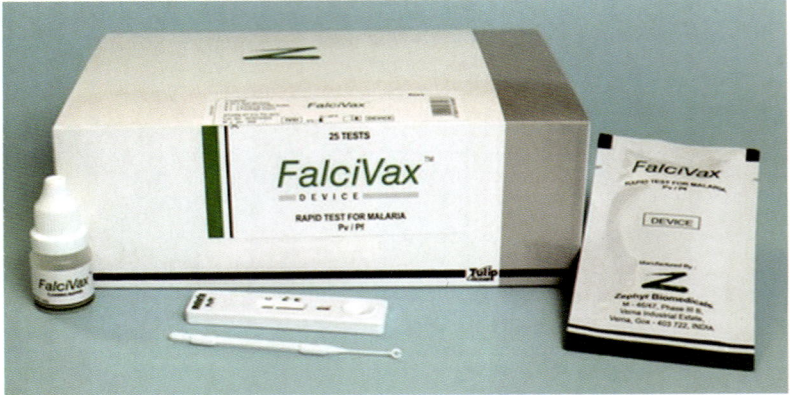

Fig. 10.10: FalciVax

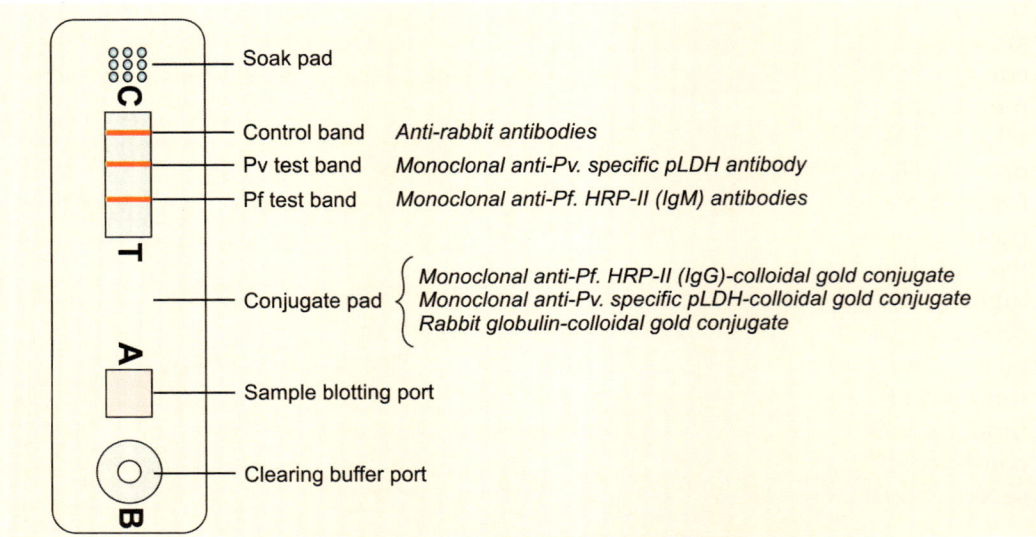

	Soak pad	
C		
	Control band	*Anti-rabbit antibodies*
	Pv test band	*Monoclonal anti-Pv. specific pLDH antibody*
	Pf test band	*Monoclonal anti-Pf. HRP-II (IgM) antibodies*
T		
	Conjugate pad	*Monoclonal anti-Pf. HRP-II (IgG)-colloidal gold conjugate* *Monoclonal anti-Pv. specific pLDH-colloidal gold conjugate* *Rabbit globulin-colloidal gold conjugate*
A		
	Sample blotting port	
	Clearing buffer port	
B		

Fig. 10.11: Design and composition of FalciVax

Interpretation

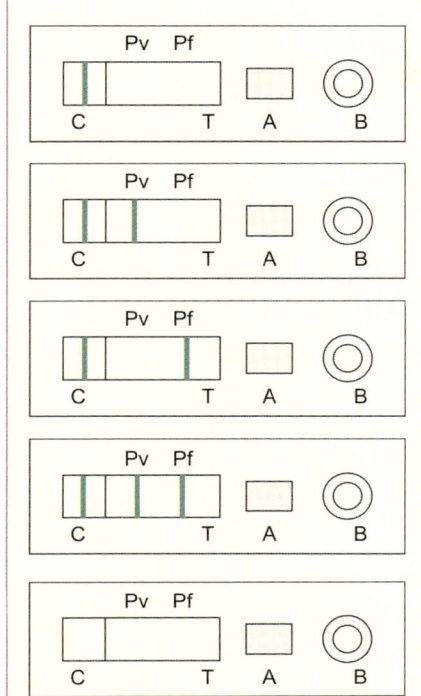

Negative for malaria: Only one pink-purple band appears in the control window 'C'.

Positive for Pv malaria: In addition to the control band, a pink-purple band also appears under the region marked 'Pv' in the test window 'T'.

Positive for Pf malaria: In addition to the control band, a pink-purple band also appears under the region marked 'Pf' in the test window 'T'.

Positive for mixed infection: In addition to the control band, two pink-purple bands appear under the regions marked 'Pf' and 'Pv' in the test window 'T'.

Invalid results: The test should be considered invalid if no bands appear on the device. Repeat the test with a new device ensuring that the test procedure has been followed accurately.

5. Rapid test for malaria Pv/Pf, e.g. Paramax 3

Test Principle: Utilizes the principle of immunochromatography. As the test sample flows through the membrane assembly of the device after addition of the clearing buffer, the colored colloidal gold conjugates of monoclonal anti-Pf. HRP-2 (IgG) antibody and monoclonal anti-pan specific pLDH antibody complexes the HRP-2/corresponding pLDH in the lysed sample. This complex moves further on the membrane to the test region where it is immobilised by the monoclonal anti-Pf. HRP-2 (IgM) antibody and/or monoclonal anti-*P. vivax* specific pLDH antibody and/or monoclonal anti-Pan specific pLDH antibody coated on the membrane leading to formation of a pink-purple colored band in the respective regions which confirms a positive test result. Absence of a colored band in the test region indicates a negative test result for the corresponding antigen. The unreacted conjugate along with the rabbit globulin-colloidal gold conjugate and unbound complex if any, move further on the membrane and are subsequently immobilised by anti-rabbit antibodies coated on the membrane at the control region, forming a pink-purple band. The control band formation is based on the 'Rabbit/anti-Rabbit globulin' system. Since it is completely independent of the analyte detection system, it facilitates formation of consistent control band signal independent of the analyte concentration. This control band serves to validate the test performance.

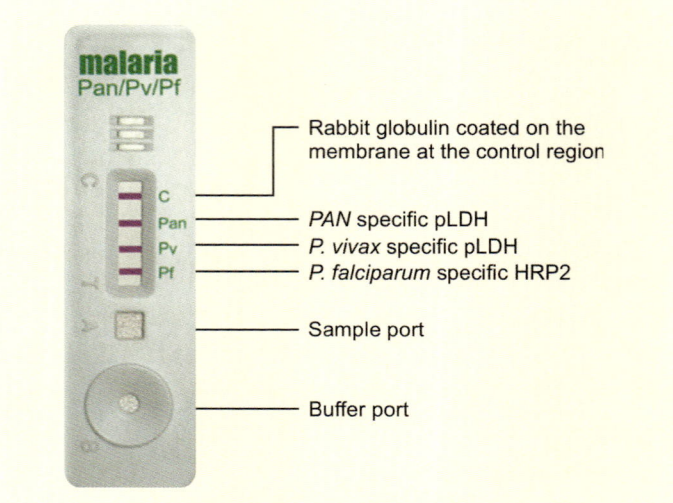

Fig. 10.12: Design and composition of Paramax 3

Interpretation

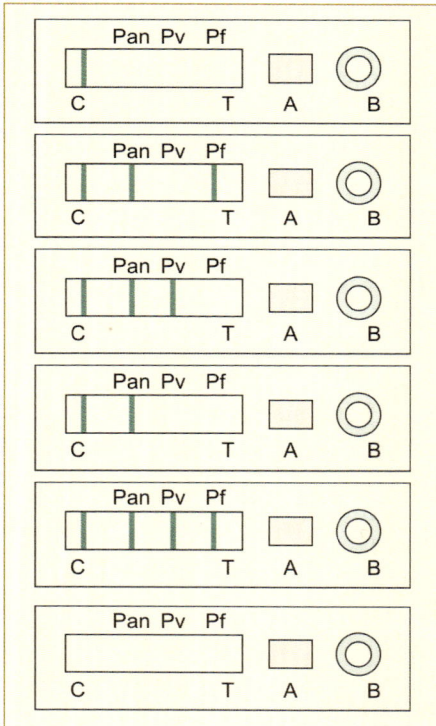

Negative for malaria: Only one pink-purple band appears at the control region 'C'.

Positive for Pf: In addition to the control band, two pink-purple bands appear at regions 'Pf' and 'Pan' respectively.

Positive for Pv: In addition to the control band, two pink-purple bands appear at regions 'Pv' and 'Pan' respectively.

Positive for other species: In addition to the control band, a pink-purple band appears only at region 'Pan'.

Positive for mixed infection: In addition to the control band, three pink-purple bands appear at regions 'Pf', 'Pv' and 'Pan' respectively.

Invalid results: The test should be considered invalid if no bands appear on the device. Repeat the test with a new device ensuring that the test procedure has been followed accurately.

2. Enzyme-linked immunosorbent assay (ELISA)

ELISA (enzyme-linked immunosorbent assay) is a Microwell based assay technique designed for detecting and quantifying substances such as peptides, proteins, antibodies and hormones. Other names, such as enzyme immunoassay (EIA), are also used to describe the same technology. In ELISA, an antigen must be immobilized on a solid surface and then complexed with an antibody that is linked to an enzyme. Detection is accomplished by assessing the conjugated enzyme activity via incubation with a substrate to produce a measureable product. The most crucial element of the detection strategy is a highly specific antibody–antigen interaction.

ELISAs are typically performed in a 96-well (or 192-well) polystyrene plates, which passively bind antibodies and proteins. Having the reactants of the ELISA immobilized to the microwell surface makes it easy to separate bound from non-bound material during the assay. This ability to wash away non-specifically bound materials makes the ELISA a powerful tool for measuring specific analytes within a crude preparation.

ELISA formats

ELISAs can be performed with a number of modifications to the basic procedure. The key step, immobilization of the antigen of interest, can be accomplished by direct adsorption to the assay plate or indirectly via a capture antibody that has been attached to the plate. The antigen is then detected either directly (labelled primary antibody) or indirectly (labelled secondary antibody). The most powerful ELISA assay format is the sandwich assay. This type of capture assay is called a "sandwich" assay because the analyte to be measured is bound between two primary antibodies—the capture antibody and the detection antibody. The sandwich format is used because it is sensitive and robust.

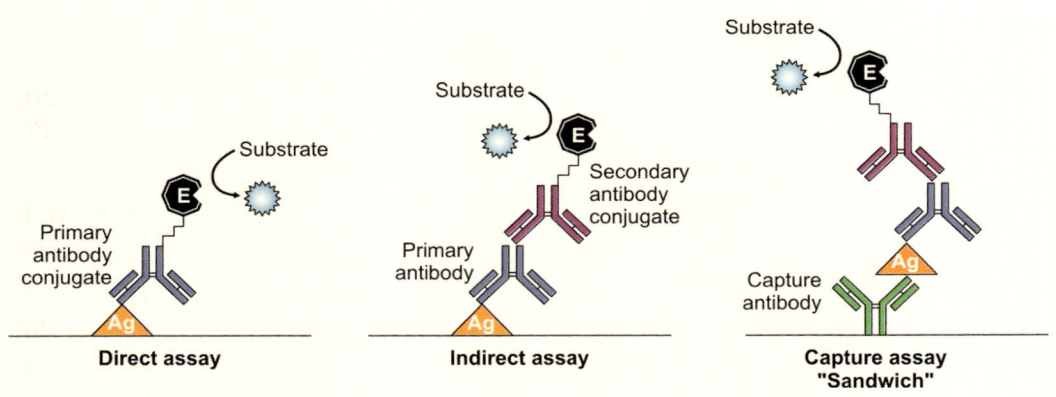

Fig. 10.13: Diagram of common ELISA formats (direct vs. sandwich assays). In the assay, the antigen of interest is immobilized by direct adsorption to the assay plate or by first attaching a capture antibody to the plate surface. Detection of the antigen can then be performed using an enzyme-conjugated primary antibody (direct detection) or a matched set of unlabeled primary and conjugated secondary antibodies (indirect detection).

Irrespective of the method by which an antigen is captured on the plate (by direct adsorption to the surface or through a pre-coated "capture" antibody, as in a sandwich ELISA), it is the detection step (as either direct or indirect detection) that largely determines the sensitivity of an ELISA.

The direct detection method uses a labelled primary antibody that reacts directly with the antigen. Direct detection can be performed with an antigen that is directly immobilized on the assay plate or with the capture assay format. Direct detection while not widely used in ELISA is quite common for immunohistochemically staining of tissues and cells.

The indirect detection method uses a labelled secondary antibody for detection and is the most popular format for ELISA. The secondary antibody has specificity for the primary antibody. In a sandwich ELISA, it is critical that the secondary antibody be specific for the detection of primary antibody only (and not the capture antibody) or the assay will not be specific for the antigen. Generally, this is achieved by using capture and primary antibodies from different host species (e.g. mouse IgG and rabbit IgG, respectively). For sandwich assays, it is beneficial to use secondary antibodies that have been cross-adsorbed to remove any secondary antibodies that might have affinity for the capture antibody.

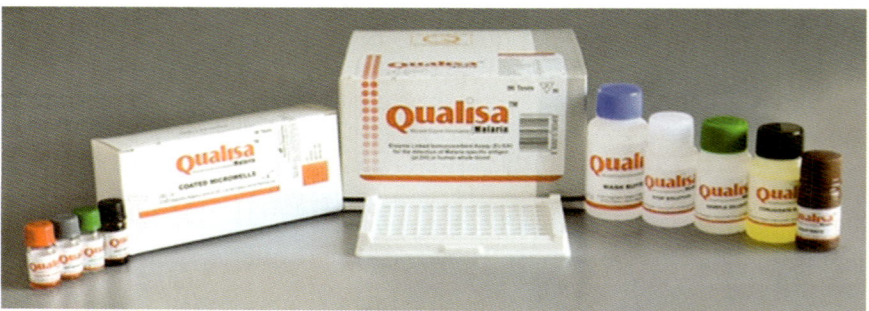

Fig. 10.14: Qualisa

There are some examples given below of ELISA for routine malaria diagnosis by antigen detection, e.g. enzyme linked immunosorbent assay (ELISA) for the detection of malaria specific antigen (pLDH) in human blood, e.g. Qualisa Malaria.

Test Principle: Agglutinating sera for Pan Malaria specific pLDH is coated onto the wells of the microtiter strips. Samples are pipetted into the wells for binding to the agglutinating sera for Pan Malaria specific pLDH. After extensive washing to remove unbound material, pLDH is recognized by the addition of a biotinylated-agglutinating sera for pan malaria specific pLDH. After removal of excess biotinylated-agglutinating sera for pan malaria specific pLDH, streptavidin-peroxidase is added. Following a final washing, peroxidase activity is quantified using the substrate solution based on 3, 3′, 5, 5′-tetramethylbenzidine (TMB) and hydrogen peroxide (H_2O_2). The intensity of the colour reaction is measured at 450 nm after acidification and is directly proportional to the concentration of pLDH in the samples.

Interpretation of results
(1) Samples with absorbance value less than the cut off value are considered non-reactive by Qualisa Malaria and are considered negative for malaria.
(2) Samples with absorbance value equal to or greater than cut off value are considered reactive by Qualisa malaria ELISA kit. The original sample should be retested in duplicate. Initially reactive sample that do not react in either of duplicate are considered negative for malaria. Initially reactive sample that reacts in either or both duplicates are considered repeatedly reactive.
(3) If a sample is repeatedly reactive the probability of malaria infection is high, especially with patients at high risk or high absorbance values. Such samples should be retested with microscopy of thick smear and thin blood films.

(4) In case of samples with high OD, there are possibilities of black precipitate formation after the addition of stop solution. This will not interfere with the interpretation of results.

3. Chemiluminescence immune assay (CLIA)

The term *Chemiluminescence* was first coined by Leichardt Weidman (1888). Chemiluminescence, which is the phenomenon observed when the vibronically excited product of an exoergic reaction relaxes to its ground state with emission of photons, can be defined in simplistic terms: Chemical reactions that emit light. The chemical reaction produces energy in sufficient amount (approximately 300 kJ mol 1 for blue light emission and 150 kJ mol 1 for red light emission) to induce the transition of an electron from its ground state to an excited electronic state. This electronic transition is often accompanied by vibrational and rotational changes in the molecule.

In organic molecules, transitions from a π bonding to a π^* anti-bonding orbital ($\pi\rightarrow\pi^*$) or from a non-bonding to an anti-bonding orbital ($n\rightarrow\pi^*$) are most frequently encountered. Return of the electron to the ground state with emission of a photon is thus called chemiluminescence. The excited molecule can also lose energy by undergoing chemical reactions, by collisional deactivation, internal conversion or inter-system crossing. These radiation less processes are undesirable from an analytical point of view when they compete with chemiluminescence.

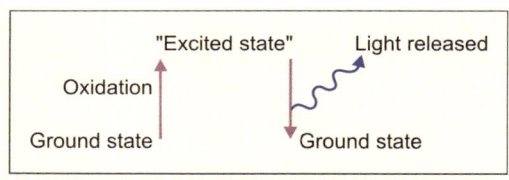

Fig. 10.15: Chemiluminescence

or

When two molecules react chemically so that there is a release of energy (an exothermic reaction), that energy sometimes manifests itself not as heat but as light. This occurs because the energy excites the product molecules into which it has been funnelled. A molecule in this excited state either relaxes to the ground state, with the

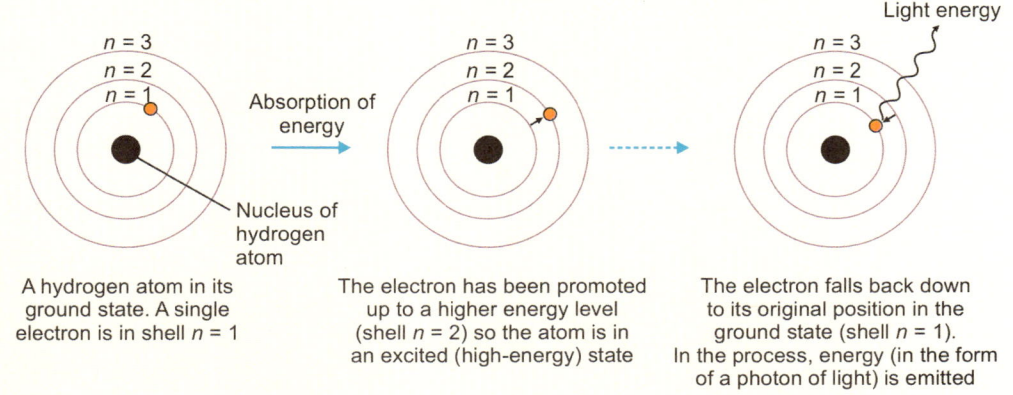

Fig. 10.16: Exothermic reaction

direct emission of light, or transfers its energy to a second molecule, which becomes the light emitter. This process is referred to as chemiluminescence.

$$A + B \rightarrow AB^* \rightarrow Products + Light$$

Chemiluminescent reactions can be grouped into three types:

1. Chemical reactions using synthetic compounds and usually involving a highly oxidized species such as a peroxide are commonly termed chemiluminescent reactions.
2. Light-emitting reactions arising from a living organism, such as the firefly or jelly-fish, are commonly termed bioluminescent reactions.
3. Light-emitting reactions which take place by the use of electrical current are designated electro-chemiluminescent reactions.

Chemiluminescent and bioluminescent reactions usually involve the cleavage or fragmentation of the O-O bond, an organic peroxide compound. Peroxides, especially cyclic peroxides, are prevalent in light emitting reactions because the relatively weak peroxide bond is easily cleaved and the resulting molecular reorganization liberates a large amount of energy.

Principle of CLIA

In the presence of complimentary antigen and antibody, the paratopes of the antibody binds to the epitope of the antigen to form an antigen–antibody or an immune complex. Estimating the levels of such immune complex by use of labelled antibodies form the basis of CLIA. It involves use of stationary solid phase coated either with the antigen or antibody of interest. Addition of conjugate and post-incubation, which ensures intact immune complexes are formed, substrate is added. This results in generation

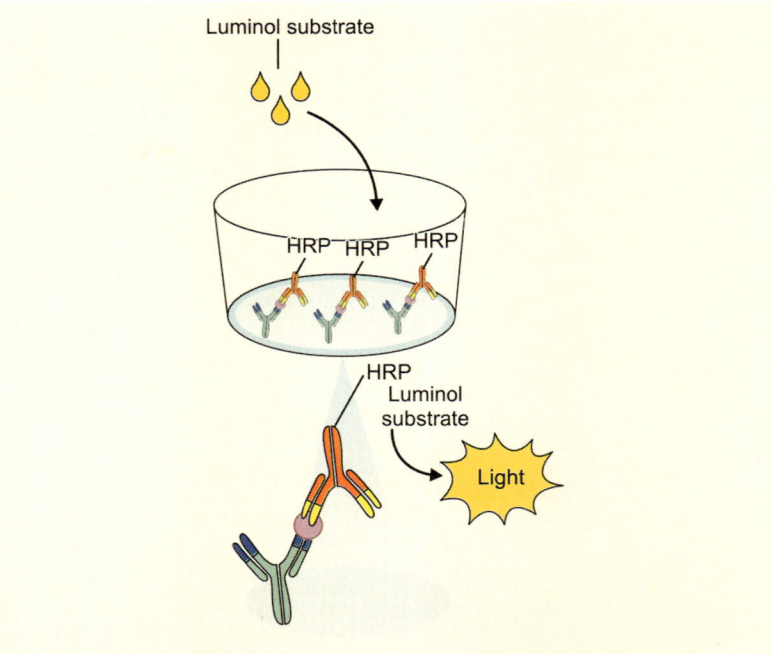

Fig. 10.17: : Diagrammatic representation of principle of CLIA

of light, the intensity of which is directly proportional to the amount of labelled complexes present and which indirectly aids in quantification of the analyte of interest. The intensity of light is measured in terms of relative light units. For example, chemiluminescence assay for the detection of malaria specific antigen (pLDH) in human blood.

For example, Electra Mal Ag—The Electra MAL Ag CLIA assay is for use on Electra SA and Electra FA analysers'. Electra MAL Ag CLIA works on the principle of chemiluminescence wherein light is produced by a chemical reaction from a substance as it returns from an electronically excited state to the ground state. When catalysed by HRP, the oxidation of luminol by hydrogen peroxide produces an electronically excited form of 3-aminiphthalate which on relaxation emits light with maximum intensity at $\lambda = 425$ nm.

TM Electra MAL Ag CLIA micro-well strips are coated with agglutinating sera for pan malaria specific pLDH. Samples are pipetted into the wells for binding to the agglutinating sera for pan malaria specific pLDH. After extensive washing to remove unbound material, pLDH is recognized by the addition of a biotinylated-agglutinating serum for pan malaria specific pLDH. After removal of excess biotinylated-agglutinating sera for pan malaria specific pLDH, streptavidin-peroxidase is added. After washing wells to remove unbound enzyme, chemiluminescent substrate is added. The bound enzyme converts substrate to a reaction product that emits a photon of light.

Chemiluminescence is measured in relative light units (RLU) that is typically proportionate to the amount of analyte present in the sample. The presence or absence of analyte in the sample is determined by comparing the sample RLU with Cut-off TM which is calculated by Electra SA and Electra FA analysers' and expressed as Electra cut off index (ECI). ECI is equivalent to S/CO ratio which is calculated by using sample RLU and calculated cut off of the specific testing batch. Samples with ECI values greater than or equal to 1.00 are considered reactive and samples with ECI values less than 1.00 are considered non-reactive.

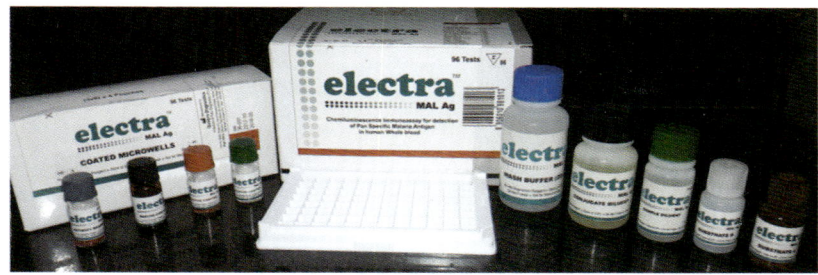

Fig. 10.18: Electra MAL Ag

Interpretation
1. Results are interpreted in ECI. This is determined by dividing the RLU of the sample by the Cut off value calculated for that specific run.
2. Samples with ECI values greater than or equal to 1.00 are considered reactive and samples with ECI values less than 1.00 are considered non-reactive.
3. Samples that are initially reactive in Electra MAL Ag CLIA should be retested in duplicate. Repeated reactivity is highly predictive malaria infection.
4. A grey zone of ± 10% is recommended.

PCRs—an Aid to Diagnose Parasitic Diseases

The Polymerase Chain Reaction (PCR) is a technique discovered by Dr. Kary B. Mullis in 1985 to synthesize multiple copies of a specific fragment of DNA from a template. The PCR reaction consists of cycling the DNA through three specific temperatures in a buffer solution consisting of the template, primers, nitrogenous bases and enzymes. PCR is now a common as well as the most indispensable technique used in medical laboratory and clinical laboratory research for a broad variety of applications including biomedical research and criminal forensics.

Principle of PCR

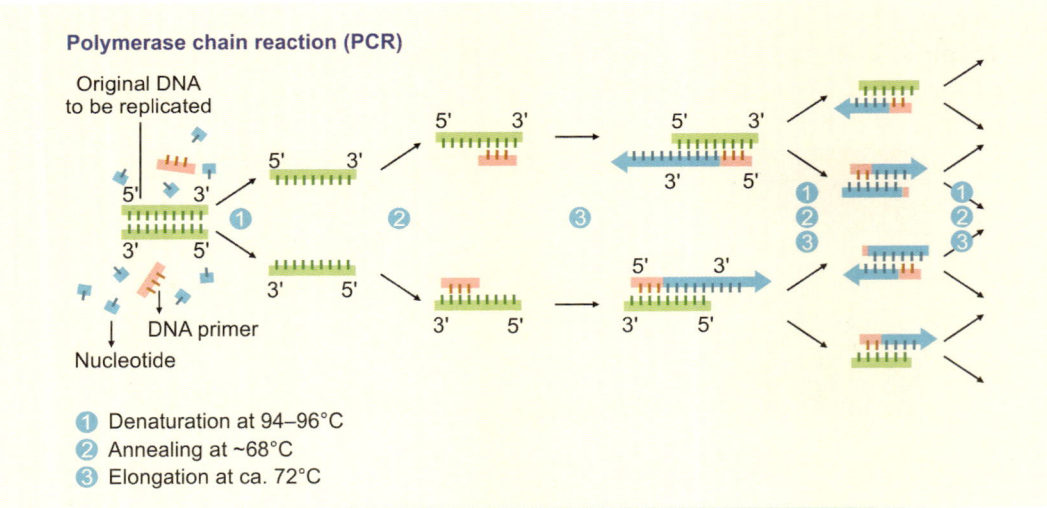

Fig. 11.1: Steps in PCR (*Courtesy*: Wikipedia)

Almost all the PCR methods are based on thermal cycling wherein the reactants in a PCR are exposed to repeated cycles of heating and cooling to allow different temperature dependent steps to proceed continuosly at the specified temperatures. PCR comprises two main reagents, namely primers and DNA polymerase. Primers or oligonucleotides are short single stranded DNA fragments having complementary sequence to that of the target DNA strand. DNA polymerase is an enzyme that helps in the addition and extension of the new DNA strand. Almost all PCR applications employ a heat-stable DNA polymerase, known as Taq polymerase, an enzyme originally isolated from the thermophilic bacterium *Thermus aquaticus*. This enzyme is a heat stable enzyme. Apart from these two main components, PCR also comprises a PCR buffer, magnesium chloride and dNTPS (deoxyribonucleotide triphosphate).

PCR consists of 3 steps:

Denaturation: Wherein the double-stranded template DNA is heated to separate it into two single strands. This is accomplished by heating the starting DNA template at 95°C.

Annealing: The temperature at which primers bind or anneal to the template DNA strand. During the annealing step the temperature is lowered from 95°C to around 58–60°C. In this step the primers will anneal to the DNA template strand.

Extension: In this step the temperature is raised to around 72°C so that the DNA polymerase can add nucleotides onto the annealed end of the primers and extends the strand to give a new strand.

These three cycling steps of denaturation, annealing and extension are repeated to around 40–45 cycles to obtain millions of copies of DNA. The number of copies doubles after each cycle.

Types of PCR

There are many types of PCR based on the various kinds of requirements.

1. **RT-PCR or Reverse Transcription PCR:** It is used to reverse-transcribe and amplify RNA to cDNA

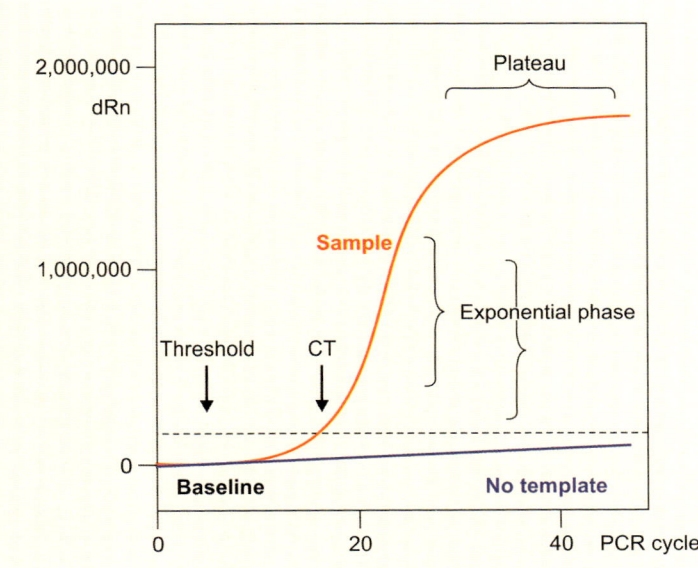

Fig. 11.2: Depiction of real time PCR plot

[*Courtesy*: NPTEL (National Programme on Technology Enhanced Learning)]

2. **Real Time PCR or Quantitative PCR (qPCR):** Real-time or quantitative PCR (qPCR) is used for the amplification of DNA in a linear manner in order to quantify absolute or relative amounts of target sequence in a sample. With the help of a fluorescent reporter, the amount of generated DNA can be measured. In qPCR, DNA amplification is monitored at each cycle of PCR. When the DNA is getting amplified logarithmically at each cycle, the amount of fluorescence increases over the basal level. The thermal cycle at which the signal exceeds the fluorescence detection threshold is known as the **Threshold cycle** (C_T) or crossing point. A standard curve of log concentration against C_T can be made by making use of multiple dilutions of a known amount of standard DNA. The quantity of DNA or cDNA in an unknown sample can thus be determined from its C_T value.

Different chemistries are used for detection by qPCR:

   (a) Use of an intercalating dye like the SYBR® Green I dye which incorporates between the base pairs of DNA. This detection method is suitable when the PCR reaction generates a specific product, as the dye is capable of intercalating into any double-stranded DNA product (Fig. 11.3).

   (b) Use of primer or short oligonucleotide specific to the target of interest, as in TaqMan® probes, Molecular Beacons™, or Scorpion primers (Fig. 11.4). In case of molecular Beacons, they are labeled with a fluorescent dye or quencher and do not exhibit any significant fluorescence in the free, unhybridized condition. But upon binding to the template, the probe becomes fluorescent as the quencher gets distanced from the fluorescent reporter. The amount of PCR product amplified is directly proportional to the amount of fluorescence.

   (c) *Taqmann probe-based detection:* While in the case of TaqMan® probes, fluorescence occurs when the dye is clipped from the probe during the polymerase extension (Fig. 11.5).

3. **Ligation-mediated PCR:** It uses small DNA oligonucleotide 'linkers' (or adaptors) that are first ligated to fragments of the target DNA.

4. **Methylation-specific PCR (MSP):** It is used to identify patterns of DNA methylation at cytosine-guanine (CpG) islands in genomic DNA.

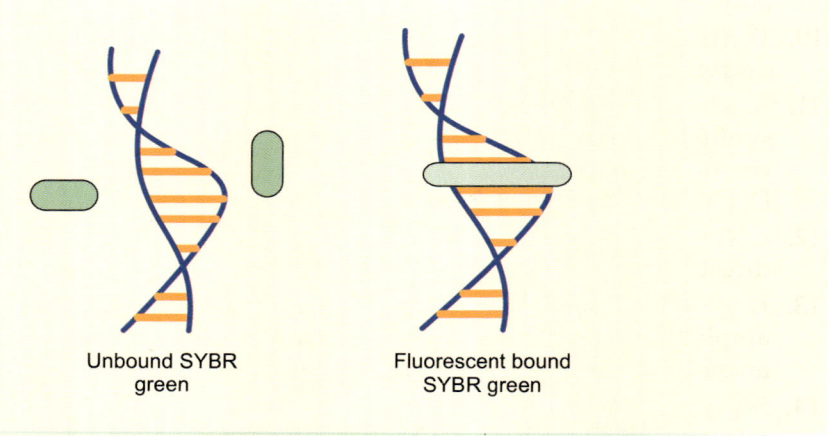

Unbound SYBR green

Fluorescent bound SYBR green

Fig. 11.3: Mechanism of attachment of SYBR green dye to DNA
[*Courtesy*: NPTEL (National Programme on Technology Enhanced Learning)]

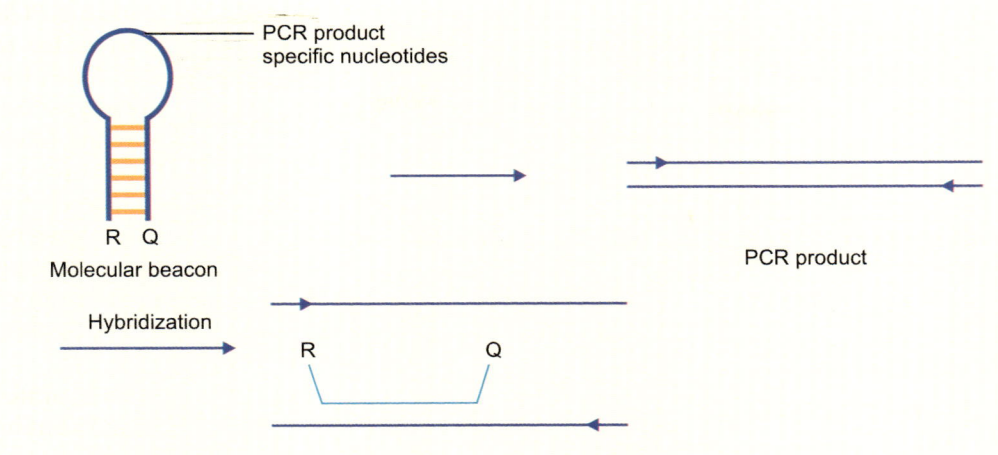

Fig. 11.4: Molecular Beacon-based PCR detection
[*Courtesy*: NPTEL (National Programme on Technology Enhanced Learning)]

5. **Multiplex-PCR:** It uses several pairs of primers annealing to different target sequences.
6. **Variable number of tandem repeats (VNTR) PCR:** It targets areas of the genome that exhibit length variation.
7. **Asymmetric PCR:** It preferentially amplifies one strand of the target DNA.
8. **Nested PCR:** It is used to increase the specificity of DNA amplification. Two sets of primers are used in two successive reactions. In the first PCR, one pair of primers is used to generate DNA products, which may contain products amplified from non-target areas. The products from the first PCR are then used as template in a second PCR, using one ('hemi-nesting') or two different primers whose binding sites are located (nested) within the first set, thus increasing specificity.
9. **Hot-start PCR:** It is a technique performed manually by heating the reaction components to the DNA melting temperature (e.g. 95 °C) before adding the polymerase.
10. **Touchdown PCR:** In this technique, the annealing temperature is gradually decreased in later cycles.
11. **Assembly PCR (also known as polymerase cycling assembly or PCA):** It is the synthesis of long DNA structures by performing PCR on a pool of long oligonucleotides with short overlapping segments, to assemble two or more pieces of DNA into one piece.
12. **Colony PCR:** It is the technique in which the bacterial colonies are screened directly by PCR, for example, the screen for correct DNA vector constructs.
13. **Digital polymerase chain reaction:** It is the technique where simultaneously amplification of thousands of samples is done, each in a separate droplet within an emulsion.
14. **Suicide PCR:** It is typically used in paleogenetics or other studies where avoiding false positives and ensuring the specificity of the amplified fragment is the highest priority. The method prescribes the use of any primer combination only once in

a PCR (hence the term "suicide"), which should never have been used in any positive control PCR reaction, and the primers should always target a genomic region never amplified before in the lab using this or any other set of primers.

15. **COLD-PCR (co-amplification at lower denaturation temperature-PCR):** It is a modified protocol that enriches variant alleles from a mixture of wildtype and mutation-containing DNA.

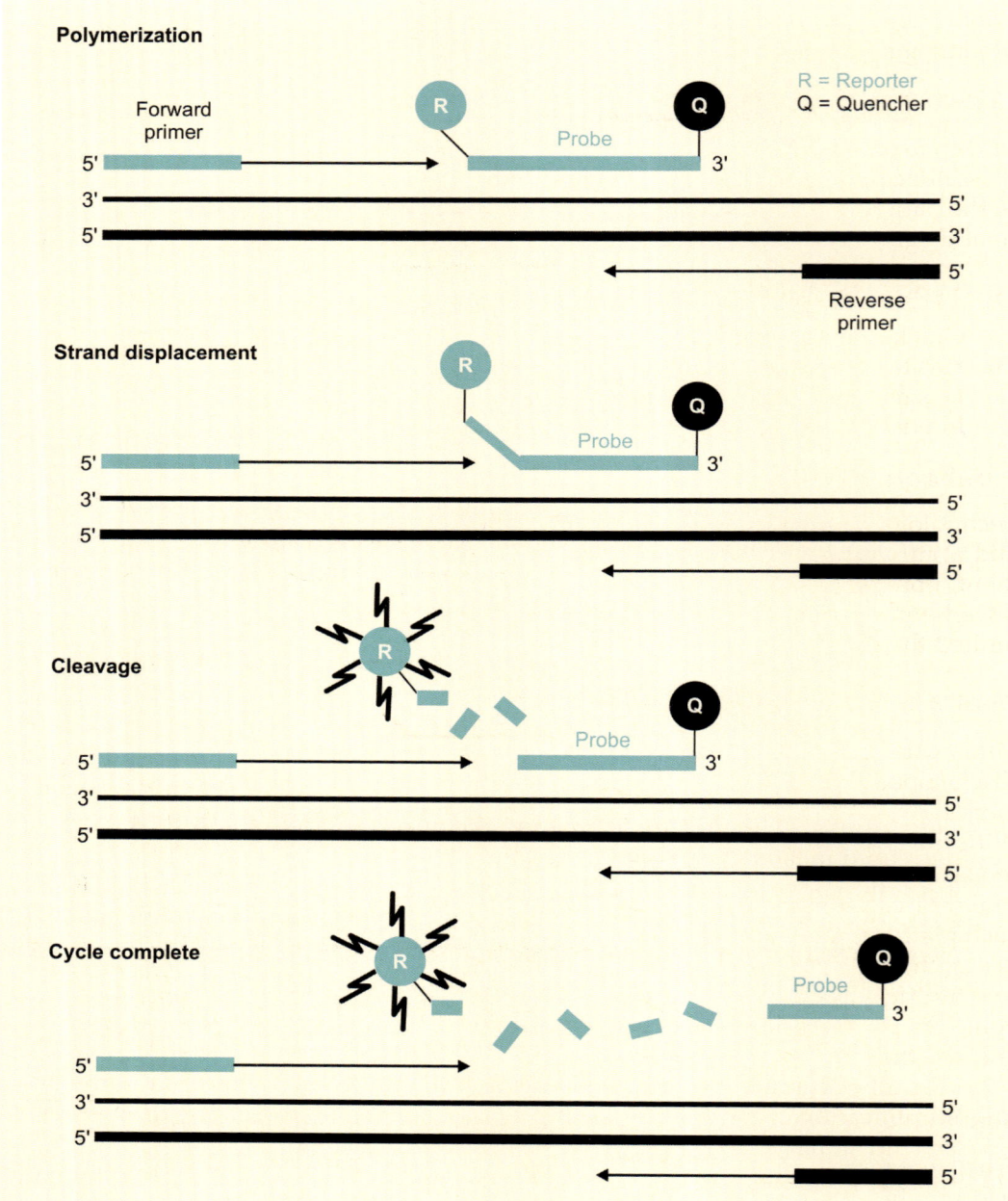

Fig. 11.5: Taqmann probe-based PCR detection (*Courtesy*: Wikipedia)

APPLICATIONS OF PCR

PCR technique has vast applications. It can be used for DNA cloning application for sequencing, gene cloning and manipulation, gene mutagenesis; construction of DNA-based phylogenies, functional analysis of genes, diagnosis and monitoring of hereditary diseases, amplification of ancient DNA, analysis of genetic fingerprints for DNA profiling (for example, in forensic science and parentage testing), and finally it has a huge impact in the detection of pathogens for infectious disease diagnosis.

Current State of Diagnosis

In the current scenario, most of the doctors are not aware of tests that can diagnose these infections on day 1 of infection. Early diagnosis helps in faster and better recovery of the patient. Presumptive/provisional diagnosis requires 24–72 hrs for results and final diagnosis. But the current requirement is for precise and quick diagnosis.

Advantages of PCR over Conventional Techniques

a. Quick, accurate, more sensitive and specific
b. Has fast turnaround time as compared to other tests such as culture
c. Has more wider application such as detecting infectious diseases, genetic testing, forensics, drug resistance, and tumor marker detection and monitoring.

Drawbacks of PCR

Technologies based upon the polymerase chain reaction (PCR) method are specific and accurate but due to other drawbacks such as the high cost of the PCR equipment, non-portability, requirement of additional infrastructure such as a need for a well-equipped lab with air conditioned facility, well-trained technician, etc has limited the usage of PCR for pathogen diagnosis.

What is the Current Requirement

Miniaturization of the PCR platform would confer advantages in terms of portability, ease of operation, reduction in instrument cost, faster turnaround times and enhancement in the availability and accessibility of PCR tests in resource-poor geographies. With the combined advantages of affordability, simplicity in operation, diagnostic sensitivity and portability, micro-PCR devices qualify as strong candidates for POC (point of care diagnosis) for wide-scale applications. Truelab™ workstation is one such platform meeting all these requirements. The ICMR (Indian Council of Medical Research) has issued a certificate of approval for the Truelab™ platform after extensive multicentric validation of the device for tuberculosis and RIF resistance detection. This platform has been installed successfully in many of the public health sector units by the Government of India.

Truelab Workstation

Truelab™ workstation is a simple hand held, battery operated, easy to carry nucleic acid amplification workstation consisting of lightweight, portable, mains / battery operated **Truelab™ Uno Dx** Real Time micro PCR Analyzer, **Trueprep™ AUTO** Sample Prep Device, room temperature stable **Truenat™** micro PCR chips and

Trueprep™ AUTO Sample Prep kits. It is a portable system for amplification and reporting of results in less than an hour. Even the peripheral laboratories with minimal infrastructure and minimally trained technician can easily perform these tests routinely in their facilities and report PCR results in less than an hour.

Truenat™ micro PCR chip is a disposable, room temperature stable, chip-based Real Time PCR test with dried down PCR reagents for performing Real Time PCR test for detection and diagnosis of specific pathogens and runs on the **Truelab™ Uno Dx** Real Time micro PCR Analyzer. It requires only 6 μL of purified DNA/RNA to be added to the reaction well for the analysis. The intelligent chip also carries test and batch related information including standard values for quantitation. The **Truenat™** micro PCR chip also stores information of used test to prevent any accidental re-use of the test.

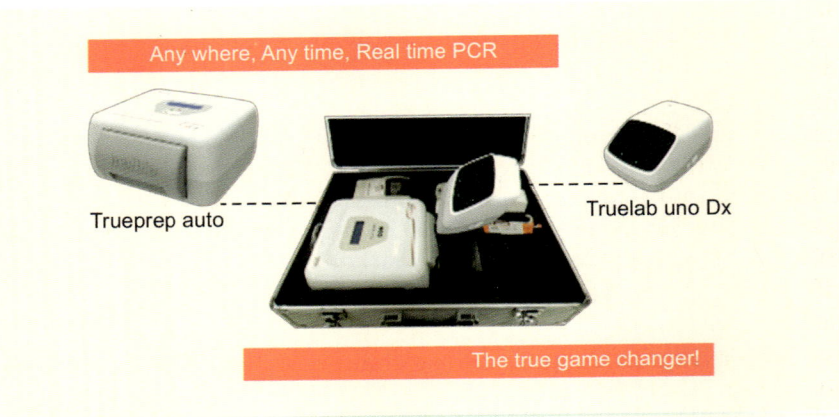

Fig. 11.6: Truelab™ workstation (*Courtesy:* Molbio diagnostics)

List of tests available using Truelab™ platform			
MTB	Dengue/Chikungunya	NG	HAV
MTB plus	Dengue	Trichomonas	HEV
MTB RIF	Chikungunya	GBS	HIB
MTB INH	Zika	MRSA	PA
MTB FQ	Malaria PV/PF	Influenza A/B	Rabies
MTB/NTM	Salmonella	HLA-B27	*Streptococus pneumoniae*
HIV 1	HPV	Nipah	*Neisseria meningitides* (Nm)
HBV	CT/NG	H3N2/H1N1	Nm/SP
HCV	CT	H1N1	Staph/PA
			Staph/MRSA

Types of Parasitic Infections that can be Diagnosed by PCR

PCR can be used for the diagnosis of parasites such as malaria (*Plasmodium falciparum, Plasmodium vivax*), Leishmania, *Toxoplasma gondii*, etc.

Standard Operation Procedure (SOP) for Detection of Malaria Pf/Pv on Truelab™ Platform

1. Intended use

Truenat™ Malaria Pf/Pv is a chip-based Real Time Polymerase Chain Reaction (qPCR) test for the quantitative detection and diagnosis of *Plasmodium falciparum* Pf and Pv in human blood specimen and aids in the diagnosis of infection with malaria caused by *Plasmodium falciparum* and *Plasmodium vivax*. Truenat™ malaria Pf/Pv runs on Treulab™ Uno Dx real time micro PCR analyzer.

2. Introduction

Malaria is a life-threatening disease caused by the protozoan parasite, *Plasmodium falciparum*/ *Plasmodium vivax* which is transmitted via the bite of an infected female Anopheles mosquito. In the human body, the parasites multiply in the liver, and then infect red blood cells. *Plasmodium falciparum* is known to cause the most dangerous malignant malaria which has the highest rate of complications and mortality. Early and accurate diagnosis of Falciparum malaria is necessary to initiate appropriate treatment, check transmission of the disease and prevent death. Microscopic examination of stained blood smears is still considered as the "gold standard" for detection of malaria parasitemia. However, in comparison to PCR methods, these are reported to be only 80–90% sensitive. Nested PCR and real time PCR present higher sensitivity and specificity to malaria diagnosis compared to light microscopy. However, PCR or Real Time PCR tests have so far been restricted to centralized reference laboratories as they require skilled manpower and elaborate infrastructure. Also the turnaround time for results could take a few days.

Truenat™ Malaria Pf/Pv is a disposable, room temperature stable, chip-based Real Time PCR test with dried down PCR reagents for performing Real Time PCR test for detection and diagnosis of Pf/Pv Malaria and runs on the Truelab™ Uno Dx Real Time micro PCR Analyzer. It requires only 6 µL of purified DNA to be added to the reaction well for the analysis. The intelligent chip also carries test and batch related information including standard values for quantitation. The Truenat™ Malaria Pf/Pv chip also stores information of used test to prevent any accidental re-use of the test.

The Truelab™ Uno Dx Real Time micro PCR Analyzer enables decentralization and near patient diagnosis and detection of Pf/Pv malaria by making real time PCR technology rapid, simple, robust and user friendly and offering "sample to result" capability even at resource limited settings. This is achieved through a combination of lightweight, portable, mains/ battery operated Truelab™ Uno Dx Real Time micro PCR Analyzer and Trueprep™ AUTO Sample Prep Device and room temperature stable Truenat™ micro PCR chips and Trueprep™ AUTO Sample Prep kits so that even the peripheral laboratories with minimal infrastructure and minimally trained technician can easily perform these tests routinely in their facilities and report PCR results in less than an hour. Moreover, with these devices PCR testing can also be initiated in the field level, on site.

3. Principle of the test

Truenat™ Malaria Pf/Pv works on the principle of Real Time Polymerase Chain Reaction (real time PCR) based on Taqman chemistry. Truenat™ Malaria Pf/Pv is a disposable, room temperature stable, micro PCR chip with dried down PCR reagents for performing Real Time PCR test for Pf/Pv and runs on the **Truelab™ Real Time micro PCR Analyzer**. It requires only 6 µL of purified DNA/RNA to be added to the reaction well for the analysis. The **Truenat™ Malaria Pf/Pv** chip is then inserted in the **Truelab™ Uno Dx Real Time micro PCR Analyzer** where further thermal cycling takes place. The intelligent chip also carries test and batch related information. The **Truenat™ Malaria Pf/Pv** chip also stores information of used chips to prevent any accidental re-use of the chip.

A positive amplification causes the dual labeled fluorescent probe in the **Truenat™ Malaria Pf/Pv** chip to release the fluorophore in an exponential manner which is then captured by the built-in opto-electronic sensor and displayed as amplification curve on the analyzer screen, on a real time basis during the test run. The cycle threshold (Ct) is defined as the number of amplification cycles required for the fluorescent signal to cross the threshold (i.e. exceed the background signal). Ct levels are inversely proportional to the amount of target nucleic acid in the sample (i.e. the lower the Ct level, the greater is the amount of target nucleic acid in the sample). In the case of negative samples, amplification does not occur and a horizontal amplification curve is displayed on the screen during the test run. At the end of the test run, Pf/Pv "DETECTED" or "NOT DETECTED" result is displayed. Based on the detection of the internal positive control (IPC), the validity of the test run is also displayed. The IPC is a full process control that undergoes all the processes the specimen undergoes—from extraction to amplification, thereby validating the test run from sample to result. Absence of or shift of IPC Ct beyond a pre-set range in case of negative samples invalidates the test run. While IPC will co-amplify in most positive cases also, in some specimen having a high target load, the IPC may not amplify, however, the test run is still considered valid. The results can be printed using the **Truelab™ micro PCR printer** or transferred to the lab computer/ or any remote computer via Wifi network or GPRS network. Up to 5000 test results can be stored on the analyzer for future recall and reference.

4. Contents of the Truenat™ Malaria Pf/Pv Kit

A. Individually sealed pouches, each containing
   1. **Truenat™ Malaria Pf/Pv** micro PCR chip.
   2. DNAse and RNAse free pipette tip.
   3. Desiccant pouch.

REF	601020005	601020020
σ	5T	20T

B. Package Insert

5. Contents of the Trueprep™ AUTO Universal Sample Pre-treatment Pack (only for Trueprep™ AUTO users)

   1. Lysis buffer.
   2. Disposable transfer pipette (graduated).

6. Storage and stability

Truenat™ Malaria Pf/Pv is stable for one year from the date of manufacture if stored between 2° and 30°C. It is also stable for up to 1 month at temperatures up to 40°C. Avoid exposure to light or elevated temperatures (above recommended levels).

Trueprep™ AUTO Universal Sample Pre-Treatment Pack is stable for 2 years from the date of manufacture if stored between 2° and 30°C. It is also stable for 4 weeks at temperatures up to 45°C. Do not freeze.

7. Materials required

Truelab™ Real Time micro PCR Workstation along with Truenat™ micro PCR chips and **Trueprep™ AUTO** Sample Prep kits

8. Specimen preparation for extraction with Trueprep™ Auto

Truenat™ Malaria Pf/Pv requires purified nucleic acids from blood specimen that are extracted using the **Trueprep™ AUTO** Universal Cartridge based Sample Prep Device and **Trueprep™ AUTO** Universal Cartridge based Sample Prep kit. Sample must be pre-treated using **Trueprep™ AUTO** Universal Sample Pre-treatment pack. Transfer 250 µl of blood specimen using the transfer pipette provided into the Lysis buffer tube provided and mix well.

9. Sample storage and transportation

Sample pre-treatment decontaminates the specimen and makes it ready for storage/transportation/extraction. The specimen in this form is stable for up to 3 days at 40°C and 1 week at 30°C.

Nucleic acid extraction: Use entire content from the Lysis Buffer tube containing specimen for further procedure with the **Trueprep™ AUTO** Universal Cartridge Based Sample Prep Device and **Trueprep™ AUTO** Universal Cartridge Based Sample Prep Kit.

10. Safety precautions

1. For *in vitro* diagnostic use only.
2. Bring all reagents and specimen to room temperature (20–30°C) before use.
3. Do not use kit beyond expiry date.
4. Carefully read the User Manuals and package inserts of all the components of the Truelab™ Real Time micro PCR System before use.
5. All materials of human origin should be handled though potentially infectious
6. Do not pipette any material by mouth.
7. Do not eat, drink, smoke, apply cosmetics or handle contact lenses in the area where testing is done.
8. Use protective clothing and wear disposable gloves when handling samples and while performing sample extraction.

11. Procedural precautions

1. Check all packages before using the kit. Damage to the packaging does not prevent the contents of the kit from being used. However, if the outer packaging is damaged the user must confirm that individual components of the kit are intact before using them.

2. Do not perform the test in the presence of reactive vapours (e.g. from sodium hypochlorite, acids, alkalis or aldehydes) or dust.
3. While retrieving the **Truenat™ Malaria Pf/Pv micro PCR** and the DNAse and RNAse free pipette tip from the pouch, ensure that neither bare hands nor gloves that have been used for previous tests run are used.

12. Procedural limitations

1. Optimal performance of this test requires appropriate specimen collection, handling, storage and transport to the test site.
2. Though very rare, mutations within the highly conserved regions of the target genome where the **Truenat™** assay primers and/or probe bind may result in the under-quantitation of or a failure to detect the presence of the concerned pathogen.
3. The instruments and assay procedures are designed to minimize the risk of contamination by PCR amplification products. However, it is essential to follow good laboratory practices and ensure careful adherence to the procedures specified in this package insert for avoiding nucleic acid contamination from previous amplifications, positive controls, or specimens.
4. A specimen for which the **Truenat™** assay reports "Not Detected" cannot be concluded to be negative for the concerned pathogen. As with any diagnostic test, results from the **Truenat™** assay should be interpreted in the context of other clinical and laboratory findings.

13. Cleaning and decontamination

1. Spills of potentially infectious material should be cleaned up immediately with absorbent paper tissue and the contaminated area should be decontaminated with disinfectants such as 0.5% freshly prepared sodium hypochlorite [10 times dilution of 5% sodium hypochlorite (household bleach)] before continuing work.
2. Sodium hypochlorite should not be used on an acid-containing spill unless the spill-area is wiped dry first. Materials used to clean spills, including gloves, should be disposed off as potentially bio-hazardous waste, e.g. in a biohazard waste container.

14. Test procedure

Step 1: Sample prep using Trueprep™ AUTO

Trueprep™ AUTO Cartridge based universal sample prep device

Testing for infectious diseases by detecting the pathogen's nucleic acid amplification methods is a highly specific and sensitive diagnostic tool. The PCR process necessitates the extraction and purification of nucleic acids from clinical specimens to free it from potential inhibitors. The **Trueprep™ AUTO Cartridge based universal sample prep device** together with **Trueprep™ AUTO sample prep Kit** provides an easy method of nucleic acid extraction and purification.

Trueprep™ AUTO sample prep device is light weight and portable. It operates on mains and/or re-chargeable battery. It is capable of performing 16 sample extractions with one recharge and is fully automatic, with minimal hands on time.

The cartridge based extraction process is quick, reliable and efficient and does not require highly skilled personnel to carry out the extraction process. All the waste from processing of the sample is contained within the cartridge dump area thus posing no risk from potentially hazardous material.

The device has a universal protocol and can work with all kinds of samples such as sputum, whole blood, serum, plasma, tissue, stool, other body fluid samples, swabs and culture specimen.

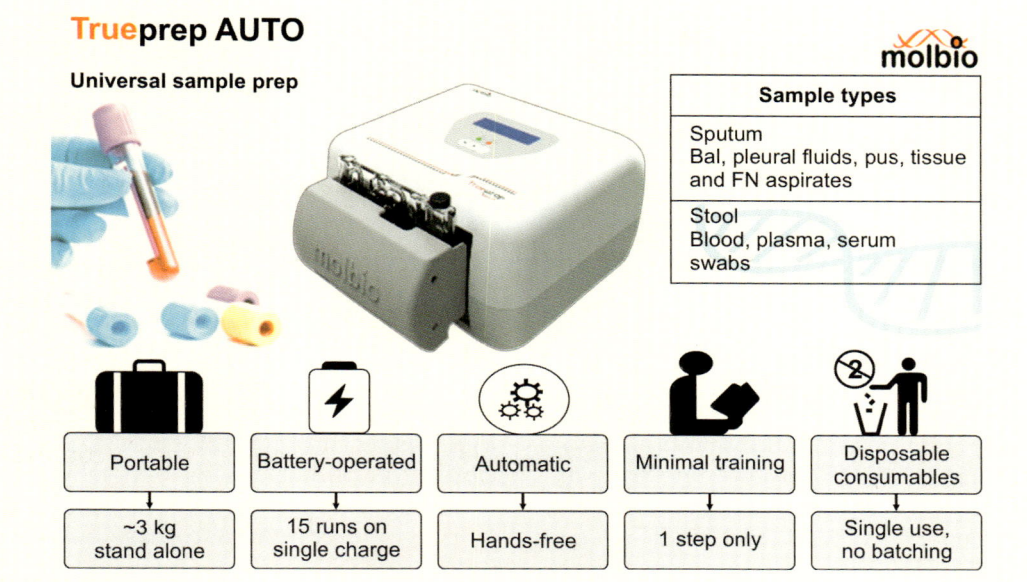

Fig. 11.7: Trueprep™ AUTO sample prep device (*Courtesy:* Molbio diagnostics)

Operating procedure

The **Trueprep™ AUTO** is electromechanical system pre-programmed to sequentially heat, mix and add reagents to the contents of the cartridge placed in the cartridge holder and has a 2-line LCD screen that displays the status.

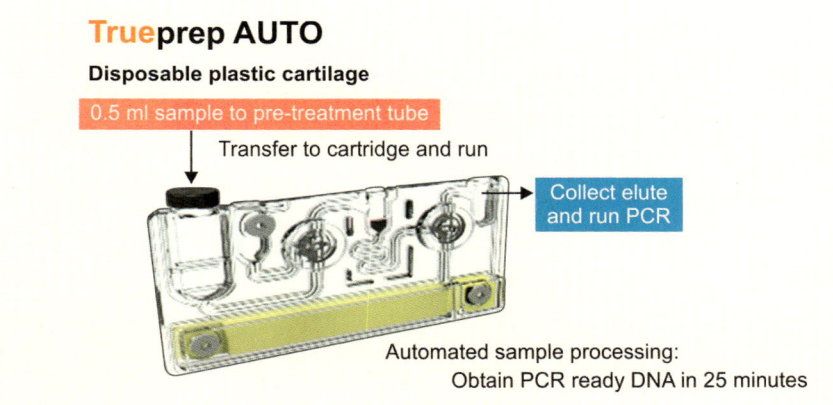

Fig. 11.8: Trueprep™ AUTO sample prep cartridge (*Courtesy:* Molbio diagnostics)

Specimen pre-treated with the lysis reagent is added to the sample chamber of the cartridge which is then placed in the cartridge holder of the device. Sample processing is initiated upon pressing the start button on the device, through an automatic pre-programmed process wherein nucleic acids released by chemical and thermal lysis of cells bind to the proprietary matrix in the matrix chamber. In subsequent steps, the captured nucleic acids are washed with buffers to remove the PCR inhibitors and finally eluted from the matrix using the elution buffer. At the end the cartridge is automatically ejected and the elute, containing purified nucleic acids is then collected from the elute chamber for further analysis.

Step 2: PCR on Truelab™ Uno Dx Real Time micro PCR Analyzer using Truenat™ Malaria Pf/Pv chips

Truelab Uno Dx Real Time Quantitative microPCR Analyzer

The **Truelab™ Uno Dx** is a revolutionary portable and battery-operated PCR analyzer. It houses a touch screen for user interaction, a sliding chip tray for the **Truenat™ Malaria Pf/Pv** microchip, optical detection systems and electronic components that control all aspects of the system. It is infrastructure independent, portable—light weight and rugged system which runs on AC/Battery power with 8 hours back up. It is based on real-time detection and has built-in network data transfer ability. It requires minimal training and easy to use, disposable, individually packed, disease specific chips. It has the data transfer capability using leveraging penetration of mobile network-print, SMS, Wi-Fi, GSM/GPRS and bluetooth transfers. It also has automated disease surveillance capability helping to identify new disease hot-spots quickly. It enables fast, accurate and reliable near-care disease testing.

Operating procedure

1. Switch on the **Truelab™** Analyzer.
2. Proceed to step 3.

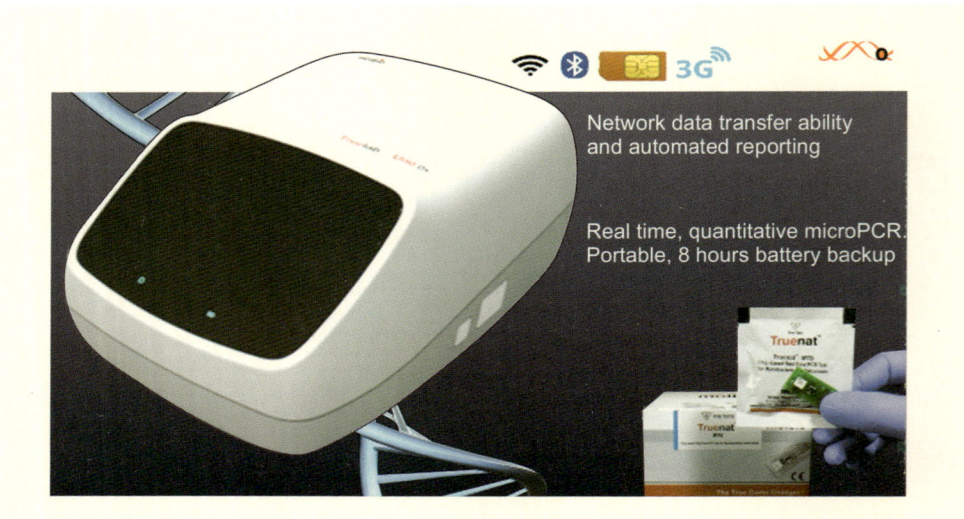

Fig. 11.9: Truelab™ Uno Dx (*Courtesy:* Molbio diagnostics)

3. Select user and enter password.
4. Select the test profile for "MALARIA Pf/Pv" on the Analyzer screen.
5. Enter the patient details as prompted in the **Truelab™** Analyzer screen.
6. Press Start Reaction.
7. Press the eject button to open the chip tray.
8. Open a pouch of **Truenat™ Malaria Pf/Pv** and retrieve the chip-based Real Time PCR test.
9. Label the chip with the patient ID using a marker pen at the space provided on the back side of the chip.
10. Place the **Truenat™ Malaria Pf/Pv** chip-based Real Time PCR test on the chip tray without touching the white reaction well. The reaction well should be facing up and away from the analyzer. Gently press the chip to ensure that it is seated in the chip tray properly.
11. Using the filter barrier tip provided in the pouch, pipette 6 µL of the purified DNA from the Elute Collection Tube into the centre of the white reaction well. Take care not to scratch the internal well surface and not to spill elute on the outside of the well.
12. Slide the chip tray containing the **Truenat™ Malaria Pf/Pv** chip-based Real Time PCR test loaded with the sample, into the **Truelab™ Analyzer**.
13. Press **Done** on the "Please Load Sample" Alert message.
14. Read the result from the screen.
15. Take out the **Truenat™ Malaria Pf/Pv** chip-based Real Time PCR test at end of the test and dispose it off as per the section on "Disposal and Destruction" (Section 15).
16. Turn on **Truelab™** micro PCR printer and select print on the screen for printing out hard copy of the results. Test results are automatically stored and can be retrieved any time later. (Refer to the **Truelab™ Analyzer** manual).
17. Switch off the **Truelab™ Analyzer**.

Truenat™ Malaria PvPf					
Center			Operator	Service	
Profile	Malaria PvPf		Date	Fri 10 Aug 2018 11:59	
Lot	ML005	Expiry Date	05-20	Sample	Blood
Patient Details					
Name	A5L1		ID	A5L1	
Age		Gender	Male	Referred By	test
Result					
Malaria Pv	21.2	Control	27.14	Malaria Pf	18.5
Run Status	Valid				
Malaria Pv			DETECTED	2.0×10^{06} P/uL	
Malaria Pf			DETECTED	1.2×10^{07} P/uL	
Print	SMS	Email	Share	Back	

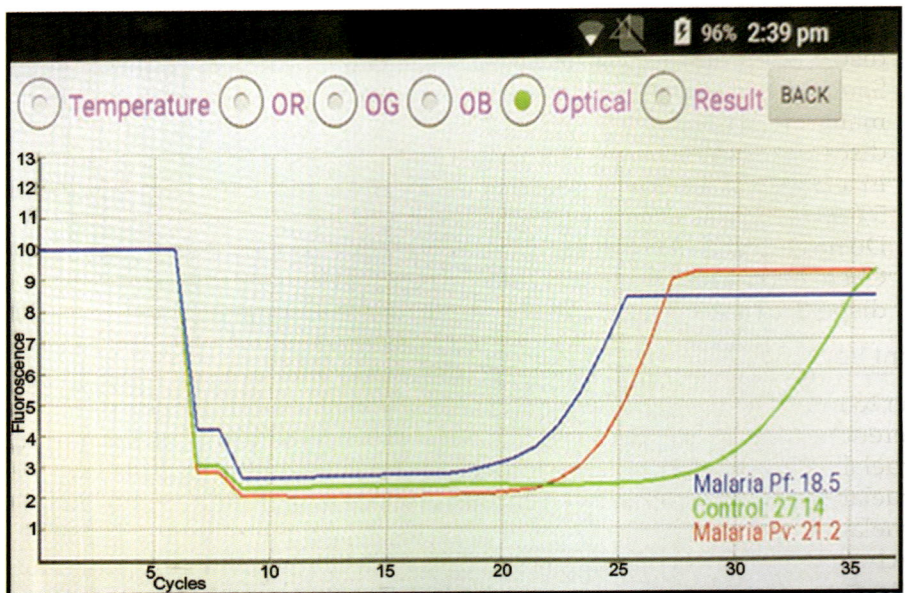

18. **Results and interpretations:** Amplification curves are displayed on the Truelab™ Real Time micro PCR Analyzer screen to indicate the progress of the test. Both the target and the internal positive control (IPC)* curves will take a steep, exponential path when the fluorescence crosses the threshold value in case of positive samples. The Ct will depend on the number of parasite genomes in the sample. The target curve will remain horizontal throughout the test duration and the IPC curve will take an exponential path in case of negative samples. In case the IPC curve remains horizontal in a negative sample, the test is considered as Invalid. At the end of the test run, the results screen will display "DETECTED" for positive result or "NOT DETECTED" for negative result. The result screen would also display the Ct value and the parasites per µL (P/µL) for positive specimen. The result screen also displays the validity of the test run as "VALID" or "INVALID". Invalid samples have to be repeated with fresh specimen from the sample preparation stage. *While IPC will co-amplify in most positive cases also, in some specimen having a high target load, the IPC may not amplify, however, the test run is still considered valid.

19. **Quality control procedures:** To ensure that the Truelab™ Real Time micro PCR Analyzer is working accurately, run positive and negative controls from time to time. The Truenat™ Universal Control Kit containing Positive Control and Negative Control must be ordered separately. It is advisable to run controls under the following circumstances:
    - Whenever a new shipment of test kits is received.
    - When opening a new test kit lot.
    - If the temperature of the storage area falls outside of 2–30°C.
    - By each new user prior to performing testing on clinical specimen.

20. **Disposal and destruction**
    1. Submerge the used **Truenat™ Malaria Pf/Pv** micro PCR chip in freshly prepared 0.5% sodium hypochlorite solution for 30 minutes before disposal as per the standard medical waste disposal guidelines.

2. Disinfect the solutions and / or solid waste containing biological samples before discarding them according to local regulations.
3. Samples and reagents of human and animal origin, as well as contaminated materials, disposables, neutralized acids and other waste materials must be discarded according to local regulations after decontamination by immersion in a freshly prepared 0.5% of sodium hypochlorite for 30 minutes (1 volume of 5% sodium hypochlorite for 10 volumes of contaminated fluid or water).
4. Do not autoclave materials or solutions containing sodium hypochlorite.
5. Chemicals should be handled in accordance with Good Laboratory Practice and disposed off according to the local regulations.

Different Versions of Truelab

In order to meet the increased sample throughout requirements Truelab™ is available in different versions:
(a) Truelab™Uno: Single chip
(b) Truelab™ Duo: Two chips
(c) Truelab™ Quattro: Four chips

Conclusion: Truelab workstation is a revolution in the field of infectious as well as parasitic disease diagnosis.

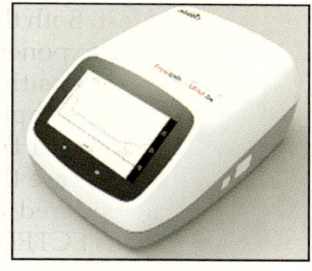   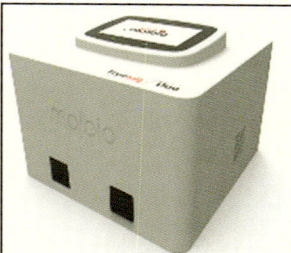   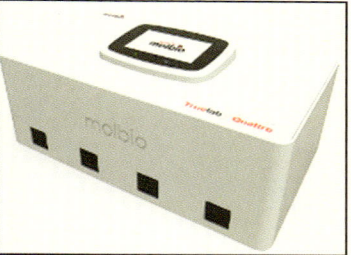

Truelab™ Uno   Truelab™ Duo   Truelab™ Quattro

Fig. 11.10: Various versions of Truelab™ (*Courtesy*: Molbio diagnostics)

BIBLIOGRAPHY

1. Andrade et. al. (2010). Towards a precise test for malaria diagnosis in the Brazilian Amazon: comparison among field microscopy, a rapid diagnostic test, nested PCR, and a computational expert system based on artificial neural networks. Malaria Journal 2010, 9: 117.
2. Angela R. Porta and Edward Enners. (2012). Determining Annealing Temperatures for Polymerase Chain Reaction. The American Biology Teacher, 74(4), 256–60.
3. Bartlett, J. M. S.; Stirling, D. (2003). "A Short History of the Polymerase Chain Reaction". *PCR Protocols. Methods in Molecular Biology*. Methods in Molecular Biology. **226** (2nd ed.). pp. 3–6.
4. J., Ninfa, Alexander; P., Ballou, David (2004). *Fundamental laboratory approaches for biochemistry and biotechnology*. Wiley.
5. "Kary B. Mullis – Nobel Lecture: The Polymerase Chain Reaction".
6. Khairnar K, et al. (2009) Multiplex real-time quantitative PCR, microscopy and rapid diagnostic immuno-chromatographic tests for the detection of *Plasmodium spp*: performance, limit of detection analysis and quality assurance. Malar J 2009, 8:284.
7. Marchand RP, et. al. (2011) Co-infections of *Plasmodium knowlesi*, *P. falciparum*, and *P. vivax* among Humans and Anopheles Mosquitoes, Southern Vietnam. Emerg Infect Dis. Jul 2011; 17(7):1232–9

8. Moody A. (2002) Rapid diagnostic tests for malaria parasites. Clin Microbiol Rev 2002; 15:66–78.
9. Mullis, Kary B. et al. "Process for amplifying, detecting, and/or-cloning nucleic acid sequences" U.S. Patent 4,683,195
10. Perlmann, P. et. al. (2000). Malaria blood-stage infection and its control by the immune system. Folia biologica 46 (6): 210–8.
11. Rich, S. M. et al (2009) The origin of malignant malaria. Proceedings of the National Academy of Sciences 106(35): 14902–7
12. Saiki, R.; Scharf, S.; Faloona, F.; Mullis, K.; Horn, G.; Erlich, H.; Arnheim, N. (1985). "Enzymatic amplification of beta-globin genomic sequences and restriction site analysis for diagnosis of sickle cell anemia". *Science*. **230** (4732): 1350–4.
13. Saiki, R.; Gelfand, D.; Stoffel, S.; Scharf, S.; Higuchi, R.; Horn, G.; Mullis, K.; Erlich, H. (1988). "Primer-directed enzymatic amplification of DNA with a thermostable DNA polymerase. *Science*. **239** (4839): 487–91.
14. Shokoples S.E. et al. (2009). Multiplexed real-time PCR assay for discrimination of *Plasmodium species with* improved sensitivity for mixed infections. J Clin Microbiol 2009, 47:975–80. WHO-FIND-CDC Malaria RDTProduct Testing Methods Manual (Version 1)- 05/2008.

Therapy of Parasitic Infections

AMOEBICIDAL DRUGS

For Luminal/Intestinal Amoebiasis

1. **Berberine (25 mg tablets):** 25–50 mg 2–3 times a day orally. Not used these days. Is contraindicated in cardiac patients, in debilitated patients, in patients with poor respiratory reserve. Side effects include respiratory depression, cardiovascular collapse.

2. **Bialamicol (250 mg tablet):** 250–500 mg thrice daily orally for 5 days. If needed the course may be repeated a month later. Not so commonly used. Side effects include nausea, vomiting, skin rash.

3. **Broxyquinoline (200–500 mg tablet/capsule):** 250–500 mg three times a day orally for 2–3 weeks. Usually given in conjunction with iodochlorhydroxyquinoline. To be avoided in patients with neurological deficit. Side effects include rarely and possibly optic atrophy in the form of subacute myelo-optic neuropathy.

4. **Carbarsone (250 mg capsule):** 250 mg 2–3 times a day orally for 10 days; course can be repeated after a week. This is now an outdated antiamoebic. Contraindicated in hepatic damage, renal damage, cardiovascular disease and optic neuritis. Side effect include urticaria, GIT disturbance, hepatitis.

5. **Di-Iodohydroxyquinoline (300 mg tablet):** 600 mg thrice daily orally for 10–20 days. It should not be used in non-specific diarrhoea, possibility of development of optic neuropathy. Contraindicated in patients allergic to iodine. Often used in conjunction with other antiamoebics like metronidazole. Side effects include skin rash, abdominal discomfort, diarrhoea, headache, pruritus ani, thyroid enlargement, visual disturbances, optic neuritis, furunculosis.

6. **Diloxanide (500 mg tablet):** 500 mg thrice daily orally for 10 days. In children 20 mg/kg body weight orally for 10 days. May be beneficial in acute amoebic dysentry. Another course may be repeated if felt necessary. Side effects include vomiting, pruritus, urticaria, flatulence, transient albu minima.

7. **Emetine Bismuth Iodide (200 mg enteric coated tablet/capsule):** 200 mg once a day orally for 10–12 days. Bed rest advisable. Hospitalisation is ideal. Careful watch on cardiac toxicity needed. Often given in conjunction with tetracycline/diloxanide in acute amoebic dysentery. Side effects include nausea, vomiting, diarrhoea.

Note: Dosages are adult dosages, where not mentioned

8. **Etofamide (200 mg capsule):** 20 mg/kg body weight once daily orally for 3–6 days. It is poorly absorbed from intestine. Side effects include nausea, headache.

9. **Glycobiarsol (500 mg tablet):** 500 mg thrice daily orally for 7–10 days, may be repeated after 2 weeks. Other safer drugs are available. Contraindicated in severe cardiovascular diseases, optic neuritis, hampered renal or hepatic function. Side effects include vomiting, epigastric distress, diarrhoea, intense thirst, tingling sensation in extremites, neuritis, nephritis, dermatitis, pigmentation.

10. **Halquinol (250 mg tablet):** 250–500 mg 3–4 times a day orally for 5 days. Course may repeated after a month. Avoid multiple courses. Side effects include nausea, vomiting, headache, dizziness, dysuria, skin rash, pruritus, rarely neuropathy and optic atrophy.

11. **Iodochlorhydroxyquin (250 mg tablet):** 250 mg 3–4 times a day orally for 7–10 days. Contraindicated in hyperthyroidism, iodine intolerance, impaired renal/hepatic damage. Often used in conjunction with other antiamoebic drugs. Side effects include iodism in susceptible patients, optic neuropathy, sensory disturbances.

12. **Ornidazole (500 mg tablet):** 500 mg twice daily for 5–10 days. Contraindicated in active neurological disorders. Claimed not to induce alcohol intolerance. Side effects include GIT disturbances, dizziness, muscle weakness, drowsiness, skin reactions.

13. **Paromomycin (250 mg capsule):** 25–35 mg/kg body weight. Avoid in patients with renal damage. Side effects include GIT upset, diarrhoea.

14. **Phanquone (50 mg tablet):** 50–100 mg thrice daily orally for 5–10 days. May be repeated after 15 days. Often given in conjunction with other antiamoebics. Side effects are diminished if taken with meals. Side effects include nausea, vomiting, burning sensation in stomach, transient dizziness, dark coloured urine.

For Extraintestinal Amoebiasis Only

Chloroquine (250 mg tablets equivalent to 150 mg base): 300 mg twice daily. Use with caution in patients with impaired hepatic/renal function, psoriasis, GIT upset, neurological and haematological disorders, history of porphyria and in alcoholics. Do not give in conjunction with gold salts, phenylbutazone, triamcinolone. Avoid use in pregnancy. Side effects include haedache, nausea, vomiting, diarrhoea, abdominal cramp, pruritus, rash, ECG changes, hypotension, blurring of vision, rarely corneal opacity, pigment deposits in cornea/retina, alopecia, photosensitvity, blood dyscrasias.

For luminal and extraluminal amoebiasis

1. **Dehydroemetine (60 mg/ml ampoule):** 60 mg deep subcutaneous or intramuscular injection once a day for 7–10 days. May be repeated after two weeks. In children 1 mg/kg body weight/day. Contraindicated in pregnancy and in patients with cardiac/renal disorders; should not be given to patient who have received emetine during the last six weeks. It can be given in conjunction with other amoebicides. It is less toxic than emetine. Side effects include hypotesion, T wave changes in ECG, allergic reaction, depression, painful injection.

2. **Niridazole (100–150 mg tablet):** 25 mg/kg body weight once daily orally for 7–10 days. Avoid in hepatic damage, epilepsy and psychotic disorders. Should not be given with isoniazid. Side effects include agitation, confusion, hallucination, transient ECG changes, oligospennia, haemolytic anaemia, abdominal

discomfort, nausea, vomiting, diarrhoea, anorexia, haedache, skin rash, paraes-thesia, high coloured urine.

3. **Emetine (60 mg/ml ampoule):** 60 mg once a day subcutaneous or intramuscular injection for 10 days. May be repeated after 6 weeks. Contraindicated in cardiac/renal diseases. Avoid in pregnancy and in children. Use with caution in debilitated patients, ECG monitoring during treatment is recommended. Safer drugs are available now. Bedrest, preferably hospitalisation during therapy is essential. Side effects include painful injection, local stiffness, nausea, vomiting, diarrhoea, dizziness, headache, muscle weakness, urticaria, purpuric rash, precordial pain, palpitation, dyspnoea, hypotension, T. wave changes in ECG.

4. **Metronidazole** (200, 400 mg tablets, 100 mg/ml ampoule) 200–400 mg thrice daily orally for 7–10 days. If necessary IV infusion can also be given. It is a widely used antiamoebic agent. Dependable and reasonably safe. Regular check up of blood counts is advisable. Avoid alcohol; contraindicated in CNS disorders and blood dyscrasia. Avoid during first trimester of pregnancy. Reduce dosage in patients with hepatic disease. It increases anticoagulant effect of warfarin. Side effects include nausea, anorexia, diarrhoea, epigastric distress, metallic taste, headache, vomiting, glossitis, stomatitis, skin rash, ataxia, paraesthesia, intolerance to alcohol, reversible neutropenia.

5. **Nimorazole (500 mg tablet):** 500 mg twice daily for 5 days orally. Avoid alcohol consumption during treatment. Keep watch on blood counts. Use with caution in patients with hepatic disease. Side effects include nausea, anorexia, vomiting and dizziness.

6. **Tinidazole (300 mg tablet):** 600 mg twice daily for 5 days orally or 2 gm once a day orally for 3 days. Contraindicated in neurological diseases and blood dyscrasias. Avoid in prenancy and lactating mother. Side effects include nausea, dizziness, headache, dryness of mouth.

7. Newer safer variants like Satronidazole (300 mg tablet to be taken twice daily orally) are also available currently.

Indirect-acting luminal amoebicide

These destroy intestinal bacteria upon which the parasite is dependent for its growth. Tetracycline (oxytetracycline or terramycin and chlortetracycline). Adult dose 250 mg given orally at 6 hourly intervals for 7–12 days. Often prescribed with other amoebicides.

Drugs for Giardiasis

1. **Broxyquinoline:** Same as for amoebiasis.
2. **Di-iodohydroxyquin:** Same as for amoebiasis
3. **Furazolidone (100 mg tablet):** 100 mg 4 times a day orally for 3–5 days. Contra-indicated in hypertension, psychoses. It increases effects of sympathomimetic agents and antidepressant drugs. Avoid use of cheese, alcohol and tyramine during treatment. Side effects include headache, nausea, vomiting, skin rash, haemolytic anaemia, aganulocytosis, alcohol intolerance.
4. **Glycobiarsol:** As for amoebiasis
5. **Metronidazole:** As for amoebiasis
6. **Tinidazole:** 150 mg twice a day for 7 days orally.

7. **Mepacrine (100 mg tablet):** One tablet thrice daily for 3–5 days. For children half a tablet twice daily for 3 days.
8. **Chloroquine:** 300 mg base, once daily for 5 days orally.

Drugs for Trichomoniasis

Ideally both, the husband and the wife, should be treated
1. **Metronidazole:** 200 mg thrice daily for 7 days, may be repeated after 4–6 weeks.
2. **Tinidazole:** 150 mg twice a day for 7 days orally.
   Other drugs that can be used are Quinacrine, Furazolidine, Glycobiarsol, Natamycin, Nimorazole, Orridazole, Quinidochlor, Satronidazole
   Locally applicable pessaries to be inserted into vagina are also used besides systemic medicines.

Drugs for Trypanosomiasis

1. **Benznidazole (100 mg capsule):** 3.5–7 mg/kg body weight once a day for 30–60 days. Start with lower dose. Useful for acute Chagas' disease. It is effective in acute stage only. Therapeutic efficacy in chronic cases is doubtful. Side effect include nausea, vomiting, abdominal pain, skin rash and peripheral neuritis.
2. **Melarsoprol (Mel. B) (3.6% solution in propylene glycol, vial):** 3–6 mg/kg body weight slow intravenous injection daily for 3–4 days. To be repeated after 7 days used as a trypanocidal drug in meningoencephalitic stage of African typanosomiasis. It is an extremely irritating drug. Avoid extravasation. Patient should remain in bed and should not be fed orally for several hours after injection. Hospitalisation of patient is ideal. It is contraindicated during epidemics of influenza, hepatic or renal damage. It is effective even it tryparsamide resistant cases. It can cause haemolytic anaemia in patients with G6PD deficiency. May precipitate erythema nodosum in leprotics. Side effects include fever, encephalopathy, nausea, vomiting, abdominal colic, hypersensitive reaction, agranulocytosis, haemolytic anaemia, peripheral neuropathy, diarrhoea, cardiac arrhythmia, dermatitis, hepatic damage.
3. **Mel. W.** Dosage same as Mel-B but is a water soluble form and can be given intramuscularly. A series of 3–4 days course is given, each daily dose is at a level of 3.6 mg/kg body weight. If necessary can be repeated after a couple of weeks. Rest of the effects same as Mel. B.
4. **Pentamidine:** (dry powder 0.3 gm/vial): 3–4 mg/kg body weight of base by intramuscular injection daily or on alternate days for 10 days. Freshly prepared solution is to be used and be protected from light. Has been used as prophylactic agent in endemic regions. Not useful when CNS is involved by *Trypanosoma rhodesiense*. Side effects include dyspnoea, palpitation, dizziness, fainting, headache, vomiting, pancreatitis, hypoglycaemia (sometimes paradoxical hyperglycemia), renal and hepatic dysfunction.
5. **Nitrofurazone** (500 mg tablet) 1500 mg daily orally (3 divided doses) for 10 days. Course may be repeated after a week (check the progress of the disease by periodic examination of CSF). For children the dose is 30 mg/kg body weight daily in divided doses. The drug is of value in cases refractory to other recognised trypanocides. Side effects include nausea, vomiting, polyneuritis, joint pains, allergic reactions, haemolytic anaemia in G6PD deficient individuals.

6. **Tryparsamide (1 gm vial):** 1–2 gm subcutaneous, intramuscular or intravenous infusion at intervals of 5 to 7 days (total 6–24 g). Useful in African Trypanosomiasis. Always use freshly prepared solution. Keep a close watch on visual function. Contraindicated in retinal diseases optic atrophy and neurosyphilis. Melarsoprol is now preferred over tryparsamide but it can be used with pentamidine or suramin when the condition of the patient is low. Side effects include dizziness, tinnitus, nausea, vomiting, headache, allergic reaction, liver damage, visual defect and even blindness, dermatitis.

7. **Suramin (1 gm vial):** Dissolve this in 10 ml of distilled water and inject intravenously (can be given intramuscularly also). Initial dose should be less (200–500 mg) and thereafter 1 gm every week for 10 weeks. Toxic symptoms include renal damage, polyneuritis and dermatitis.

Antileishmaniasis Drugs

1. **Urea stibamine** (Vial, powder 100 mg/ml) 100–200 mg intravenous injection on alternate days. One course is of 3 g. Freshly prepared solution should be used. Discard if the colour has changed.

2. **Neostibosan:** For adult the daily dose is 0.1 to 0.3 g either intravenously (5% solution) or intramuscularly (25% solution). The course of treatment consists of 8–12 injections. A total of 2.7 to 4 g of the compound is necessary to effect a cure. The number of injections varies in different endemic areas; in India 12, China 18, Mediterranean areas and Sudan 24 injections are generally needed.

3. **Stibogluconate** (vial, 60 ml, 33%) 6 ml (33%) intramuscular injection once a day for 7–10 days may be given for a longer period; may also be locally infiltrated in oriental sore. Avoid in renal or hepatic damage, cardiac patients; less toxic than antimony sodium tartarate, keep a close watch on cardiovascular parameters including ECG changes. Side effects include nausea, vomiting, rarely cardiac toxicity, bradycardia, abdominal pain, pruritus, skin rash.

4. **Sodium stibogluconate** (ampoule, 6 ml, 330 mg/ml, equivalent to 100 mg/ml of pentavalent antimony) 6 ml intramuscular or intravenous injection once a day for 6–10 days. May be repeated after 30 days. In Oriental sore local infiltration (2 ml) around the lesion. Reduce dose in debilitated patients; ECG monitoring during therapy needed. Side effects include pain at injection site, myalgia, joint stiffness, ECG abnormalities, renal/hepatic dysfunction.

5. **Pentaniidine:** As for trypanosomiasis

6. **Hydroxystilbarnidine** (vial, 250 mg) 250 mg intravenous injection (over 2–3 hours) on alternate days, may be given intramuscularly. During administration protect solution from light. Use freshly prepared solution. Intramuscular route is painful. Contraindicated in impaired hepatic and renal function. Side effects include sudden hypotension, nausea, vomiting, dizziness, tachycardia, breathlessness, pruritus, thrombophlebitis, malaise, anorexia, paraesthesia.

7. **Meglumine Antinionate** (ampoule, 1 gm): 100 mg/kg body weight by deep intramuscular injection daily for 10–12 days. Course may be repeated after 6 weeks. Contraindicated in renal and cardiac damage, rheumatoid arthritis, avoid in CNS and GIT disorders. Avoid repeated courses. Toxic effects of antimony compounds like cardiotoxicity (hypotension, arrhythmias, T wave inversion) may be expected. Agranulocytosis has been reported.

For Oriental Sore and Espundia

Pentavalent preparations of antimony are the drugs of choice. In resistant cases one can use pyrimethamine and amphotericin B. Pyrimethamine is given in 3 courses with a rest period of 8 days in between the courses. For the first two courses 50 mg daily for ten days, and for the third 25 mg daily for ten days. Folic acid should be given simultaneously.

In purely cutaneous lesion a single intramuscular injection of cycloguanil pamote in doses of 5 mg base/kg has been found to be effective.

Treatment of Resistant Cases of Kala-Azar

These cases need higher doses of antimony for longer periods; two or three courses may be repeated at fortnightly intervals. Sometimes change to another antimony compound helps. Pentamidine is the drug of choice. Amphtoericin B is also used in resistant cases of kala-azar, this, however, is a highly toxic drug. In drug-resistant cases splenectomy followed by specific chemotherapy. Amphotericin-B is administered in the dose of 0.1 mg/kg of body weight daily by slow intravenous infusion, well diluted in 0.5 litre 5% dextrose (given over 6 hours). It may be increased to 0.25 mg/kg of body weight. Total dose should not go beyond 2 g.

Antimalarial Drugs (also see relevant chapters on malaria discussed earlier)

For Acute Attack

Chloroquine-sensitive infection

1. **Amodiaquine (Tablet, 200 mg):** For acute attack 600 mg on first day followed by 400 mg/day orally for 2 days. [For prophylaxis—400 mg orally/week]. On long-term therapy skin discolouration (bluish-gray) and corneal deposits may occur but they slowly disappear. Regular vision check up during therapy is advisable. Side effects include nausea, vomiting, diarrhoea, lethargy, vertigo, insomnia. Rarely agranulocytosis, neuropathy, hepatitis, dryness of mouth, constipation, blurring of vision. Increased incidence of seizures, corneal opacity, pigmentation of finger nails and skin.

2. **Chloroquine (Tablets, 250 mg equivalent to 150 mg base and ampoule of 5 ml with 40 mg/ml as base):** For acute attack of malaria 600 mg of base stat followed by 300 mg after 6–8 hours and 150 mg twice daily for two days orally. In cerebral malaria 200 mg intramuscular or intravenous injection thrice a day. Use with caution in patient with impaired hepatic/renal function, psoriasis, GIT or neurological or haematological disorders, history of porphyria and in alcoholics. Should not be used in conjunction with gold salts, phenylbutazone and triamcinolone. It is superior and safer than quinine. Avoid chloroquine and quinine together. Regular ophthalmological examination advised for patients on long in term therapy. Avoid use in pregnancy. Side effects include headche, nausea, vomiting, diarrhoea, abdominal cramps, pruritus, rash, ECG changes, hypotension, blurring of vision, rarely corneal opacity, pigment deposits in cornea/retina, alopecia, photosensitivity, blood dyscrasias.

3. **Hydroxychloroquine (Tablet, 200 mg):** As a suppressive 400 mg/week orally. As a curative 800 mg followed by 400 mg after 8 hours and 200 mg twice a day orally. It is contraindicated in hepatic damage. Avoid in cases of porphyria, psoriasis

and hypersensitive patients. Regular ophthalmic check-up during treatment is necessary. Side effects include nausea, vomiting, headache, diarrhoea, abdominal pain, pruritus, skin rash, corneal deposits, retinopathy, cardio-vascular depression.

Chloroquine resistant infection

1. **Dapsone (25 mg, tablet):** 25 mg once a day (to be given with pyrimethamine) dosage can be gradually increased if needed. Use with caution in pulmonary, cardiac patients. Do blood counts regularly. Side effects include hemolytic anaemia, anorexia, nausea, vomiting, dizziness, headache, tachycardia, nervousness, insomnia, neuropathy, fever, agranulocytosis, pruritus, psychosis.
2. **Mefloquine (250 mg):** 1–1.5 gm orally single dose. Widespread use not indicated. Avoid use in women of child bearing age and in children. Side effects include nausea, vomiting, dizziness, disorientation, hallucination, depression, diarrhoea, weakness, headache.
3. **Quinine (Tablet or capsule 100 and 300 mg; ampoule 10 ml of 3%):** For suppression of malaria: 300–600 mg orally once a day; for treatment of acute attack 1.2–2 gram orally in 3–4 divided doses for 7–10 days. Intravenous administration, if needed, must be given slowly (300–600 mg at a rate not more than 25 mg/minute) Contraindicated in haemoglobinuria, optic neuritis and in hypersensitive patients, use with caution in cardiac disease and in pregnancy. May enhance the effect of anticoagulants. Acidification of urine by ammonium chloride increases its excretion in urine. Side effects include headache, nausea, fever, vomiting, confusion, tinnitus, hypotension, deafness, blindness, haemolytic anaemia, abortion in pregnant ladies, black-water fever.
4. **Sulphadoxine/Pyrimethamine** (Sulphadoxine 500 mg + pyrimethamine 25 mg, tablet) used for chloroquine resistant malaria. For prophylaxis 2 tablets, for children 1–2 tablets at intervals of one month. For treatment 2–3 tablets in single dose. Children 20 mg/kg body weight sulphadoxinc and 1 mg/kg body weight pyrimethamine as a single dose. Contraindications are hypersensitivity to sulphonamides, severe liver or renal dysfunction, blood dyscrasias, neonates, pregnancy, lactation. Special precautions include regular blood counts during long-term prophylaxis and G6PD deficiency.

For prophylaxis

1. **Chlorproguanil (Tablet, 20 mg):** 20 mg once a week orally. After leaving endemic zone more effective than proguanil and longer duration of action are the main advantages. Side effects include vomiting, epigastric distress, resistance may occur.
2. **Cycloguanil** (Ampoule, 350 mg) 5–6 mg/kg body weight deep intramuscular injection once in four months. Therapeutic status overtaken by safer and more effective drugs. It is a metabolic product of proguanil. It has minimal side effects but anorexia, nausea and vomiting may occur.
3. **Mefloquine:** Discussed earlier
4. **Pamaquine:** (Tablet, 10 mg) 10–20 mg thrice daily orally for 5 days. It has been superseded by primaquine. It has a synergistic beneficial effect with quinine (pamaquine effective against gametes and quinine against asexual erythrocytic stage of parasite). Side effects include epigastric distress, nausea, cyanosis, acute

haemolytic anaemia, methaelmoglobinemia; rarely jaundice, liver damage and cardiac irregularities.

5. **Pentaquine (Tablet 60 mg):** 60 mg once a day orally for 14 days. Is less toxic than pamaquin but toxicity reduces widespread use. It has low margin of safety. Side effects include headache, abdominal pain, anorexia, diarrhoea, methaemoglobinemia, postural syncope, haemolytic anaemia.

6. **Primaquine (Tablet 7.5 mg base):** 7.5 mg base twice a day for 14 days orally (preceded by a course of chloroquine for acute attack of malaria). Caution in patients with granulocytopaenia, watch for methaemoglobinemia. Avoid bone marrow depressant with primaquine therapy. Mepacrine increases toxicity of primaquine. Side effects include nausea, abdominal pain, vomiting, jaundice, methaemoglobinemia, bone marrow depression, haemolytic anaemia in patients with G6PD deficiency.

7. **Quinocide (Tablet, 30 mg):** 30 mg once daily orally for 14 days. Use with caution in patients with anaemia and bleeding disorders. Side effects include haemolytic anaemia and abdominal cramps.

Drugs for Balantidiasis

1. **Oxytetracycline:** Course consists of 500 mg of the drug administered orally to adults at 6 hourly intervals for a period of 7–10 days.
2. **Carbarsone and Diodoquin:** Discussed earlier with drugs for amoebiasis.

Intestinal Anthelmintics

These drugs can either kill the worms (vermicide) or help in their expulsion (vermifuge).
Basic principles of therapy of intestinal halminthiasis
  A. Establish a specific diagnosis. Multiple worms may be present with or without protozoal infection.
  First treat problem causing greater signs and symptoms.
  B. Establish the presence/absence of other systemic diseases. As most of the antihelmintic drugs are not well tolerated by alcoholics, therefore, use with utmost care and direct the patient to refrain from taking alcohol.
  C. With currently available drugs purgation is often not needed.
  D. Examine all stool samples the next day for any expelled worms.
  E. Always assess stool sample as a follow-up measure and if necessary give a second course of treatment.

1. **Mebendazole** (Tablet 100 mg, Suspension 100 mg/ml): For threadworn 100 mg orally to be repeated after 2 weeks; For hookworm, ascariasis and trichuriasis 100 mg twice daily for 3 days. No fasting or purging is required. Avoid in patients with severe liver damage, pregnancy and in patients with a history of allergy to mebendazole. Side effects include nausea, vomiting, transient abdominal pain and diarrhoea. Rarely allergic reactions, allopecia, reversible neutropenia, pruritus, drowsiness, headache, eosinophilia, anaemia, impaired liver function.

2. **Piperazine** (Tablet 250–500 mg, syrup 100 mg/ml). For ascariasis 75 mg/kg body weight (maximum permissible dose is 3.5 gm/day) orally for 2 days. For oxyuriasis 65 mg/kg body weight (maximum 2 gm) in 2 divided doses orally daily for 7 days. No fasting/enema needed. Contraindicated in pregnancy, epilepsy and neurological disorders. Caution required in renal dysfunction. Simultaneous

treatment of other family members is desirable. Course may be repeated after 1–2 weeks. Side effects include GIT upset, pruritus, transient paresthesia, headache, urticaria. Rarely neurotoxicity (nystagmus, ataxia, weakness, tremor, convulsions) may occur.

3. **Pyrantel Parnoate** (Tablet 250 mg, suspension 50 mg of base/ml) 10 mg/kg body weight orally as single dose. Maximum dose 1 gm. Used for oxyuriasis, ankylostomiasis and ascariasis. Avoid in children under 2 years of age, in impaired liver function and in pregnancy. Mutually antagonistic to piperazine. Side effects include mild GIT upset, headache, dizziness, weakness, fever, drowsiness insomnia, skin rash, elevated SGOT level.

4. **Thiabendazole** (Tablet 500 mg, suspension 500 mg/5 ml): 25 mg/kg body weight orally twice a day for pinworm and for 2 days for other infestations. It is used for *S. stercoralis*, Ascariasis, Anklyostomiasis, Enterobiasis. Avoid in heapatic and renal disease. Hypersensitive type of reaction may occur. Avoid driving or operation of machines. Caution in diabetics and in patients with renal lithiasis. May increase aminophylline concentration in blood. Side effects include hepatotoxicity, diminished mental alertness, anorexia, nausea, vomiting, dizziness, pruritus, giddiness, headache, numbness, hypoglycemia, crystalluria.

5. **Albendazole** (400 mg tablet, suspension 200 mg/5 ml): Used for single or mixed infections with roundworms, whipworms, threadworms, hookworms, tapeworms, strongyloidiasis and hydatid cysts. Dosage for children 1–2 years 200 mg as a single dose. Adults and children above 2 years 400 mg as a single dose. Strongyloidiasis, Taeniasis, *H. nana* infections—give 400 mg once daily for 3 consecutive days. Hydatid disease—400 mg twice daily with meals for 28 days. Therapy may be repeated after 2 weeks interval for a total of 3 cycles. Contraindication—pregnancy. Take special precautions in women of childbearing age, administer within 7 days of start of normal menstruation. Perform liver function tests every 2 weeks during high dose treatment of hydatid disease. *This by far is the best and most broad-spectromed antihelminthic drug.*

6. **Pyrviniuni** (Tablet 50 mg, suspension 10 mg/ml): For threadworm infestation— 5 mg/kg body weight single dose orally, may be repeated after 2–3 weeks; for strongyloidiasis 5 mg/kg body weight daily orally for 5–7 day. Use is avoided because of availability of more potent and safer drugs. Avoid chewing of tablet. Side effects include dark red coloured stool and vomitus (if vomiting occurs), nausea, diarrhoea, allergic reactions and photosensitivity.

7. **Levamisole** (Tablet, 50 mg, 150 mg) Adults 150 mg single dose; children 50 mg single dose. In case of severe hookworm infestation repeat dose after 1–7 days, is useful for roundworms, hookworms, and mixed infestations. It should not be administered with lipophilic agent.

8. **Tetramisol** (Tablet 150 mg, usually given with phenophthalein added 60 mg): For children dose is 50 mg of tetramisole. Dosage in adults is 150 mg and for children 50 mg as single dose, can be repeated after 12 hours. Useful for ascariasis, ancylostomiasis, necatoriasis. It should not be given with lipophilic agents.

9. **Bephenium** (5 gm packet of granules): Dosage is 5 gm single dose orally on empty stomach and food withheld for 2 hours, may be repeated after 3 days in severe cases. Useful in hookworm infestation and ascariasis. Purgation is not needed. Dosage should be reduced to half in children below 20 kg; deworming

should be followed by treatment of co-existing anaemia. Side effects include nausea, diarrhoea, vomiting, headache and vertigo.

10. **Betoscanate** (capsule 50 mg): 150 mg single dose orally or three doses of 100 mg each 12 hours apart orally. Used for hookworm infestation. Usually single dose/course suffices, can be repeated after 2 months if needed. Not very commonly used. Other safer drugs are available. Side effects include nausea, vomiting, anorexia, abdominal pain, headache, dizziness, diarrhoea.

11. **Carbon Tetrachloride** (capsule 2–4 ml): 2–4 ml as a single dose in the morning in empty stomach. Used for hookworm infestation. Has also been used for tapeworm infestation. It is an obsolete antihelmintic. It is highly toxic.

12. **Chenopodium Oil** (capsule 0.6 ml) Obsolete drug.

13. **Tetrachlorethylene** (capsule 1 ml): 0.1 ml/kg body weight with a maximum of 5 ml orally as a single dose, can be repeated after 7 days. Has been used for ancylostomiasis and intestinal flukes. Contraindicated in liver damage, ulceration of GIT, anaemia, lactating mothers. Avoid alcohol. Purgative may increase toxicity. Avoid fat and alcohol one day before and after the drug. In mixed infections ascariasis should be treated first before tetrachlorethylene therapy. Side effects include drowsiness, giddiness, nausea, vomiting, liver damage, kidney damage, hypotension, cardiac arrhythmias. Rarely dependence may occur.

Anti-Dracunculosis Drugs

1. **Metronidazole:** Discussed earlier.
2. **Thiabendazole:** Discussed earlier.
3. **Niridazole (Tablet 100–500 mg):** 25 mg/kg body weight once a day orally for 7 days in dracunculosis and for 10 days in schistosomiasis. Rest discussed under amoebicides.

Anti-Filarial Drugs

1. **Carbarsone:** Discussed under amoebicides.
2. **Iverniectin:** (Capsule 1 mg) 100–150 µg/kg body weight orally as a single dose. Used as an antifilarial agent in onchocerciasis. Contraindicated in pregnancy. Avoid in lactating mothers and in children. Effect lasts for more than a year. Long duration of action is the main advantage. Side effects include fever, headache, pruritus, myalgia, lymph node tenderness, mild transient hypotension and insomnia.
3. **Diethylcarbamazine** (Tablet 50, 100 mg): 2 mg/kg body weight thrice daily orally for 2–3 weeks. Used in filariasis, tropical pulmonary eosinophilia and in onchocerciasis. In the tretment of onchocerciasis start therapy with lower doses, corticosteroids may be added to reduce side effects which include headache, malaise, weakness, anorexia, nausea, vomiting, joint pains, skin rash, enlarged tender lymph nodes and proteinuria.

Drugs for Intestinal Cestode Infestation

1. **Quinacrine (Tablet 100 mg):** Adult dose is 1 gm. Two tablets of 100 mg are given with a little water, every 10 minutes, till 1 gm is given. Along with the drug, sodium bicarbonate 10 g may be added. A saline purgative 2 hours after last dose and phenobarbitone 100 mg half an hour before administration of the

drug are to be given. For *T. solium* infestation drug can be given through RyJe's tube straight into the duodenum. The patient is given semi-liquid diet on the day before treatment and a saline purgative is given in the afternoon. It is effective against *D. latum, T. saginata, T. solium* and *H. diminuta* infection. The drug does not kill the parasite but loosens its hold and the intact parasite stained yellow is voided within a couple of hours. All stools passed within 24 hours after the administration of drug should be saved and examined carefully for the minute scolex of the worm. Intramuscular injection of 0.5 ml pituitrin 1 to 1½ hours after administration of quinacrine helps to expel the tapeworm whose hold has been loosened by qunacrine. Side effects include headache, dizziness, vomiting, blood dyscrasias urticaria, yellow skin, blue-black discolouration of nails, toxic psychosis.

2. **Dichlorphen** (Tablet 2 mg): 2 mg thrice a day orally for a day. Useful in *T. solium, T. saginata* and *D. latum* infestations. Contraindicated in late pregnancy, impaired liver function, and severe heart disease. Avoid alcohol. Side effects include nausea, vomiting, urticaria, intestinal colicky pain, rarely jaundice, allergic contact dermatitis.

3. **Niclosamide** (Tablet 500 mg): After fasting 2–4 tablets to be chewed and swallowed. In *H. nana* infestation 2 gm on first day and the one gram once a day orally for 6 days after breakfast. May be repeated after a month. Is useful for treating and is the drug of choice for *T. solium* and *T. saginata, D. latum* and *H. nana* infestations. Purging is essential in *T. solium* infestation as there is risk of cysticercosis. Almost devoid of side effects, nausea, abdominal discomfort/pain may occur.

4. **Bethional:** Given in Taeniasis orally, in a single dose of 2 g followed by a saline purgative after 2 hours.

5. **Praziquantel** (Tablet 600 mg): 40 mg/kg body weight orally (single dose) used in cysticercosis. *See* details under anti-schistosoma drugs.

Schistosomicidal Drugs

1. **Hycanthone** (Vial, powder 200 mg/vial): 3 mg/kg body weight deep intramuscular injection. May be repeated after 3 months. Is an outdated drug, other safer drugs available. Has carcinogenic potential too.

2. **Lucanthone** (Tablet 1 g): 1 g twice a day orally for 3 days. Useful against *S. haematobium*. Contraindicated in pregnancy, hepatic damage, acute bacterial infections, history of sensitivity to lucanthone. Avoid simultaneous use of hepatotoxic drugs (phenothiazines and MAO inhibitors) to these patients. Side effects include nausea, vomiting, headache, dizziness, abdominal pain, rarely liver damage, convulsions and yellow discolouration of skin.

3. **Metrifonate** (Capsule 250 mg): 5–15 mg/kg body weight orally three times at a gap of two weeks each (half the dose for prophylaxis) especially useful against *S. haematobium*. Neuromuscular blocking effect of drugs may be modified during next 48 hours after metrifonate. Avoid inhalation. Side effects include vertigo, lassitude, nausea, colic, vomiting, abdominal pain, pruritus, eosinophilia, fever and adenopathy.

4. **Niridazole:** (Tablet 100–500 mg): 25 mg/kg body weight once a day orally for 7 days for dracunculosis and for 10 days in schistosomiasis. See under amoebicides for rest.

5. **Oxamniquine** (capsule 250 mg): 15 mg/kg body weight orally as a single dose or twice for two days. Especially used for *S. mansoni*. In epileptic patients it may precipitate epileptic attacks. Not effective against *S. haematobium*. Side effects include dizziness, drowsiness, high coloured urine, eosinophilia, myalgia, headache, diarrhoea, insomnia.

6. **Praziquantel** (tablet 600 mg): 40 mg/kg body weight orally (single dose) for *S. mansoni* and *S. haemotobium* infection, 30 mg/kg in 2 divided doses (one day only) for *S. japonicum* infection orally (swallowed with water after meals). It is also useful for cysticercosis. It is the drug of choice for schistosomiasis. Side effects include abdominal pain, headache, dizziness, skin rash, fever and nausea.

7. **Stibocapitate** (vial, powder, 500 mg/vial): 500 mg intramuscular injection once or twice (total 2.5 grams). Especially useful for *S. haematobium*. Contraindicated in cardiac patients and hepatic diseases. Better tolerated than antimony sodium tartarate. Side effects include painful injection, nausea, vomiting, metallic taste, diarrhoea, substernal pain, lassitude and extrasystoles.

8. **Stibophen** (ampoule 5 ml, 6%): 100 mg on first day intramuscular injection or intravenously 200 mg on second day, 300 mg on third day and then on alternate days (total dose being 2.4–4.5 g grams). Useful in schistosomiasis. Avoid in patients with impaired liver function. Use of old J3 ampoules may enhance toxicity. Side effects include nausea, vomiting, bradycardia, epigastric pain, haemolytic anaemia and liver damage.

Drugs for Fascioliasis

1. **Emetine:** Dosage is 1 mg/kg/day daily as IM injection till a total dose of 60 mg/day is given.

2. **Bithionol:** 30–50 mg/kg body weight per day in 3 divided doses orally for 10–15 days. Side effects include mild and transient nausea, vomiting, abdominal pain and diarrhoea. Also good against paragonimiasis and clonorchiasis.

Drugs for Clonorchiasis

1. **Antimony compounds:** Sodium antimonyl tartar emetic and stibophen have been found effective in reducing the number of worms in biliary passages and also the egg output in the faeces.

2. **Bithionol:** Mentioned earlier.

3. **Chloroquine:** 10.4 mg/kg body weight for up to 39 days. Total amount given varies from about 20 to 40 g.

Drugs for Paragonimiasis

1. **Emetine:** 65 mg intramuscularly for 10–12 days.
2. **Chloroquine:** 250 mg twice daily for 2 months.
3. **Bithionol:** Same as for fascioliasis.

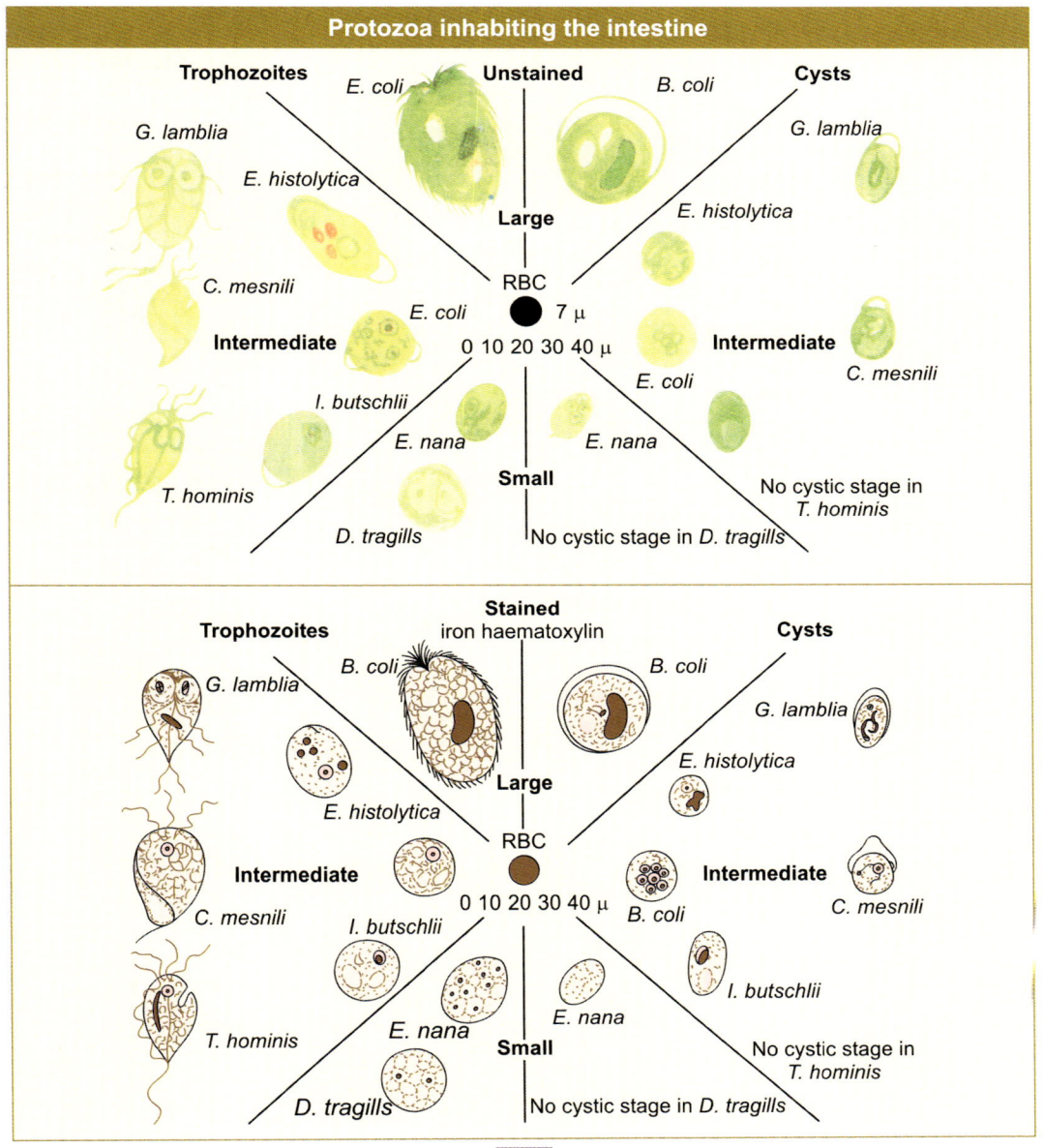

Protozoa inhabiting the intestine

Unstained

Trophozoites — E. coli — B. coli — Cysts

G. lamblia — G. lamblia

E. histolytica — E. histolytica

C. mesnili

Large

RBC — 7 μ

E. coli — 0 10 20 30 40 μ

Intermediate — Intermediate

E. coli — C. mesnili

I. butschlii

E. nana — E. nana

T. hominis — No cystic stage in T. hominis

Small

D. tragills — No cystic stage in D. tragills

Stained
iron haematoxylin

Trophozoites — B. coli — B. coli — Cysts

G. lamblia — G. lamblia

E. histolytica — E. histolytica

Intermediate — **Large** — Intermediate

RBC

C. mesnili — 0 10 20 30 40 μ — C. mesnili

I. butschlii — B. coli

E. nana — I. butschlii

E. nana

T. hominis — No cystic stage in T. hominis

D. tragills — **Small** — No cystic stage in D. tragills

Morphological differentiations

Toxoplasma in pseudocysts
in various cells

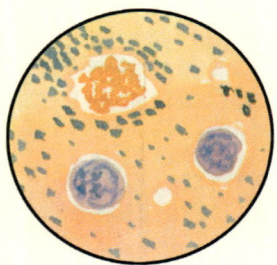

**Exoerythrocytic schizonts
of Plasmodium**
in liver cells

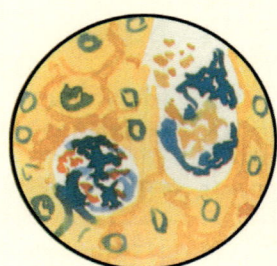

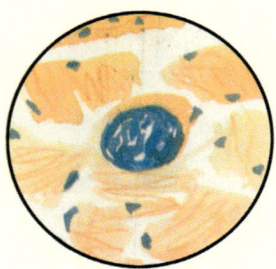

Sarcocystis lindemanni
in human muscle

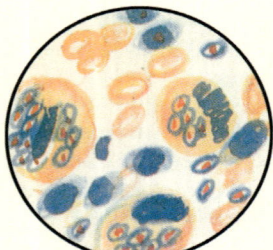

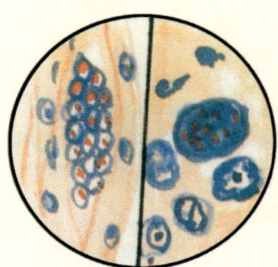

**Leishman donovan bodies
in RE cells**
in visceral leishmaniasis

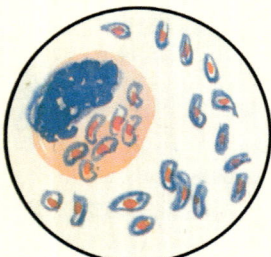

**Leishmanial forms of
*Trypanosoma cruzi***
in myocardial and CNS cells

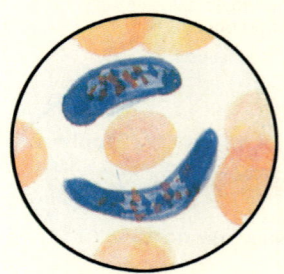

Toxoplasma gondii
Not in blood

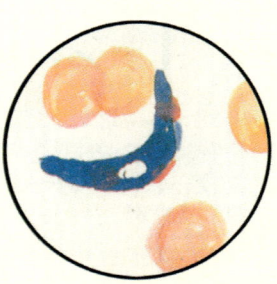

Ookinete of Plasmodium
in mosquito's stomach

Gametocytes of *P. falciparum*
in blood

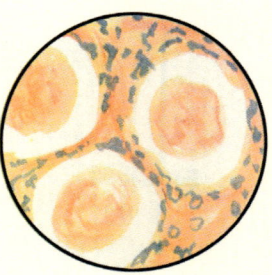

***Pneumocystis carinii* in lung**

Metazoans

Nematodes

Heads

A. lumbricoides	E. vermicularis	A. duodenale	N. americanus	W. bancrofti
Three lips	Bulbous oesophagus	Buccal capsule with 2 pairs of teeth	Buccal capsule plates	Bluntly rounded

Tails

A. duodenale
Bursa with dorsal ray-shallow cleft-tips tridigitate

N. americanus
Bursa with dorsal ray-deep cleft-tips bifid
Spicule fused and barbed

T. trichiura
Head attenuated form tails

Larvae

Rhabditiform

Bulbous oesophagus

Strongyloides— rhabditiform larva
Short buccal cavity— long oesophagus

D. medinensis

Filariform

Straight oesophagus

Ancylostome— rhabditiform larva long buccal cavity— short oesphagus

Mirofilaria sheathed

W. bancrofti

Nuclei do not reach tip of tails

Loa loa

Nuclei reach tip to tail

B. malayi

Long sheath—two discrete nuclei in tip of tail

In tissue

T. spiralis in muscle

O. volvulus in subcutaneous tissue

Microfilaria unsheathed

D. perstans
Nuclei to tip of tail

M. ozzardi
Nuclei almost to tip of tail

D. streptocerca

Tail blunt-curved like "shepherds crook"

O. volvulus

Not found in blood

Cestodes

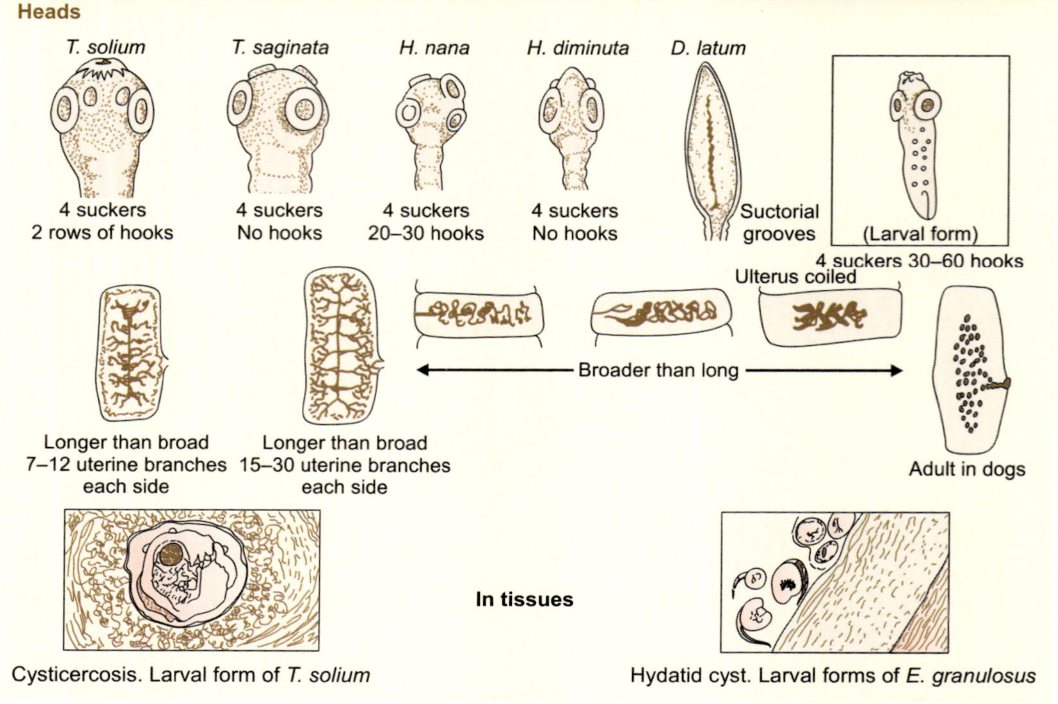

Heads

T. solium	T. saginata	H. nana	H. diminuta	D. latum
4 suckers 2 rows of hooks	4 suckers No hooks	4 suckers 20–30 hooks	4 suckers No hooks	Suctorial grooves

(Larval form)

4 suckers 30–60 hooks

Uterus coiled

Longer than broad 7–12 uterine branches each side

Longer than broad 15–30 uterine branches each side

← Broader than long →

Adult in dogs

In tissues

Cysticercosis. Larval form of *T. solium*

Hydatid cyst. Larval forms of *E. granulosus*

Trematodes

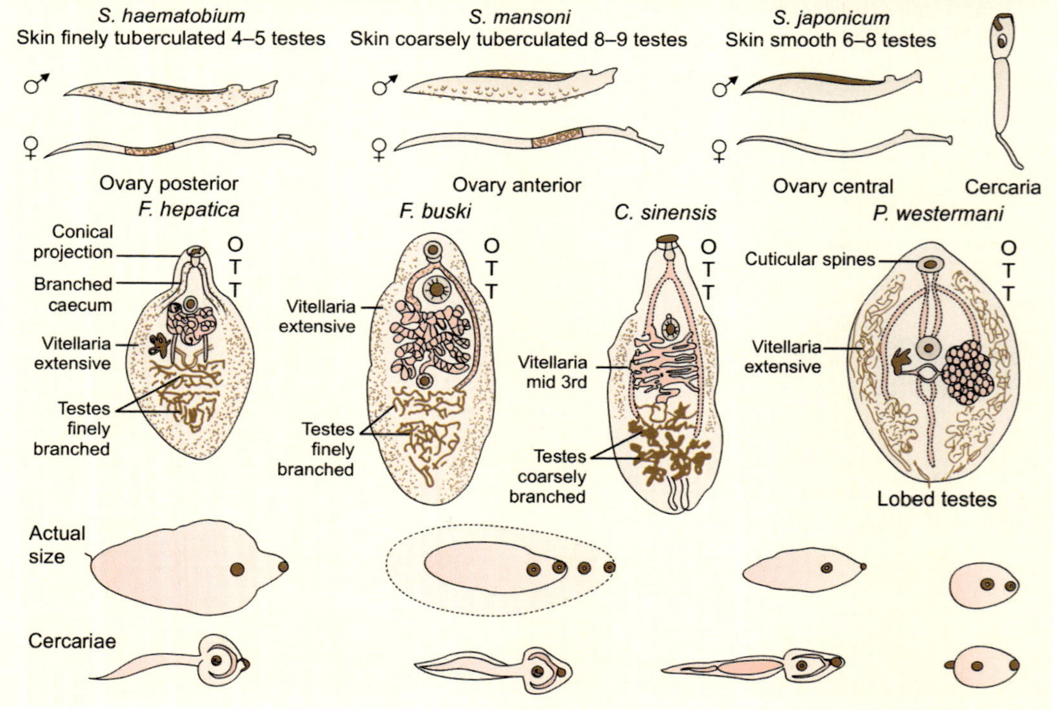

S. haematobium
Skin finely tuberculated 4–5 testes

S. mansoni
Skin coarsely tuberculated 8–9 testes

S. japonicum
Skin smooth 6–8 testes

♂ ♀

Ovary posterior

Ovary anterior

Ovary central

Cercaria

F. hepatica

Conical projection
Branched caecum
Vitellaria extensive
Testes finely branched

O T T

F. buski

Vitellaria extensive
Testes finely branched

O T T

C. sinensis

Vitellaria mid 3rd
Testes coarsely branched

O T T

P. westermani

Cuticular spines
Vitellaria extensive
Lobed testes

O T T

Actual size

Cercariae

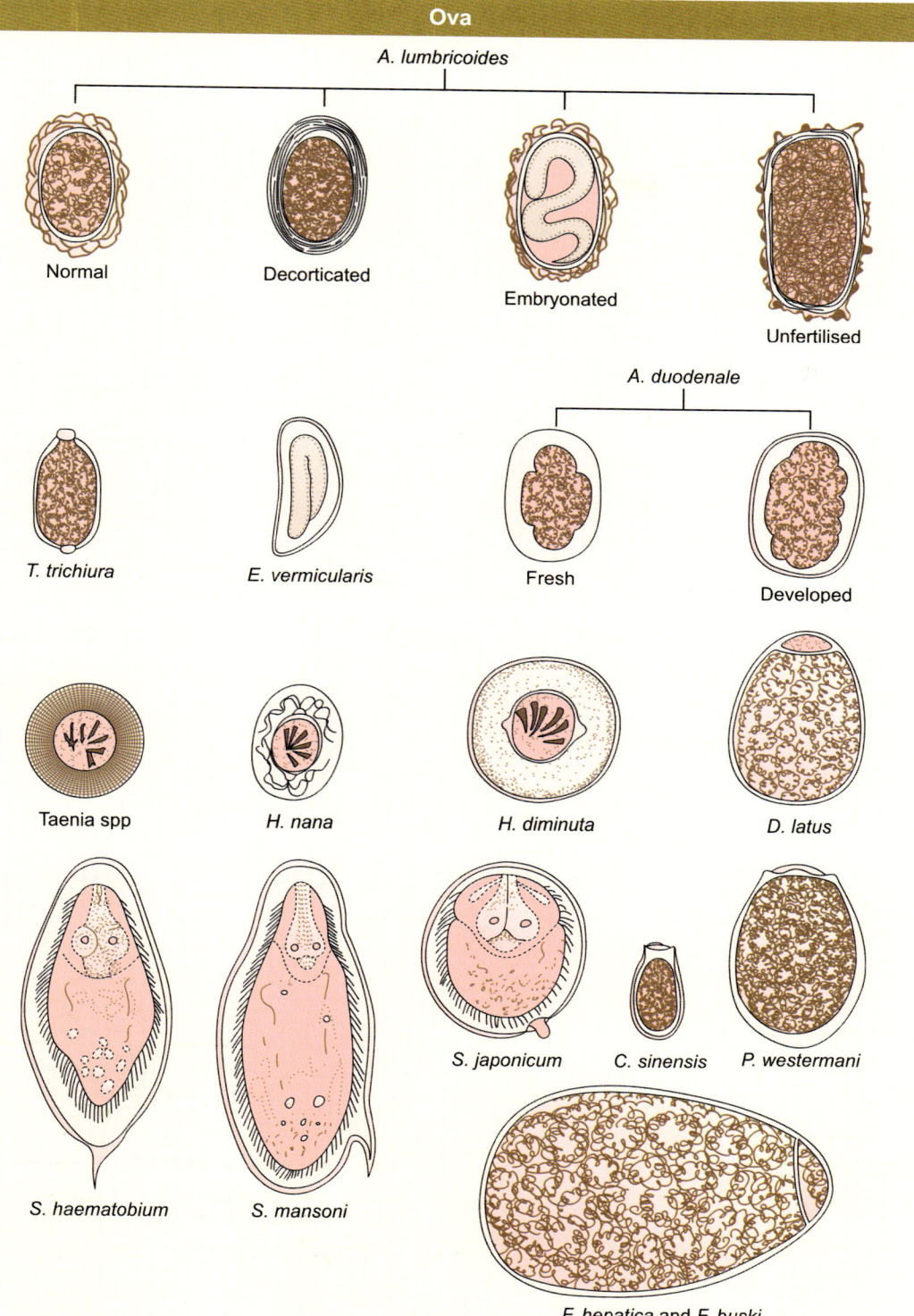

Ova

A. lumbricoides

Normal   Decorticated   Embryonated   Unfertilised

A. duodenale

T. trichiura   E. vermicularis   Fresh   Developed

Taenia spp   H. nana   H. diminuta   D. latus

S. haematobium   S. mansoni   S. japonicum   C. sinensis   P. westermani

F. hepatica and F. buski

Ova of the less common or less important worms

Cestoda

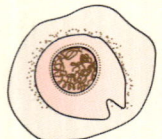
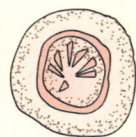
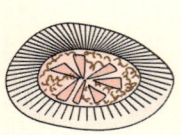
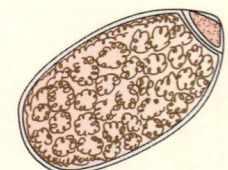

Bertiella studeri   Dipylidium caninum   Multiceps multiceps   Echinostoma ilocanum

Trematoda

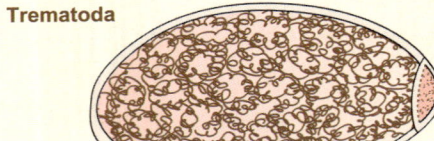
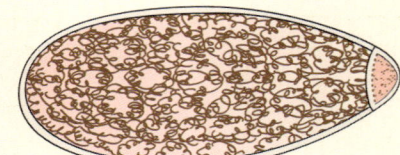

Fasciola gigantica   Gongylonema pulchrum

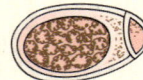
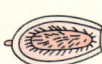
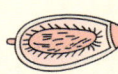
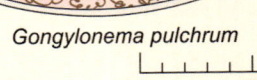

0   50   100 μ

Dicrocelium   Spisthorchis   Heterophyes   Metagcnimus
denditricum   felineus   heterophyes   yokagawai

Nematoda

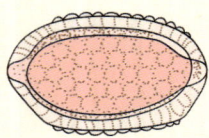
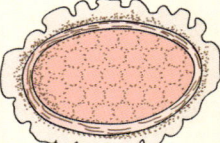
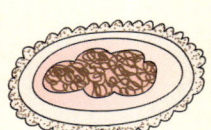
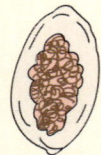

Capiliaria hepatica   Dioctophyma renale   Syngamus laryngeus   Trichostrongylus spp.

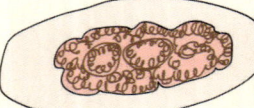
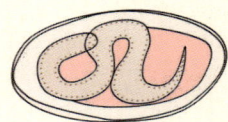
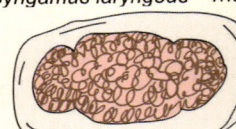
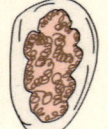

Oesophagostomum   Metastrongylus   Ternidens   Haemonchus
apiostomomum   elongatus   deminutus   contortus
(like hookworm)

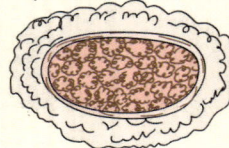
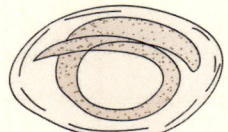
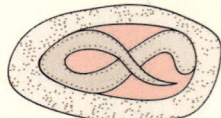

Toxocara spp.   Physaloptera caucasica   Gastrodiscoiders hominis
(ova in dogs and cats)

Miscellaneous worms

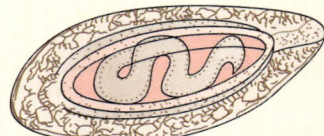
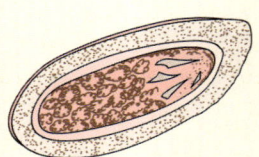

Macracanthorhynchus hirudinaceus   Moniliformis moniliformis

Pathogenesis and pathology of worm infections

Factors

Generally DO NOT MULTIPLY IN MAN	Generally NOT IN INTIMATE TISSUE CONTACT
Repeated or massive attacks before effects are apparent	Immunity response poor

Offence and Defence

Metabolities (Alive) Decomposition products (Dead)	Size Mechanical pressure and obstructive effects	Excitation of local tissue reaction	Absorption of nourishment

General effects	*Local tissue effects*

1. General effects

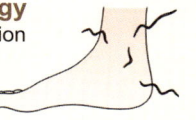

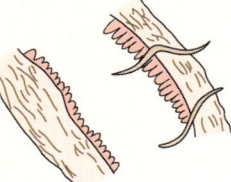

	Ascariasis	Clinico-pathological correlation
Toxaemia and Allergy Acute during larval invasion e.g. Ancylostomiasis	Trichiniasis	Fever Eosinophilia Urticaria Katayama fever
Ova invasion CHRONIC ILL-DEFINED Can occur in any heavy work infection	Schistosomiasis	Irregular fever Eosinophilia, Urticaria nervous disturbance especially in child

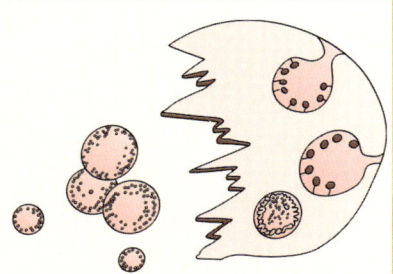

Anaphylaxis Rupture of cysts, e.g. hydatid disease	Acute anaphylactic shock

Malnutrition
e.g. Large taperowm infections
Heavy nematode infections, etc.

Anaemia Loss of blood	Hookworm infections	Loss of weight Fatigue

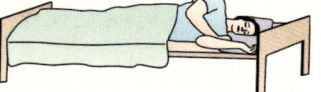

Decreased General Resistance In any prolonged heavy infection	Anaemia with sequelae Intercurrent disease

2. Local effects   **A. General**

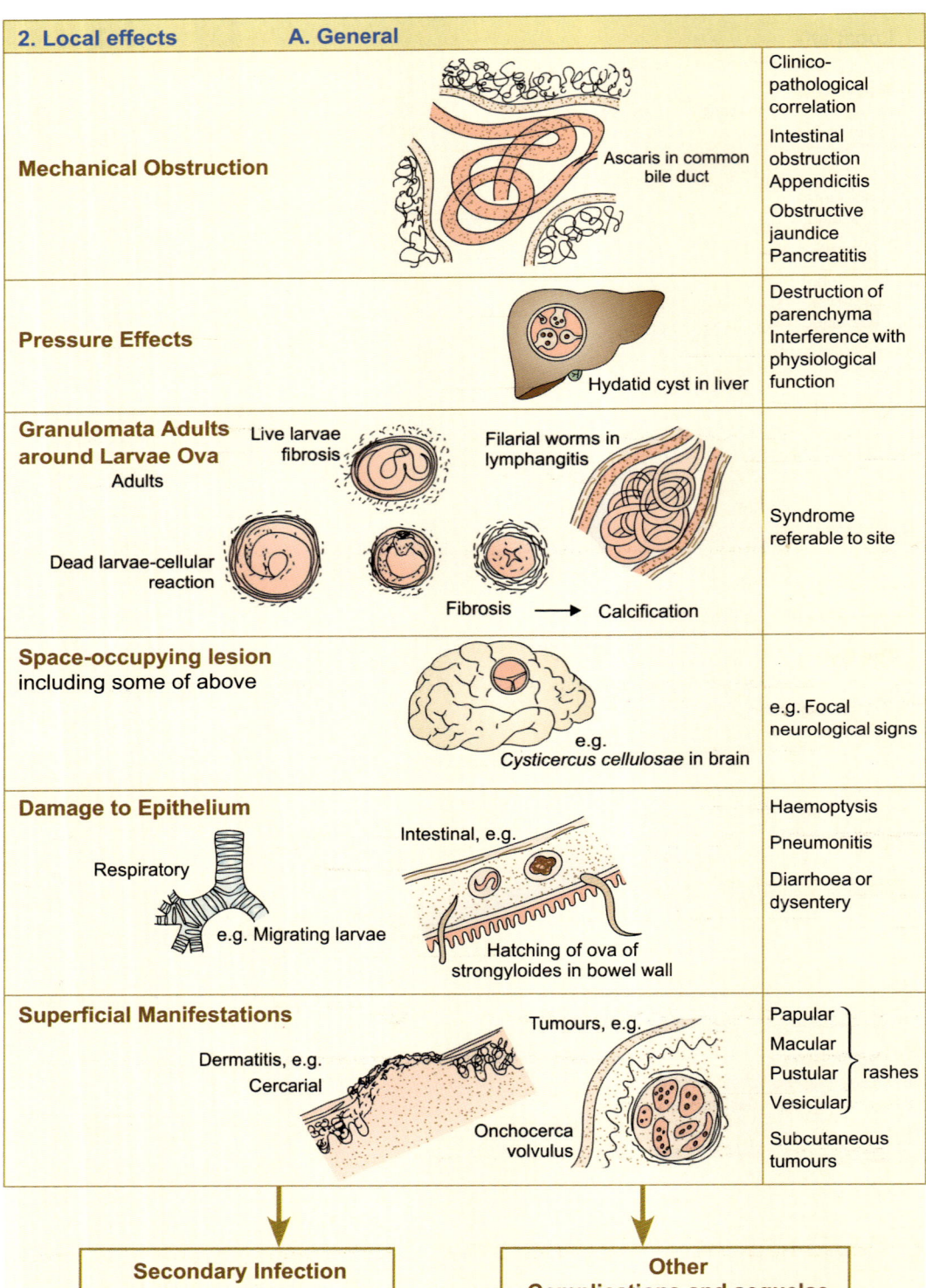

Section	Diagram labels	Clinico-pathological correlation
Mechanical Obstruction	Ascaris in common bile duct	Intestinal obstruction Appendicitis · Obstructive jaundice Pancreatitis
Pressure Effects	Hydatid cyst in liver	Destruction of parenchyma Interference with physiological function
Granulomata Adults around Larvae Ova Adults	Live larvae fibrosis · Filarial worms in lymphangitis · Dead larvae-cellular reaction · Fibrosis → Calcification	Syndrome referable to site
Space-occupying lesion including some of above	e.g. *Cysticercus cellulosae* in brain	e.g. Focal neurological signs
Damage to Epithelium	Respiratory e.g. Migrating larvae · Intestinal, e.g. Hatching of ova of strongyloides in bowel wall	Haemoptysis · Pneumonitis · Diarrhoea or dysentery
Superficial Manifestations	Dermatitis, e.g. Cercarial · Tumours, e.g. *Onchocerca volvulus*	Papular · Macular · Pustular · Vesicular ⎫ rashes · Subcutaneous tumours

Secondary Infection   **Other Complications and sequelae**

Local effects	B. Particular		
The Brain and Spinal Cord	Cestoda	**LARVAE**	Clinico-pathological correlation

Granuloma round ectopic ova

Living larvae in fibrous capsule

Fibrous or Calcified nodule

Granuloma round dead larvae

		CYSTICEROUS CELLULOSAE (*T. solium*) COENURUS CEREBRALIS (Multiceps spp) HYDATID (*E. granulosus*)	Focal neurological signs, e.g. epilepsy
	Nematoda	VISCERAL LARVA MIGRANS Especially TOXOCARA spp. Ascaris lumbricoides Strongyloides steporalls	Space occupying lesions
	Trematoda	ECTOPIC OVA *Schistosoma mansoni* and *japonicum* *Fasciola hepatica* *Heterophyes heterophyes* *Metagonimus yokogowai*	
The Eye	Nematoda	Adults *Loa loa* *Thelazia callipaeda* *Dirofilaria conjunctivae*	Irritation Conjunctivitis Keratitis Eye tumour Blindness

Adults under conjunctiva

invasion of larvae

		Larvae Mf. of Onchocerca volvulus VISCERAL LARVA MIGRANS e.g. *Toxocara canis*	
The Mouth and Pharynx	Nematoda	*Gongylonema pulchrum*	Irritation

Adults in mucosa

Adults in lumen

	Trematoda	Spurious infection with *Fascicola hepatica* (Halzoun)	Irritation Haemoptysis

Local effects of worm infection (*Contd.*)

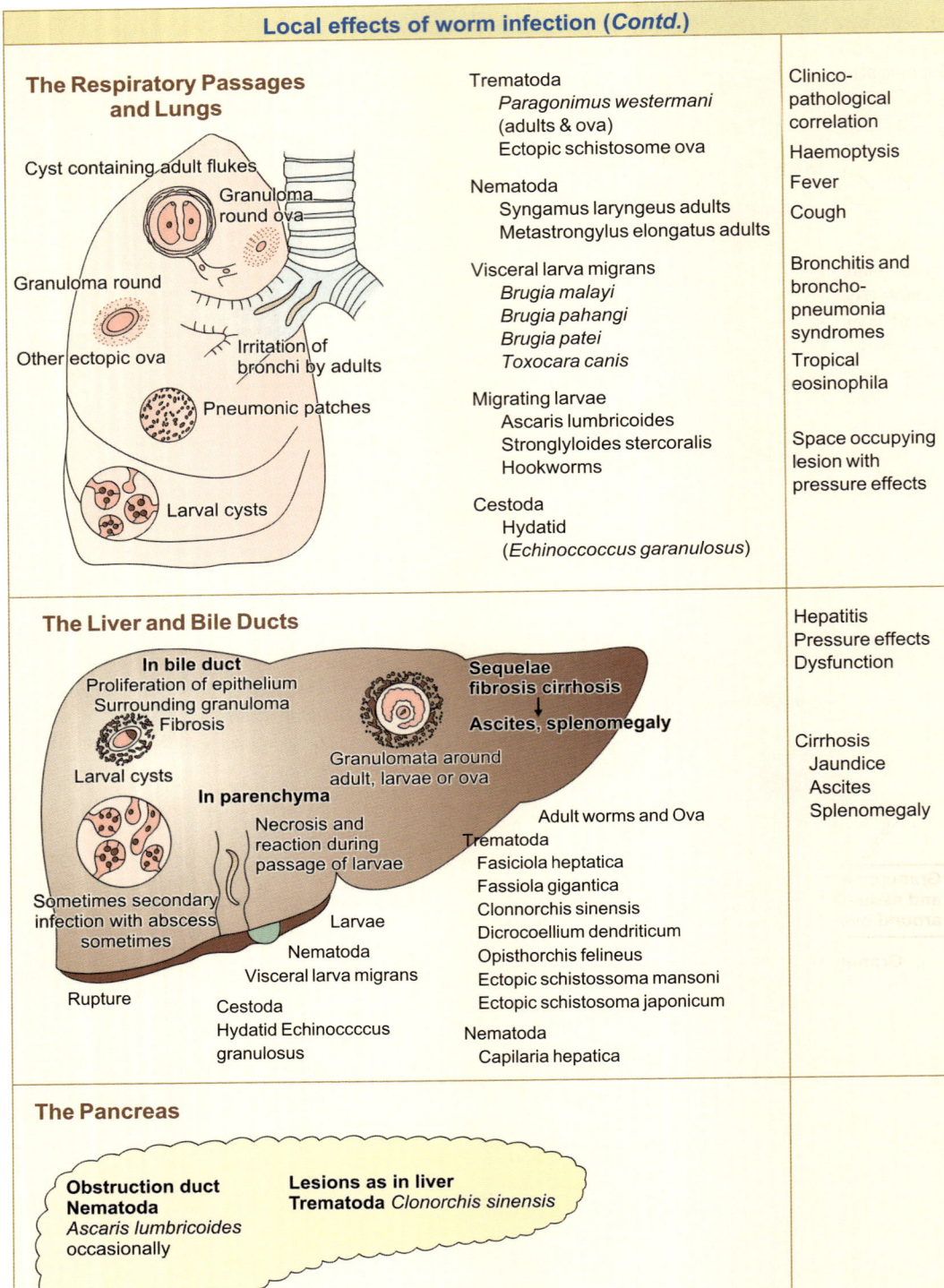

The Respiratory Passages and Lungs

Cyst containing adult flukes

Granuloma round ova

Granuloma round

Other ectopic ova

Irritation of bronchi by adults

Pneumonic patches

Larval cysts

Trematoda
  Paragonimus westermani (adults & ova)
  Ectopic schistosome ova

Nematoda
  Syngamus laryngeus adults
  Metastrongylus elongatus adults

Visceral larva migrans
  Brugia malayi
  Brugia pahangi
  Brugia patei
  Toxocara canis

Migrating larvae
  Ascaris lumbricoides
  Stronglyloides stercoralis
  Hookworms

Cestoda
  Hydatid
  (*Echinoccoccus garanulosus*)

Clinico-pathological correlation

Haemoptysis

Fever

Cough

Bronchitis and broncho-pneumonia syndromes

Tropical eosinophila

Space occupying lesion with pressure effects

The Liver and Bile Ducts

In bile duct
Proliferation of epithelium
Surrounding granuloma
  Fibrosis

Larval cysts

In parenchyma
Necrosis and reaction during passage of larvae

Sometimes secondary infection with abscess sometimes

Rupture

Sequelae fibrosis cirrhosis
↓
Ascites, splenomegaly

Granulomata around adult, larvae or ova

Larvae

Adult worms and Ova
Trematoda
  Fasiciola heptatica
  Fassiola gigantica
  Clonnorchis sinensis
  Dicrocoellium dendriticum
  Opisthorchis felineus
  Ectopic schistossoma mansoni
  Ectopic schistosoma japonicum

Nematoda
Visceral larva migrans

Cestoda
Hydatid Echinoccccus granulosus

Nematoda
  Capilaria hepatica

Hepatitis
Pressure effects
Dysfunction

Cirrhosis
  Jaundice
  Ascites
  Splenomegaly

The Pancreas

Obstruction duct
Nematoda
Ascaris lumbricoides occasionally

Lesions as in liver
Trematoda *Clonorchis sinensis*

Pancreatitis

Local effects of worm infection (*Contd.*)

The Intestinal Tract

Superficial mucosal irritation absorption of nutriment occasionally obstruction

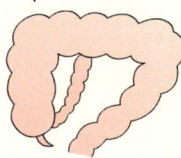

Nematoda
Ascaris lumbricoides
Trichuris (Trichura)
Enterobus vermicularis
Mermithoid worms
Trichostrongylus spp
physoloptera, caucasica
Haemochus contortus

Trematoda
Fasciolopsis buski
Watsonus watsoni
Gastrodiscoides hominis
Haterophyes heterophyes
Metagonimus yokagawai
Echinostoma spp.

Cestoda
Taenia solium
Taenia saginata
Dibothriocephalus latum
Hymenolepis diminuta
Diplogonoportus grandis
Intermicapsifer spp. Bertisella studeria
Dipylidium canium. Raillentina spp.

Clinicopathology correlataion

IN VAST MAJORITY ASYMPTOMATIC

Vague abdominal symptoms: anorexia, indigestion, colicky pain, loss of weight, diarrhoea, appendicitis, obstruction

---

Suck blood

Nematoda
  Hookworms Ancylostoma duodenale
    Ancylostoma brazillense human strains
    Necator americanus
  Trichostrongylus spp.

Vague abdominal symptoms

Anaemia and sequelae

May absorb B$_{12}$

Cestoda
  Perianai irritation Dibothricoephalus latum
Nematoda
  Enterobius vermicularis

Megaloblastic anaemia

Pruritis ani and vulvae

Adults or larvae penetrate mucosa

Nematoda
Strongyloides stercoralis
Oviposition and hatching in wall

Trichinella spiralis
Larviposition in wall
Ternidens diminutus and

Oesophagostomum apiostomum
Encapsulated in wall
adult to lumen

Cestoda
Hymenolepis nana
Cysticercus in wall
Adult in lumen

Granulomata and sequelae around ova

Granuloma

Papilloma

Secondary infection ulcers and abscesses

Trematoda
Schistosoma mansoni (Mainly large intestine)
Schistosoma japonicum (Mainly small intestine)

Fibrosis

From colic and dysentery

To slight abdominal pain, diarrhoea

Dysentery sequelae

Diarrhoea

Obstruction illeus fistulae
(and extra into lesions)

Local effects of worm infection (*Contd.*)

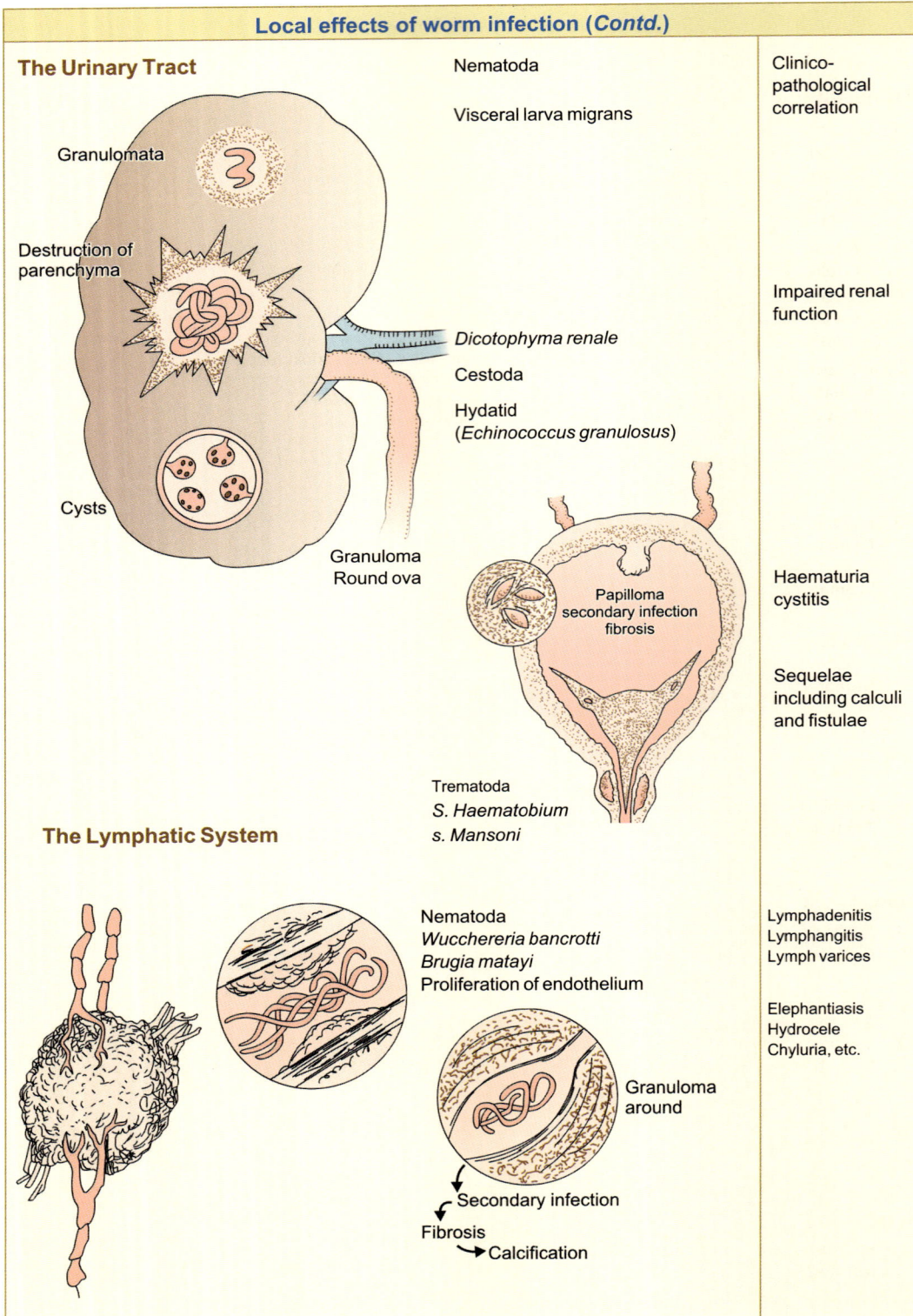

The Urinary Tract

Nematoda

Visceral larva migrans

Granulomata

Destruction of parenchyma

Dicotophyma renale

Cestoda

Hydatid
(*Echinococcus granulosus*)

Cysts

Granuloma
Round ova

Papilloma
secondary infection
fibrosis

Trematoda
S. Haematobium
s. Mansoni

The Lymphatic System

Nematoda
Wucchereria bancrotti
Brugia matayi
Proliferation of endothelium

Granuloma
around

Secondary infection

Fibrosis
Calcification

Clinico-pathological correlation

Impaired renal function

Haematuria
cystitis

Sequelae including calculi and fistulae

Lymphadenitis
Lymphangitis
Lymph varices

Elephantiasis
Hydrocele
Chyluria, etc.

Local effects of worm infection (*Contd.*)

The Circulatory System
Transient in blood

1. Larvae to pulmonary capillaries nematoda
   Ascaris lumbricoides
   Stronglyloides stercoralis
   Ancylostoma duddenale
   Ancylostoma brazillense (human strains)

   Necator americanus
   Dirofiliaria spp.
   Brugia malayi ⎫
   Brugia pahangi ⎬ A type of visceral larva migrans
   Brugia pateia ⎭

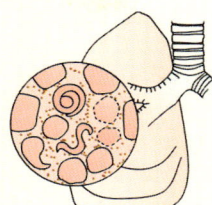

Clinico pathological correlation

Haemophysis Pneumonia sometimes Tropical eosinophilia

2. Larvae to encyst at site of predilection
   Nematoda   Trichnella spiralis
   Cestoda   Taenia solium (Cysticercus cellulosae)
            Echinococcus granulosus (hydatid)
            Multiceps spp. (Coenurus)

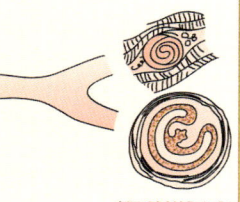

Severe constitutional symptoms in trichinosis

None *per se* with remainder

3. Larvae to mature to adults at site of predilection
   Nematoda   Wuchereria bancrofti
            Brugia malayi
   Trematoda   Ectopic Paragonimus westermani
            Ectopic Fascicola hepatica

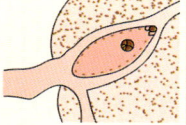

None *per se*

4. Ectopic or animal strain larvae to provoke granulomata anywhere (visceral larva migrans)
   Nematoda   **Cestoda**
            Ascaris lumbricoides   Sparganum mansoni
            Strongyloides stercorals   Sparganum proliferum
            Toxocara canis (and *cati*)
            Gnathostoma spinigerum

None *per se*

None *per se*

5. Ectopic ova to provoke granulomata anywhere
   Trematoda
            Schistosoma mansoni   Heterophyes heterophyes
            Schistosoma japonicum   Metagonimus spp.

None *per se*

More permanent in blood

1. Adults live in circulatory system
   Nematoda Sometimes Dirofiliara spp. **Trematoda**
            in heart   Schistosoma haematobium
                                   Schistosoma mansoni
                                   Schistosoma Japonicum

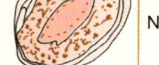

None *per se*

2. Larvae circulate in blood
   Nematoda   Wuchereria bancrofti
            Brugia malayi
            Loa loa
            Dipetalonemia streptocerca
            Dipetalonema perstans
            Mansonella ozzardi
            Diroifilaria spp.

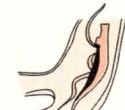

May be responsible for some general constitutional symptoms

Myocarditis and heart failure

In Myocardium
   Larvae provoking granulomata and myocarditis
   Nemtoda
            Trichinella spralis
            Occasionally other ectopic larvae or ova

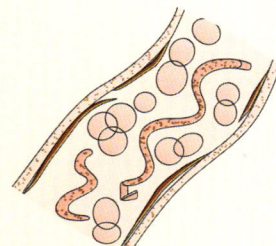

Local effects of worm infection (*Contd.*)

The Skin and Subcutaneous Tissue

			Clinico-pathological correlation
Penetration by invading larvae	**Nematoda** ***Strongyloides stercoralis*** ***Ancylostoma duodenale*** *A. brazillense* (human strains) ***Necator americanusa***		Pretchial dermatitis

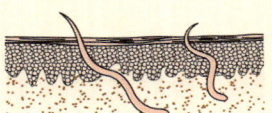

To blood stream	*A. brazillense* (animal strains) *A. caninum*	cutaneous larva migrans	Swimmer's itch Creeping eruption

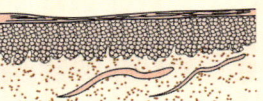

	Trematoda Schistosoma spp. (human strains) Schistosoma spp. (animal strains)		Little effect Cercanal dermatitis
Arrest in epidermis	**Nematoda** Filarial larvae *Wuchereria bancrotti* *Brugia malayi*		None *per se* or slight dermatitis Calabar swelling Fibrotic tumour M F dermatitis

Site of Predilection of Adult

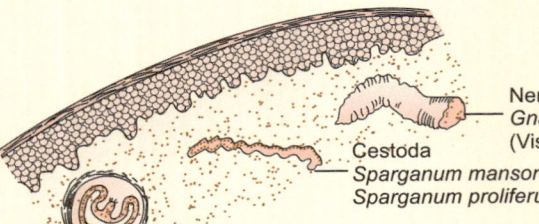

—— Fleeting swelling			Ulcer
—— Fibrosis around	LOA LOA		
—— Dermatitis from MF	Onchocerca volvulus		
—— Inflammation			
Presents through skin	*Dracunculus medinensisa*		

Inhabited by Ectopic Larvae

		Swelling
		Irritation
		Infection

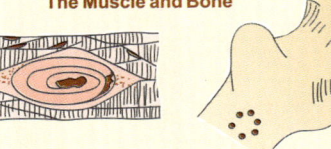

Nematoda
 Gnathostoma spinigerum
 (Visceral larva migrans)

Cestoda
 Sparganum mansoni
 Sparganum proliferum

Cestoda
 Cysticercus cellulose (*Taenia solium*)

Nematoda

Irritation by Adult

		Pruritis ani and vulvae

The Muscle and Bone

Nematoda Trichinella Spiralis	Cestoda Cysticerus cellulosae (*Taenia solium*) Sparganum spp. Hydatid (*Echinococcus granulosus*)	Pain and swelling Pain and spontaneous fractures

ROUTES OF INFECTION: THE KEY TO PREVENTION

Human infection by	Route outside body	Class	Species
Ingesting OVA	Infective ova voided in faeces, To new or same host on fingers, on dust, etc.	Nematoda	Enterobius vermicularis
		Cestoda	Hymenolepis nana Taenia solium (in human cysticerosis) Echinoodoccus granulosus (in hydatid disease)
	Immature ova voided in faeces Mature in soil To new host on vegetables, etc.	Nematoda	Trichuris trichiura Ascaris lumbricoides
Prevention of skin By Larvae			
(a) from soil	Ova voided in faeces Hatch in soil Rhabditiform then filariform larvae (infective)	Nematoda	Ancylostoma duodenale Necator americanus A. brazillense (in cutaneous larva migrans)
	Larvae voided in faeces Filariform, infective to new or same host Rhabditiform, metamorphose to filariform (infective)		⌈Strongyloides stecoralis Direct cycle I ⌊Direct cycle II Schistoma haematobiuma
(b) from water	Ova voided in urine or faeces Hatch in water to miracida Penetrate snail Develop to cercariae Liberated into water	Trematoda	Schistoma haematobium S. mansoni S. japonicum Non-human schistosomes (in cercarial dermatitis)
Larvae injected by insects			
(a) Mosquito spp	⌈Microfillariae in blood or tissue juices ingested by insect Mature in insect, now infective Injected into man	Nematoda	Wuchereria bancrofti Brugia malayi Loa loa
(b) Chrysops			
(c) Simulium			Onchocerca volvulus
(d) Culicoides spp.	Pathogenicity to man doubtful		⌈Dipelalonema perstans D. streptocerca ⌊Mansonella ozzardi
Encysted larvae eaten			
(a) In Cyclops	Larvae from skin ulcer to water Ingested by cyclops Encyst therein	Nematoda	Dracunculus medinensis
(b) In Meat Pork	Larvae liberated in intestinal wall Encyst in flesh of Same host		Trichinella spiralis
	Ova voided in faeces Ingested by pigs Encyst in flesh	Cestoda	Taenia solium (adult infection)

Contd.

Human infection by		Route outside body	Class	Species
	Beef	Ingested by cattle Encyst in flesh		*Taenia saginata*
(c) In freshwater fish	Ova voided in faeces	Mature in water Hatch to coracidium Ingested by Cyclops (etc.) Develop into procercoid Cyclops ingested by fish Encyst in muscles—pleroceroid (infective)	Cestoda	*Dibothriocephalus latus*
		Ingested by snail Hatch in snail and develop to cercariae Liberated to water Penetrate cypinoid Fish Encyst as metacercariae (infective)	Trematoda	*Clonorchis sinensis*
(d) In crustacea	Ova voided in sputum or faeces	Mature in water Penetrate snail Development to cercariae Liberated to water Penetrate Crustaceans Encyst as metacercariae (infective)		*Paragonimus westermani*
(e) On vegetation	Ova voided in faeces	Mature in soil Hatch to miracidia Penetrate snail Development to cercariae Liberated to vegetation Encyst as metacercariae (infective)		*Fasciola hepatica* *Fascicoipsis buski*
(f) In fleas	Ova voided in faeces	Ingested by fleas Develop into cysticercoid	Cestoda	*Hymenolepis dimuta*

Index

Acanthocheilonema
(*Dipetalonema*)
perstans 149
Acquired active immunity 7
autoimmune reaction 7
cellular factors 7
cell-mediated immunity
(cmi) 7
non-specific cellular
response 7
humoral factors 7
hypersensitivity reaction 8
delayed hypersensitivity 8
immediate hypersensitivity 8
premunition 8
tolerance 8
Acute amoebic dysentery—
intestinal lesions 23
chronic intestinal amoebiasis—
intestinal lesions 24
gross pathology 23
microscopic features 24
ulcer distribution 23
African trypanosomiasis,
South American
trypanosomiasis and
visceral leishmaniasis 65
Amoebic liver abscess—clinical
features 26
course of liver abscess 27
Amphistomata 209
Ancylostoma braziliense 134
Ancylostoma caninum 134
Ancylostoma duodenale 128
Angiostrongylus cantonensis 171
Anisakis marina 146
Antimalarials 94
artemether and
lumefantrine 96
artesunate 96
atovaquone and proguanil 95
chloroquine phosphate 94
class summary 94
clindamycin 95
doxycycline 95
mefloquine 95
primaquine 95
prophylaxis 96
quinidine gluconate 95
quinine 94
tafenoquine 96

tetracycline 95
Aphasmid nematodes of lesser
importance 124
Ascaridoidea 141
ascaris lumbricoides 141

Balantidiasis 67
Balantidium coli 67
classification 68
cyst 68
diagnosis 70
geographical distribution 67
habitat 67
life cycle 68
morphology 68
pathology 70
prophylaxis 70
transmission 69
treatment 70
trophozoite 68
Bertiella studeri 201
Biopsy studies 247
bone marrow aspiration 248
bone marrow biopsy 248
lymph node puncture for
kala-azar and African
trypanosomiasis 248
splenic puncture for kala-azar
diagnosis 247
Blackwater fever 97
aetiology 97
clinical features 99
clinical pathology 99
complications 99
effects of intravascular
haemolysis 98
pathogenesis 98
pathology 98
treatment 99
Blood and tissue flagellates 35
Blood examination for
parasites 240
butter solution used in the
laboratory 241
concentration methods 245
examination of blood for
microfilariae 244
field's stain 242
fixing of blood films 240
Giemsa's stain 241
Leishman's stain 241
making thick smears 240
preparation of a thin blood
film 240
staining of blood films 240

staining of thick film 242
stain preparation and
staining 241
Blood flagellates 50
Brugia malayi 148, 157

Capillaria hepatica 123
Capillaria philippinensis 123
Cestoda 174
classification of 180
life cycle 178
Cestodes of lesser
significance 200
Chagas' disease 60
Chilomastix mesnili 34
Ciliatea 67
Ciliates 67
Ciliophora 67
Class cestoda 173
general features 174
Classification in brief of medically
important protozoans 11
Classification of parasites 1
Clonorchis sinensis 225
Coccidia 103
classification 103
oocyst morphology 103
Coenurus cerebralis 200
Commensalism 1
Cutaneous larva migrans 167
Cutaneous leishmaniasis (oriental
sore, chiclero's disease,
uta) 47
Cyclophyllidean tapeworms of
man 186
general characters 186
larval development 186
Cysticercus bovis 189
Cysticercus cellulosae 189

Dicrocoeliidae 208, 224
Dicrocoelium dentriticum 224
Differentiating features of
schistosome 212
Dioctophyma renale 124
Dipetalonema
(*acanthocheilonema*)
perstans 162
Dipetalonema streptocerca 149,
162
Diphyllobothrium latum 181
Diplogonoporus grandis 185
Dipylidium caninum 201
Dirofilariasis 162
Distomata 218

Dog tapeworm, hydatid worm 193
Dracunculoidea 163
Dracunculus medinensis 163
Drug prophylaxis 10

Echinococcus granulosus 193
Echinococcus multilocularis 197
Echinostomatidae 209, 233
Echinostoma species 233
Effects of parasite 5
Entamoeba histolytica 15
   complications and
      sequelae 22
   cultivation 19
   geographical distribution 16
   habitat 16
   historical 15
   life cycle 19, 20
   modes of infection 21
   morphology 16
   pathogenicity 21, 22
   pathogenic lesions 21
   reproduction 19
   reservoirs of infection 21
   role of carriers 21
   unstained preparations 17
Enterobius vermicularis 138
Eosinophilic meningoen-
   cephalitis 171
Espundia (muco-cutaneous
   leishmaniasis caused
   by *Leishmania
   brasiliensis*) 49
Examination of stool 235
   anal swab 239
   direct centrifugal floatation or
      DCF method 238
   direct smear 237
   E. histolytica—microscopic
      examination 235
   floatation method 237
   helminthic infections 237
   iodine solution 236
   Kato's cellophane-covered
      thick smear 239
   scotch cellulose tape
      method 239
   sedimentation method 238
   simple floatation method 237
   stained preparation 236
   staining methods 236
   unstained preparation 235

Fasciola gigantica 223
Fasciola hepatica 218
Fasciolidae 208, 218
Fasciolopsis buski 221
Filarial worms 148
Filariodea 146
   classification 146
   differentiating features of adult
      worms 147
   differentiating features of
      microfilariae (Mf) 147
   geographic disposition 147

Gastrodiscidae 209, 233
Gastrodiscoides hominis 233
Gastrointestinal tract
   amoebae 15
   classification 15
Giardia lamblia 32
   laboratory diagnosis 32
   life cycle 32
   morphology 32
   pathogenicity 32
   treatment 33
Gnathostoma spinigerum 165,
   167
Gongylonema pulchrum 172
Gordiid worms or hair snakes 173
Guinea worm 163

Haemonchus contortus 137
Headings 2
   geographical distribution 2
   habitat 2
   history 2
   infection reservoirs 3
   modes of infection 3
   morphology and life cycle 2
Helminthology 108
Heterophyidae 209, 228
Heterophytes heterophytes 228
Heterotrichida 67
Hookworms 133
Hosts 2
Human and animal
   trypanosomes 66
Human malarial parasites 73
   comparison of course of natural
      infection of *P. vivax* and
      P. falciparum in man 82
   developing trophozoites 77
   erythrocytic schizogony 73
   exo-erythrocytic schizogony 75
   febrile paroxysms 85
   gametogony 75
   geographical distribution 73
   habitat 73
   human cycle 73
   immature schizonts 78
   incubation period 85
   life cycle 73
   life cycle of malarial
      parasites 74
   macrogametocytes 79
   malarial infection:
      immunological
      consequences 83
   mature schizonts 78
   microgametocytes 79
   morphology of malarial
      parasites 76
   mosquito cycle 75
   other methods of
      transmission 83
   pathology 85
   pre-erythrocytic schizogony 73
   schizogony 76

spread of malaria 84
stages in thin films 77
therapeutic malaria 84
thick films 80
Hymenolepididae 198
Hymenolepis 198
Hymenolepis diminuta 200
Hymenolepis nana 199

Immunodiagnostics in
   parasitology 251
antibodies 253
antigen 251
antigen–antibody
   reactions 255
chemiluminescence immune
   assay (CLIA) 267
ELISA formats 265
enzyme-linked immunosorbent
   assay (ELISA) 264
how do antigen–antibody
   reactions help in
   diagnosis 255
immunodiagnostics 251
microscopy 256
principle of CLIA 268
rapid detection tests (RDTS) 256
rapid test for malaria (pan), e.g.
   parabank 259
rapid test for malaria (pan/pf),
   e.g. malascan plus 260
rapid test for malaria pv/pf, e.g.
   falcivax 262
rapid test for malaria pv/pf, e.g.
   paramax 3 263
rapid test for *P. falciparum*
   malaria: Paracheck
   pf 257
serology-based assays
   system 256
structure of antibodies 253
tools for diagnosis 256
types of antibodies 254
types of diagnostic tests 256
Immunological responses and
   parasites 6
Intermicapsifer spp 201
Intestinal, oral and genital
   flagellates 32
Intestinal schistosomiasis 217
Isospora 104

Laboratory cultivation 245
   cultivation of *E. histolytica* 245
   cultivation of leishmaniae 246
   cultivation of malarial
      parasite 246
   significance of culture
      technique 246
Laboratory diagnosis 8
   biopsy material/aspirates 9
   blood 8
   indirect evidences 9
   serological tests 10
   sputum 9

stool 8
urine 9
Laboratory diagnosis of
    amoebiasis 28
    amoebic hepatitis and
        abscess 29
    intestinal 28
    other extraintestinal lesions 29
Larva migrans 167
Leishmania donovani 36
    amastigote stage 37
    anaemia 42
    bone marrow 42
    clinical features 40
    cultivation 38
    diagnosis of leishmaniasis 43
    direct evidences 44
    geographical distribution 36
    habitat 36
    immunology 43
    incubation period 40
    indirect evidences 44
    intestines 42
    life cycle 39
    liver 42
    lymph nodes 42
    methods of infection 38
    morphology 36
    other methods of
        transmission 40
    pathogenesis and
        pathology 40
    pathogenicity 40
    pathogenic lesions 40
    promastigote stage 38
    prophylaxis 46
    spleen 40
    susceptible animals 38
    treatment 46
Leishmaniasis 36
    clinical classification of
        leishmaniasis 36
    generic character 36
Liquid based cytology as an aid
        to diagnose parasitic
        diseases/infestation 248
Loa loa 149, 158

*Macrocanthorhynchus
        hirudinaceus* 173
Malaria prophylaxis 99
    history 102
    medications 100
    risk factors 102
    risk management 100
    strategies 100
    vaccines 102
Mansonella ozzardi 149, 162
Mermithid worms 124
Metagonimus yokogawai 229
Metastatic lesions in
        amoebiasis 24
    extraintestinal lesions 25

gross features 26
    hepatic amoebiasis 24
    liver abscess pus 26
    microscopic features 26
Metastatic lesions in other
        organs 27
    cerebral amoebiasis 27
    cutaneous amoebiasis 27
    pulmonary amoebiasis 27
    splenic abscess 28
Metastrongylos elongastos 137
Metazoa 108
Moniliformis moniliformis 173
Multiceps 200

Necater americanus 131
Nemathelminthes 109
Nematoda 109
    classification 113
    general characteristics 109
    important terms 114
    intestinal 113
    larval stages of nematodes 110
    life cycle 110
    life cycle in general 115
    modes of infection 110
    reproductive system 109
    somatic 113
    systematic classification 113
Nematodes of lesser
        importance 172

*Oesophagostomum
        apiostomum* 136
Onchocerca volvulus 149, 159
Opisthorchiidae 208, 225
Opisthorchis felineus 227
Oriental schistosomiasis 217
Other filarial worms 162
Oxyuroidea 138

Paragonimus westermani 230
Parasitism 1
Pathogenic effects 6
Pathology of schistosomiasis 216
PCRs—an aid to diagnose
        parasitic diseases 270
    advantages 275
    applications of PCR 275
    drawbacks 275
    parasitic infections that can be
        diagnosed by PCR 276
    principle of PCR 270
    truelab workstation 275
    types of PCR 271
    what is a PCR? 270
    what is the current
        requirement 275
Pernicious malaria 86
    acute phase 87
    algid malaria: pathology 91
    biochemical changes 92
    chronic phase 88
    clinical pathology 91
    complications and
        sequelae 89

laboratory diagnosis of
        malaria 92
    liver 90
    pathogenesis 86
    pathology 87
    septicaemic malaria:
        Pathology 91
    specific organ changes 90
    treatment 94
Phylum acanthocephala (thorny
        headed worms) 173
Physaloptera caucasica 172
Plasmodium 72
    evolution of knowledge
        regarding malarial
        parasites 72
    species 72
Platyhelminthes trematoda 202
    classification 207
    general features 202
    general morphology 203
    historical aspects 207
    life cycle 205
    modes of infection 206
    systematic classification 207
Pneumocystis carinil 107
Portal of entry 3
Postkala-azar dermal
        leishmaniasis (dermal
        leishmanoid) (PKDL) 46
Practical parasitology 235
Primary amoebic menin-
        goencephalitis 30
    infections in human beings 30
    morphological features of the
        amoeba 30
Prophylaxis 10
Prophylaxis against
        amoebiasis 30
    community prophylaxis 30
    personal prophylaxis 30
Protozoa 12
    adaptation for survival 14
    definition 12
    ectoplasm 13
    endoplasm 13
    limiting cell membrane 13
    locomotor apparatus 13
    morphology 12
    nucleus 12
    physiology 12
Protozoa of uncertain status 106

Raillietine madagascarensis 201
Recapitulation 299
    cestodes 302
    nematodes 301
    ova 303
    pathogenesis and pathology of
        worm infections 305
    protozoa inhabiting the
        intestine 299
    trematodes 302
Relationships between two living
        organisms 1

Sarcocystis lindemanni 104
  classification 104
  laboratory diagnosis 105
  pathology 105
  probable life cycle 105
Scheme of study observed in this
      book 2
Schistosoma 208
Schistosoma haematobium 212
  diagnosis 214
  geographical distribution 212
  habitat 213
  investigations 214
  life cycle 213
  morphology 213
  pathology 214
  prophylaxis 215
  treatment 215
Schistosoma japonicum 216
Schistosoma mansoni 215
Schistosomatoidea 209
  general features 209
  general morphology 210
  immunity 211
  life cycle in general 210
Simeon's modification of
      Boye's and Sterenel's
      method 243
  examination of blood for
      malarial parasite 243
  mounting and preservation of
      films 243
Source of infection 3
South American
      trypanosomiasis 60
Sparganum 184
Spiruroidea 165
Sporozoa 71
Spread of parasitic infections 4
Standard operation procedure
      (SOP) for detection
      of malaria pf/pv on
      truelab 277
Strongyloidea 128
Strongyloides stercoralis 125
Symbiosis 1
Syngamus laryngeus 136
Taenia 187
Taenia saginata 187, 189
Taenia solium 187, 189
Taenidae 187
Terminology 1
Ternidens deminutus 135
Thelazia callipaeda 172
Therapeutic prophylaxis 10
Therapy of parasitic
      infections 287
  amoebicidal drugs 287
  anti-dracunculosis drugs 296
  anti-filarial drugs 296
  antileishmaniasis drugs 291
  antimalarial drugs 292

drugs for balantidiasis 294
drugs for clonorchiasis 298
drugs for fascioliasis 298
drugs for giardiasis 289
drugs for intestinal cestode
      infestation 296
drugs for paragonimiasis 298
drugs for trichomoniasis 290
drugs for trypanosomiasis 290
for extraintestinal amoebiasis
      only 288
for oriental sore and
      espundia 292
infection 309
intestinal anthelmintics 294
routes of infection: the key to
      prevention 313
schistosomicidal drugs 297
treatment of resistant cases of
      kala-azar 292
Toxoplasma gondii 106
Treatment 10
Trichinella spiralis 117
Trichinelloidea 117
Trichomonas 34
Trichostrongylus spp. 136
Trichuris trichiura (whipworm) 121
Triglotrematidae 229
Troglotrematidae 209
Trypanosoma 52
  animal trypanosomes 52
  characteristics 52
  classification 52
  method of reproduction 52
  morphology 52
Trypanosoma brucei 53
  blood and CSF 59
  chronic sleeping sickness 58
  clinically 59
  cultivation 54
  habitat 53
  laboratory diagnosis 59
  life cycle 55, 61
  life cycle: General 56
  life cycle in insect 56
  life cycle in man 56
  morphology 54
  pathogenesis and
      pathology 57
  pathogenic lesions 59
  polymorphism 54
  prophylaxis 64
  T. brucei subgroup 53
  treatment 60
  vectors and reservoirs 55
Trypanosoma cruzi 35, 60
  cultivation 60
  development in man 61
  development in reduviid
      bug 61
  geographical distribution 60
  habitat 60
  immunology 61

laboratory diagnosis 63
pathogenesis 63
pathogenesis and
      pathology 64
reservoir hosts 61
staining 60
treatment 63
Trypanosomatidae 50
  amastigote (leishmanial
      stage) 51
  choanomastigote (barley-corn
      form) 51
  epimastigote (crithidial stage) 51
  opithomastigote (trypanosome
      or trypanomorphic
      stage) 51
  promastigote (leptomonad
      form) 51
  trypomastigote (true
      trypanosome stage) 51
Trypanosomatidae: genera
      and species affecting
      man 35
Trypanosomatid flagellates 50
Urinary schistosomiasis 217
Visceral larva migrans 168
  aetiology 168
  definition 168
  due to human nematodes 169
  due to non-human
      nematodes 168
  gnathostoma spinigerum 168
  laboratory diagnosis of visceral
      larva migrans 169
  non-human filarial spp. 169
  non-human hookworms 168
  T. canis 170
  T. cati 170
  toxocara cati 170
Wuchereria bancrofti 148, 149
  classical filariasis (*W. bancrofti*)
      pathogenic lesions 154
  developmental stages of mf. in
      mosquito 152
  development in man up to an
      adult worm 152
  diagnosis 156
  differences between classical
      and occult filariasis 153
  geographical distribution 150
  habitat 150
  historical 149
  morphology 151
  occult filariasis 154
  pathogenesis 153
  pathology and clinical
      features 152
  prophylaxis 156
  treatment 156
Zoomastigophorea 50
Zoonosis 1